Essentials of Ultrasound

MICHAEL R. WILLIAMSON, M.D.

Chief, Diagnostic Ultrasound
University of New Mexico
Health Sciences Center
Department of Radiology
Albuquerque, New Mexico

W. B. SAUNDERS COMPANY
A Division of Harcourt Brace & Company
Philadelphia, London, Toronto, Montreal, Sydney, Tokyo

W. B. SAUNDERS COMPANY
A Division of Harcourt Brace & Company

The Curtis Center
Independence Square West
Philadelphia, Pennsylvania 19106

Library of Congress Cataloging-in-Publication Data

Williamson, Michael R.
    Essentials of ultrasound / Michael R. Williamson. — 1st ed.
        p.   cm.
    ISBN 0-7216-6642-6
    1. Diagnosis, Ultrasonic—Handbooks, manuals, etc.   I. Title.
    [DNLM: 1. Ultrasonography—handbooks.   WN 39 W731e 1996]
    RC78.7.U4W547   1996
    616.07′543—dc20
    DNLM/DLC   95-30946

NWST
IAKC 7555

ESSENTIALS OF ULTRASOUND   ISBN 0-7216-6642-6

Printed in the United States of America.

Last digit is the print number: 9   8   7   6   5   4   3   2   1

To Susan, Mary, Ross, Michelle, Lena, Les

ACKNOWLEDGMENTS

Thanks to Gabriela Miranda, Percy Bryant, Jonathan Briggs and Adriana Blake for their work in compiling and composing this book.

Numerous people contributed cases but special thanks go to Robert Rosenberg who collected many of the images in this book, Liz Stamm also provided several hard to find cases. Susan Williamson helped with the pediatric portions of this book.

There are also many people who at one point or another contributed to my education in ultrasound. I thank them. They are listed in alphabetical order as follows: Bert Ammann, Terry Angtuaco, Suppiah Balachandra, Buck Brewer, Charles Boyd, Dick Hattan, Michael Manco-Johnson, Grant Rees, Jeff Rose, Hemendra Shah, Whit Vick, Mark Vitter, and Jim Walsh.

Sara Langwell deserves credit for the fine drawings and the cover illustration. Erlinda Ramos, Nancy Furbush, Ina Rutenberg, Sandy Maturo, and Regina Gabaldon also helped with images.

Finally, this book would not have been possible without the support provided by Fred Mettler.

PREFACE

Essentials of Ultrasound was inspired by Mettler and Guibertau's *Essentials of Nuclear Medicine*. It is an attempt to provide a core amount of information in a compact volume. This book is directed primarily at the radiology resident but the radiologist who wants a quick review of ultrasound may also find it useful. There are comprehensive texts on ultrasound available for readers who wish more detailed information. This book is similar to *Essentials of Nuclear Medicine* in that a detailed list of references has not been provided. Instead, suggested readings for more detailed information are listed at the end of each chapter. Many residents have told me that they find the differential diagnoses listed in *Gamuts in Ultrasound* by Williamson and Williamson very useful. I have provided many of those gamuts in this book.

Finally, I have tried to include techniques that have proved to be clinically useful. Some controversial and/or seldom used techniques have been omitted.

MICHAEL R. WILLIAMSON

CONTENTS

Plate 1. Color Doppler. Transverse image of splenic vein. Flow is depicted in two colors, with red toward the transducer and green away from the transducer, even though all flow is the same direction. See Figure 1–40 on page 27.

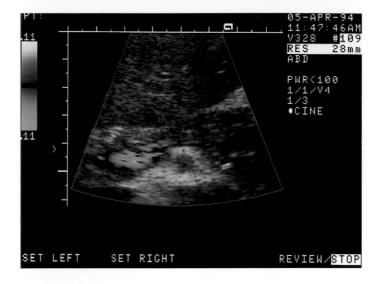

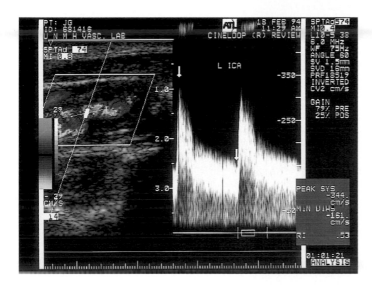

Plate 2. Color Doppler image of internal carotid artery shows obvious stenosis. Doppler spectrum shows peak systolic velocity of 344 cm/sec and end-diastolic velocity of 161 cm/sec, indicating stenosis should be at least 80 percent. See Figure 2–4 on page 34.

Plate 3. Transverse image of a teardrop-shaped hypoechoic parathyroid adenoma. This color Doppler image shows a small amount of flow. See Figure 3–3 on page 45.

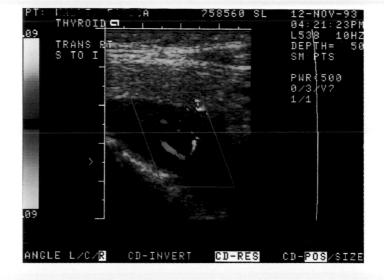

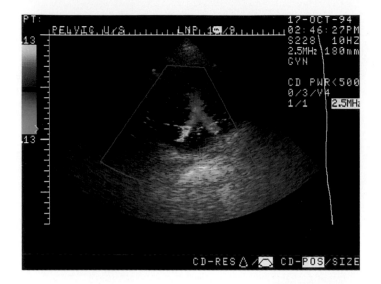

Plate 4. Transverse color Doppler image showing ureteric jets. See Figure 6–17 on page 124.

Plate 5. Color Doppler image shows enlarged epididymis (E) with increased flow consistent with epididymitis. See Figure 6–28B on page 135.

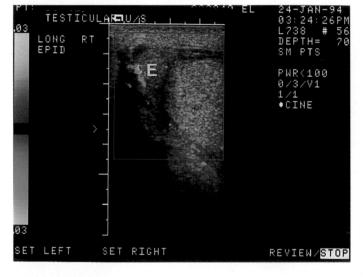

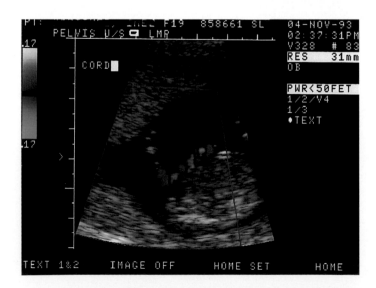

Plate 6. Coiled umbilical cord (normal). Noncoiling cord should raise concern for fetal anomalies. See Figure 8–10 on page 165.

CHAPTER 1

Physics in Ultrasound

Ultrasound Characteristics

Ultrasound waves are waves of energy similar to audible sound. The frequency of "ultra" sound waves, however, is greater than 20,000 cycles per second (hertz) and, therefore, they are not audible. Most waves used for imaging have a frequency between 2 and 10 million hertz. When sound energy moves through the human body, the molecules of the transmitting medium (the liver, for example) are slightly disturbed. The energy is transmitted from one liver molecule to an adjacent molecule, similar to the way billiard balls transmit energy from one to another when they collide. The sound energy moves through tissue in longitudinal waves and the molecules of the transmitting medium oscillate in the same direction as the wave. Ultrasound waves are usually depicted as sine waves. As a wave is passing through tissue, some molecules are pushed closer together and others are spread apart, mimicking the peaks and valleys of the sine wave. These peaks and valleys are known as areas of compression and rarefaction (Fig. 1–1).

The distance from one compression to the next band of compression (the distance between the peaks of the sine wave) is the wavelength (λ). The number of times any given molecule is compressed each second is the frequency (f) and is expressed in cycles per second or hertz (Hz) (Fig. 1–2). Sound waves are also described by their periods which is the length of time for one cycle to pass. The period of the wave is equal to the inverse of the frequency:

$$\frac{1}{\text{period(s)}} = f(\text{Hz})$$

The speed of sound in tissue is equal to the wavelength times the frequency (speed = λ × f). Wavelength and frequency are determined both by the medium and by the source of the wave.

In human tissue, ultrasound moves at an average speed of 1,540 m/sec. This speed varies depending on the type of tissue; for example, ultrasound waves move more slowly through fat. Two characteristics of the transmitting medium primarily determine the speed of sound through it: its compressibility and its density. Speed is inversely related to compressibility. The molecules in more compressible tissues are widely spaced and so transmit sound more slowly. Dense materials also do not transmit sound waves rapidly because the already tightly spaced molecules are difficult to compress. In addition, the inertia of relatively large molecules (often found in dense materials) reduces sound velocity. Therefore, sound velocity is faster in less dense and less compressible tissues.

The amplitude of a sound wave is the maximum distance each molecule is displaced compared to its normal state. Amplitude will be greater if the wave has more energy. The power of an ultrasound wave is measured in watts (w) and is the total energy generated (by the source) per second. Intensity is the amount of energy per unit area (the amount of energy passing through any given point in 1 second) across the sound beam or watt/cm². Intensity is proportional to amplitude squared so that if amplitude is doubled, intensity increases by a factor of 4. Notice that the wave front decreases in intensity as it travels through tissues partly because the energy is spread over a larger area (Fig. 1–3).

Sound intensity may also be described in terms of one sound compared to another. This is the bel system in which:

$$\log_{10}\frac{A}{B} = \text{bels}$$

1

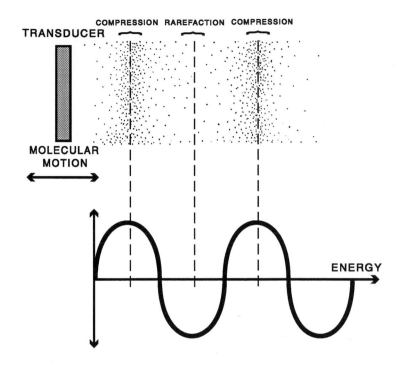

Figure 1–1. Vibrating transducer forms longitudinal waves consisting of areas of compressed molecules. In a longitudinal wave, molecular motion is in the same direction as the direction of wave propagation.

where A = intensity of the 1st sound and B = intensity of the 2nd sound.

10 decibels = 1 bel.

Therefore, a 10-decibel or 1-bel difference in sounds is equal to a tenfold difference in intensity. Two bels or 20 decibels is a 100-fold difference (Table 1–1).

As the sound wave moves through tissue, the wave front spreads out, and this is responsible for some of the decrease in intensity. Attenuation also occurs when some sound energy is absorbed and converted to heat. Two other mechanisms of attenuation are reflection and scattering. A rule of thumb is that there is 1 decibel (dB) of attenuation for each centimeter in tissue depth per megahertz (MHz) signal. For example, a 3 MHz signal will loose 3 dB of intensity for each centimeter in depth.

The amount the sound beam is reflected depends on the angle of incidence, just as when light strikes a mirror. Reflection is maximized when the sound wave strikes the interface between two types of tissue perpendicularly. If the beam is more than a few degrees away from perpendicular, reflected sound will not come back to the source and will not be detected (Fig. 1–4). The characteristics of the surface being struck also determine the amount of reflec-

tion. Large flat surfaces act like mirrors and reflect sound the best. They are called specular reflectors (Fig. 1–5). An example is the interface between kidney and liver. Rough surfaces with irregularities much less than one wavelength in size will scatter the energy in all directions and reflect only small amounts of the energy back to the source (Fig. 1–6). These are scatterers.

The amount of sound energy reflected back to the source when it is perpendicular to a specular reflector is dependent on the impedance of the tissue. Impedance, Z, is a constant for any given tissue and is equal to density (ρ) times velocity (c).

$$Z = \rho \times c$$

The amount of reflected energy (reflection coefficient; R) is expressed as:

$$R = \frac{(Z_2 - Z_1)^2}{(Z_2 + Z_1)^2}$$

where Z_2 is the second tissue and Z_1 is the first tissue at an interface. Large differences in impedance between two tissues mean lots of reflection. An example is gas, which has a much different impedance than soft tissue, leading to a near total reflection of the sound.

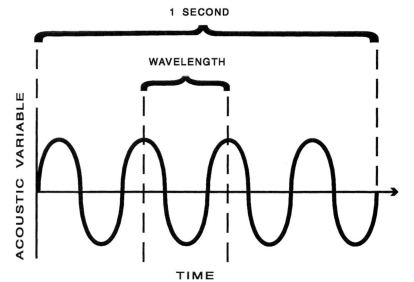

1 SECOND

WAVELENGTH

ACOUSTIC VARIABLE

TIME

Figure 1–2. This wave has a frequency of 4 Hz. The period is the time for one cycle to pass, or .25 seconds.

The sound that is not reflected, scattered, or absorbed proceeds deeper into the tissue. However, it may be refracted or bent (Fig. 1–7). This direction change occurs whenever there is a change in velocity in passing from one medium, or one tissue, to another. Snell's law states that:

$$\frac{\sin \theta_i}{\sin \theta_t} = \frac{V_1}{V_2}$$

θ_i = angle of incidence

θ_t = angle of transmission

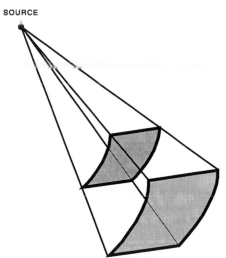

SOURCE

Figure 1–3. As the wave travels from its source, the energy is spread over a larger and larger area. This decreases the intensity at any one point.

If velocity is slower in medium 2, then the angle between the sound beam and a perpendicular will be smaller.

In diagnostic imaging, the sound is transmitted in short bursts or pulses of a few waves (Fig. 1–8). The same instrument that produced the signal, the transducer, then receives the returning wave. The pulse duration is the length of time that sound is transmitted. The time from the beginning of one pulse to the beginning of the next is the pulse repetition period (PRP). The number of pulses per second is the pulse repetition frequency (PRF). Pulse repetition period equals one over the pulse repetition frequency:

$$PRP = \frac{1}{PRF}$$

The wave period times the number of cycles in the pulse equals the pulse duration. Duty factor is the fraction of time that the sound is being transmitted. It is calculated by dividing the pulse duration by the pulse repetition period. Pulses of sound will not be as pure in frequency as continuous sound waves. They will contain mixtures of many different frequencies with a dominant frequency.

The intensity of an ultrasound beam is different at different points in space (space variation) within the sound beam. If we monitor the intensity at one given point in

Table 1–1. GAIN OR ATTENUATION VALUES IN DECIBELS FOR VARIOUS VALUES OF POWER OR INTENSITY RATIO*

GAIN OR ATTENUATION (dB)	INTENSITY OR POWER RATIO	
	Attenuation	*Gain*
1	0.79	1.3
2	0.63	1.6
3	0.50	2.0
4	0.40	2.5
5	0.32	3.2
6	0.25	4.0
7	0.20	5.0
8	0.16	6.3
9	0.13	7.9
10	0.10	10.0
15	0.032	32.0
20	0.01	100.0
25	0.003	320.0
30	0.001	1,000.0
35	0.0003	3,200.0
40	0.0001	10,000.0
45	0.00003	32,000.0
50	0.00001	100,000.0
60	0.000001	1,000,000.0
70	0.0000001	10,000,000.0
80	0.00000001	100,000,000.0
90	0.000000001	1,000,000,000.0
100	0.0000000001	10,000,000,000.0

*The ratio is output power or intensity divided by input power or intensity. In the case of attenuation, it is the fraction of power or intensity remaining.

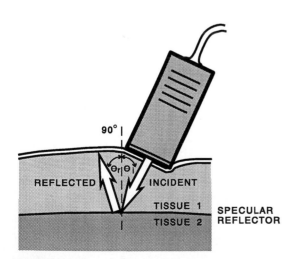

Figure 1–4. Sound reflected at the interface between tissue 1 and tissue 2 will not be detected because the transducer is too far from perpendicular. θ_i (angle of incidence) = θ_r (angle of reflection).

space, the intensity at that point will vary with time (temporal variation).

The temporal peak is the intensity when the ultrasound transducer is pulsing (Fig. 1–9). The temporal average is the average intensity on the entire cycle, including both the time when the pulse is on and when the transducer is receiving between pulses.

The spatial average is the average intensity throughout the beam and the spatial peak is the maximum intensity anywhere in the beam (Fig. 1–10).

A third measurement is the pulse average intensity (Fig. 1–9). This is the intensity when the transducer is "on" and producing sound.

Six intensities may be measured:

SPTP   Spatial peak, temporal peak
SPPA   Spatial peak, pulse average
SPTA   Spatial peak, temporal average
SATP   Spatial average, temporal peak
SAPA   Spatial average, pulse average
SATA   Spatial average, temporal average

Continuous-wave Doppler has higher intensity levels than a pulsed ultrasound im-

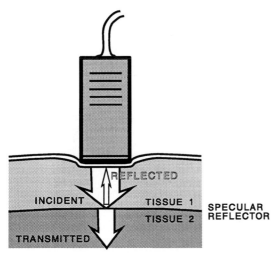

Figure 1–5. Large flat surfaces act as mirror-like (specular) reflectors, sending large amounts of sound back to the transducer.

aging instrument since the instrument is emitting sound continuously.

Transducers

The heart of the ultrasound machine is the transducer. A transducer changes energy from one form to another. In ultrasound, electric energy is changed to sound energy when current is applied to the transducer. Ultrasound transducers are piezoelectric devices. When voltage is applied to them, their shape deforms and a pressure wave is created. Conversely, if pressure (i.e., a returning ultrasound wave) is applied,

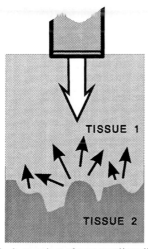

Figure 1–6. A rough surface scatters the energy.

their shape also deforms and voltage is produced. The amount of voltage produced is proportional to the intensity of the pressure applied and vice versa.

Quartz is a naturally occurring piezoelectric. Lead zirconate titanate is a ceramic commonly used in today's transducers. Transducers have a preferred vibrating frequency or operating frequency. Another term is resonance frequency. This resonance frequency is related to the transducer by the following equation:

resonance frequency

$$= \frac{\text{propagation speed in crystal} \left(\dfrac{mm}{ms}\right)}{2 \times \text{thickness (mm)}}$$

However, crystal thickness is equal to half of the wavelength so that

resonance frequency

$$= \frac{\text{propagation speed in crystal (mm/ms)}}{\lambda \text{ (mm)}}$$

Transducers have a "backing block" to absorb sound transmitted backward out of the crystal (Fig. 1–11). This material is a mixture of tungsten plus rubber or plastic held together by epoxy. The backing block has an impedance similar to that of the crystal. It also shortens the pulse and dampens vibrations in the transducer. After each pulse, the vibrations must be quenched while the transducer is in the receiving mode. Shortening the pulse length also improves axial resolution.

Transducers also have a facing block or matching layer that has an impedance between that of the crystal and tissue. This enhances sound transmission into the body. A coupling gel between the transducer housing and the patient also improves transmission. Air has a low impedance compared to the transducer. If sound leaves the transducer and strikes air, the change in impedance means much of the sound will be reflected and will not reach the patient.

Although the transducer has a resonance frequency, other frequencies of sound are also produced. Short pulses with few cycles produce a wider range of frequencies, while long pulses such as in continuous wave operation produce "purer" frequencies. Trans-

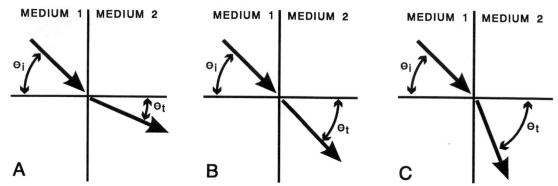

Figure 1–7. *A*, Velocity in medium 2 is slower than in medium 1. *B*, Velocity in medium 2 equals the velocity in medium 1 so there is no refraction. *C*, Velocity in medium 2 is faster than in medium 1.

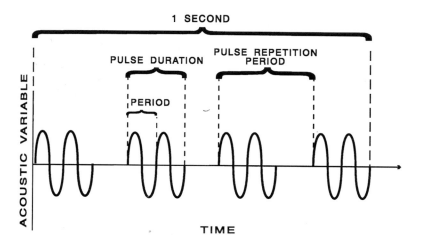

Figure 1–8. Illustration of pulse duration and pulse repetition period. In this case the pulse repetition frequency is four.

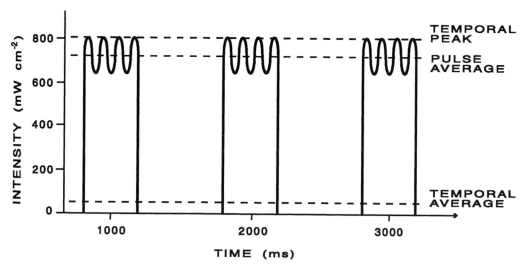

Figure 1–9. Illustration of temporal peak, pulse average, and temporal average.

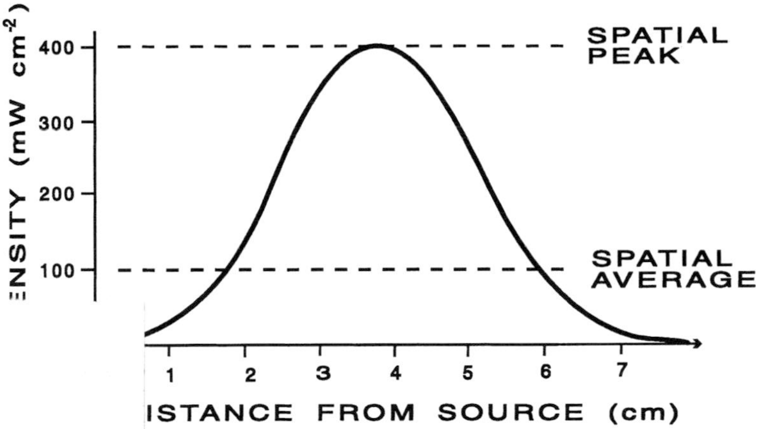

Figure 1–10. At any point in space, the intensity of the beam can be measured. The mean intensity for all points in space is the spatial average. The point in space with the highest in-

dth, cies ivi an ar- ncy The the

with and am- ctor frc h or cers id a ctor ans-

ducer has more listening time between pulses and can respond to a wider range of reflected waves.

The sound beam from a transducer is shown in Figure 1–12. The portion of the beam that is parallel or converges slightly is called the near zone or Fresnel zone. The far zone or Fraunhofer zone begins where the beam starts to diverge. The length of the Fresnel zone is dependent on the size of the transducer face and the frequency of the transducer. It is largest with large diameter transducers of high frequency. The Fresnel zone is described by:

$$\text{Fresnel zone} = \frac{r^2}{\lambda} \qquad r = \text{transducer radius} \quad \lambda = \text{sound wavelength}$$

The divergence of the beam in the far zone is also less with higher frequency transducers and large diameter transducer faces. This divergence is described by:

$$\sin \theta = 1.22 \times \frac{\lambda}{D}$$

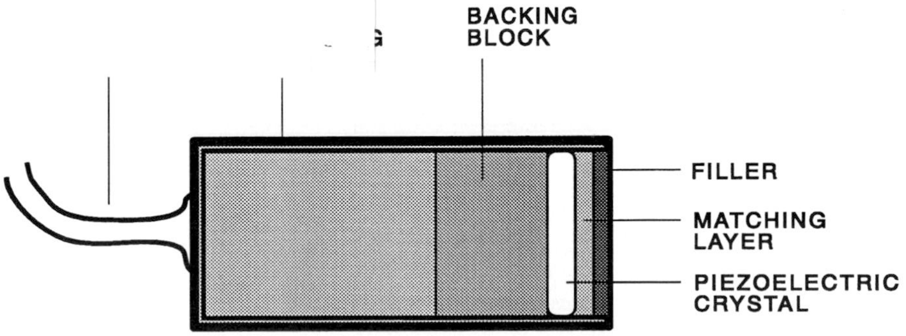

Figure 1–11. Typical transducer.

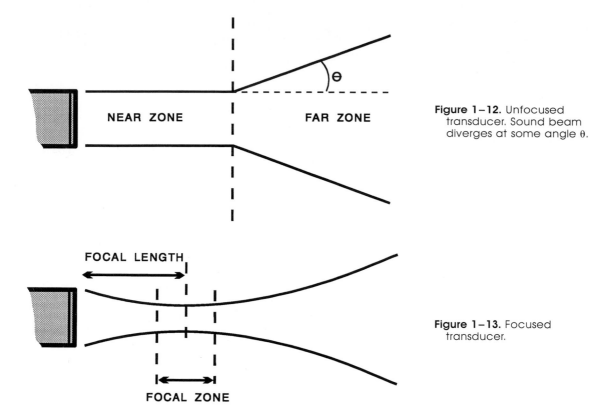

Figure 1–12. Unfocused transducer. Sound beam diverges at some angle θ.

Figure 1–13. Focused transducer.

θ = angle of divergence
λ = wavelength
D = transducer diameter

Focused transducers also may be described by focal length, the distance to the narrowest portion of the beam, and the focal zone (the distance over which the beam pattern is narrow) (Fig. 1–13). The focal zone is the portion of the beam that is some fraction of the peak intensity of the beam. The narrowest part of the beam, usually the center, is sometimes called the focal point.

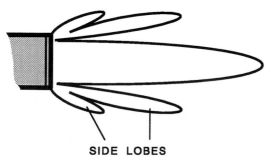

Figure 1–14. Side lobes generated by the transducer may reflect back to the transducer and produce erroneous information about the location of structures in space.

The focal length must be equal to or less than the length of the Fresnel zone for a similar unfocused transducer. Focusing of a single-element transducer may be accomplished by curving the crystal or by use of an acoustic lens. An acoustic lens has a different impedance than the transducer crystal and so bends the sound.

Small amounts of sound may radiate at sharp angles from the transducer face. These are called side lobes and can produce erroneous information about the location of objects in the image because the computer in the ultrasound machine assumes that echoes returning to the transducer were sent out from the transducer along the main beam in a straight line (Fig. 1–14).

TYPES OF TRANSDUCERS

Transducers are either mechanical or electronic.

Mechanical transducers sweep the beam of sound rapidly through the tissues many times each second. The transducers may either oscillate back and forth or a group of three transducers in a single housing may be rotated continuously (Fig. 1–15). Each of

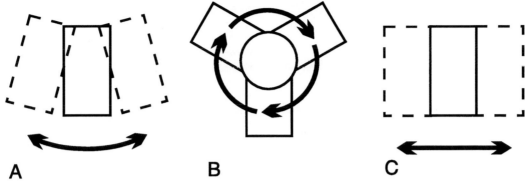

Figure 1–15. Types of transducer. *A,* Single element may oscillate continuously; *B,* three transducers rotate and each emits sound only when it rotates to the front of the transducer housing; *C,* a linear translating transducer.

the three transducers fires only when it rotates to the front surface of the transducer housing. These transducers create an image that is shaped like a piece of pie and are called sector scanners.

Electronic array transducers contain multiple crystals or elements that are activated sequentially. An annular array transducer has multiple circular elements arranged concentrically. Annular array transducers have an equal degree of focusing and resolution in both planes perpendicular to the direction of the beam.

Linear array transducers consist of a group of small rectangular elements placed side by side (Fig. 1–16A). There may be a hundred or more elements. These elements

are fired in groups so five or six elements fire simultaneously and create a beam that seems as though it is coming from a single element (but is focused) (Fig. 1–16B). This is also called a switched array. To maximize the Fresnel zone length and maintain resolution, it is important to use as large an element as possible because Fresnel zone length is proportional to the radius squared of the transducer. A group of five or six small elements together can generate a long Fresnel zone. Linear array elements are focused in the slice thickness plane by an acoustic lens with a different impedance than the individual elements. Focusing in the long axis of the array is done by firing outer elements earlier than inner elements.

Figure 1–16. *A,* Linear array transducer. *B,* Outer elements are fired before inner elements, resulting in focused beam.

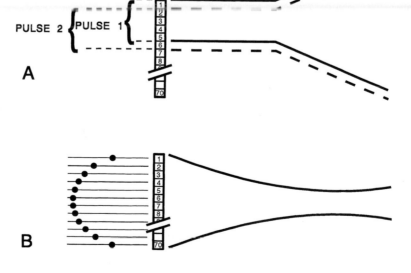

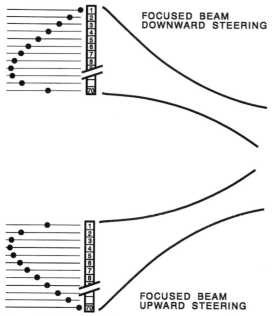

FOCUSED BEAM
DOWNWARD STEERING

FOCUSED BEAM
UPWARD STEERING

Figure 1–17. By varying the order of firing of the transducer elements, the beam can be steered. In the upper drawing element 1 is fired first. In the lower drawing element 70 is fired first.

The waves from the elements meet and reinforce each other, resulting in a focused beam. The time delay between firing of outer and inner elements determines the point of focus and can be adjusted on some transducers. The image created by linear array transducers is rectangular in shape.

Phased array transducers also consist of multiple elements side by side. The entire group of elements is fired almost, but not quite, simultaneously. Small time delays between the firings of elements focus and steer the beam from one side to the other (Fig. 1–17). Side lobe artifacts were mentioned earlier as the propagation of sound out of the path of the main beam. Array transducers have grating lobes that are several waves summed and act as a single wave moving off axis from the transducer. These can produce artifacts.

IMAGE CREATION

The transducer is placed against the patient with a thin layer of coupling gel to provide a transducer-patient connection. A transmitter circuit or pulsar circuit applies a short voltage pulse to the electrodes of the transducer crystal. The crystal starts vibrat-

ing and sends out a sound pulse of short duration, typically three cycles. The sound travels into the patient, where it is partially reflected and partially transmitted by the tissues it encounters. The reflected energy travels back to the transducer and causes the crystal to vibrate. These vibrations are changed into electric current by the crystal and then amplified.

The receiver circuit can determine the amplitude of the returned sound wave and the total travel time because it tracks when the sound was transmitted and when it returned. By knowing travel time, the depth of the reflecting tissue can be calculated using 1,540 meters/second as the sound velocity. The amplitude of the returned sound wave determines the shade of gray that should be assigned. Very weak echoes will be given a shade near the black end of the gray scale while strong echoes will be given a shade near the white end of the scale.

Each time the transducer pulses, a single line of information of an image results (Fig. 1–18). Each image or frame is made up of enough lines to produce adequate resolution, typically 128. Twenty to 30 images per second are necessary to minimize flicker. Thus, 24 images per second times 128 lines means the transducer might have a pulse repetition frequency (PRF) of 3,072 pulses per second. More images per second or more lines per image means that the PRF must be higher. If the PRF is higher, there is less time between pulses for receiving and less time for the sound to travel to a reflector and return, so that depth penetration becomes less.

A device called a digital scan convertor is usually used. This device stores information received from the transducer concerning the returning echoes. Numbers representing the amplitude of the echo are stored in a memory location corresponding to the location in space of each pixel. These numbers can then be used to generate a television image. The stored number representing amplitude is then assigned a shade of gray. Many current systems have 256 shades of gray. These are known as 8-bit systems. Each bit can be represented by 0 or 1 in the binary system. A 1-bit system could have 0 or 1 and therefore only two shades of gray. A 2-bit system can have 00, 01, 10, or 11 and four shades of gray. A 7-bit system can have 128 combinations of 0 or 1

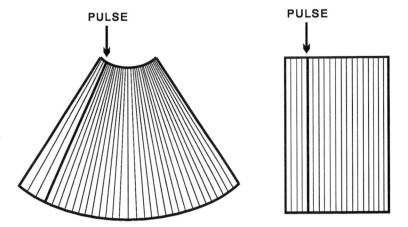

Figure 1–18. Each line of either a sector image or rectangular image results from one transducer pulse.

and an 8-bit system could have 256 shades of gray. Manufacturers may influence gray scale assignment by their preprocessing and postprocessing algorithms. Preprocessing controls the way in which numbers corresponding to amplitude are handled and manipulated before they are stored in memory. Postprocessing allows manipulation of amplitude data after storage.

Information from a digital scan convertor can be displayed in different modes. In "A" mode (amplitude), a graphic representation of the signal is used in which spike height corresponds to echo amplitude and depth is represented by distance along the horizontal axis (Fig. 1–19). "A" mode is still used in ophthalmology.

"B" mode (brightness mode) depicts the amplitude information in the form of dots. The brightness of each dot will be assigned one of the shades of gray. Higher amplitude will be displayed as a brighter shade of gray. This is commonly used in diagnostic imaging. "M" mode (motion) uses a roll of paper to record motion of the dots. Depth into the patient is represented by the vertical distance. Echo amplitudes are used to vary the brightness of each dot just as in the B mode.

The term B scan usually refers to a fixed-arm scanner used to "build up" scan information by repeatedly passing the transducer over the patient and storing the information. These are now seldom used.

Images are displayed on a television monitor. This is a cathode ray tube with a scanning electron beam. Five hundred twenty-five lines are scanned by the electron beam, with the even numbered lines scanned first. This $262\frac{1}{2}$-line scan produces a field. Odd lines are then scanned, producing a second field. All 525 lines make an image, but the image is produced in two parts. A frame rate of 30 frames per second uses 60 fields (and really 60 images) per second to reduce flicker.

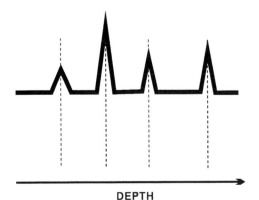

DEPTH

Figure 1–19. "A" mode; spike height corresponds to reflector strength. Position along the baseline reflects depth.

RESOLUTION

Resolution depends on two characteristics of visual acuity: detail and contrast. Linear resolution determines how far apart two reflectors must be so that they are seen as separate dots; contrast resolution determines how much difference there must be in the amplitude of two echoes before they are assigned different levels of gray. Whether or not the human eye can resolve two structures depends on types of resolution and the intrinsic ability of the individual eye to see contrast and detail.

Linear resolution in ultrasound must be divided further into depth (or axial) resolution along the direction of sound travel and lateral (transverse) resolution. Axial resolution is dependent upon the spatial pulse length. Two reflectors must be separated by one half the spatial pulse length to be seen as two dots (Fig. 1–20).

Axial resolution

$$= \frac{1}{2} \times \text{spatial pulse length}$$

Higher frequency transducers produce shorter waves that translate into a shorter pulse length and better resolution. The penalty is poor depth penetration of the beam.

Lateral resolution is equal to the diameter of the beam (Fig. 1–21). Beam diameter varies with the distance from the transducer. Small transducers help with lateral resolution, but a small transducer has a short Fresnel zone so that the improved lateral resolution is good only over a short distance into the patient. Focused transducers can help with this problem.

Contrast resolution depends upon the dynamic range of the entire ultrasound system and the number of shades of gray available. The dynamic range is the range of signal amplitudes that can be handled by the system, from the highest amplitude signal to the lowest (above noise). This is a ratio expressed in the decibel scale. A wide dynamic range means that two echoes must differ by only a small amount to be assigned different shades of gray.

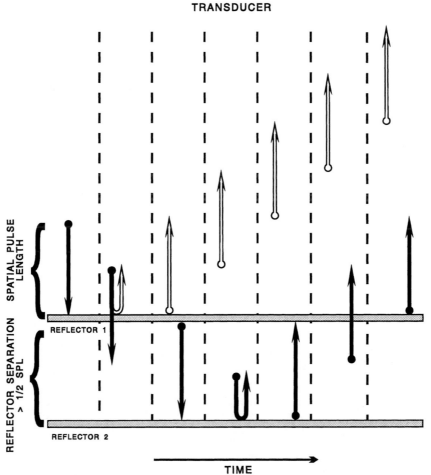

Figure 1–20. Reflector 1 and reflector 2 must be separated by at least $\frac{1}{2}$ spatial pulse length to be seen as separate. (Modified from Kremkau F. Diagnostic Ultrasound: Principles, Instruments, and Exercises, 3rd ed. Philadelphia, WB Saunders, 1989, with permission.)

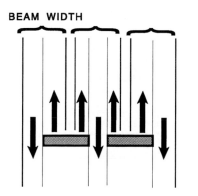

SEPARATE REFLECTORS ARE NOT RESOLVED

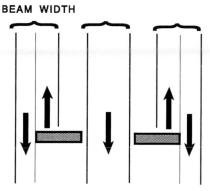

SEPARATE REFLECTORS ARE RESOLVED

Figure 1–21. Lateral resolution: two objects must be separated by one beam width to be resolved. (Modified from Kremkau F. Diagnostic Ultrasound: Principles, Instruments, and Exercises, 3rd ed. Philadelphia, WB Saunders, 1989, with permission.)

MACHINE CONTROLS

Overall "gain" is adjustable and refers to overall amplification. The time gain compensation (TGC) is a way of compensating for attenuation of sound by tissue. Echoes returning from deep within the body are amplified many more times than superficial echoes. The intent is to display a homogeneous organ (such as liver) with the same echo intensity in the near field as in the far field. This can be adjusted manually by controls on the machine (Fig. 1–22).

The frame rate also can sometimes be controlled manually. A faster frame rate means less depth penetration or fewer lines per frame because the pulse repetition frequency must be increased.

Depth, too, is controlled by the operator. Imaging at greater depth means a slower PRF and, therefore, a slower frame rate or fewer lines per image.

ARTIFACTS

As indicated, ultrasound is based on the assumption that the sound goes straight out from the transducer and returns straight back to the transducer. A second assumption is that the velocity of sound in tissue is 1,540 meters per second. The time of travel from transducer to reflector and back is used to calculate the distance between reflector and transducer. Most artifacts occur in circumstances where one of these two assumptions is not true.

Violation of the assumption that sound goes straight from transducer to reflector and straight back produces several types of artifacts:

1. Multipath artifacts occur when sound is reflected from multiple surfaces and takes a longer time to return to the transducer than it should. This causes the image to appear deeper than it is (Fig. 1–23A). The comet tail (ring down) artifact (Fig. 1–23B) is similar and is probably caused by many short reverberations within a cluster of air bubbles or other closely spaced reflectors. The result is that additional echoes are shown at a greater depth than the offending reflector.

   The mirror image artifact is another result of a multipath artifact (Fig. 1–23C). The sound beam is reflected off the diaphragm (arrows). The extra distance traveled by the sound beam results in echoes that are written deep to the diaphragm. The liver (star) is depicted above the diaphragm.

2. Reverberation artifacts are similar and occur when sound bounces back and forth between two reflectors or between one reflector and the transducer (Fig. 1–24). The extra time spent bouncing results in additional echoes deeper than the reflector on the image.

3. Refraction artifacts occur when the sound beam is bent at an interface between two types of tissue and can result in echoes that are incorrectly positioned. Refraction along the edge of a

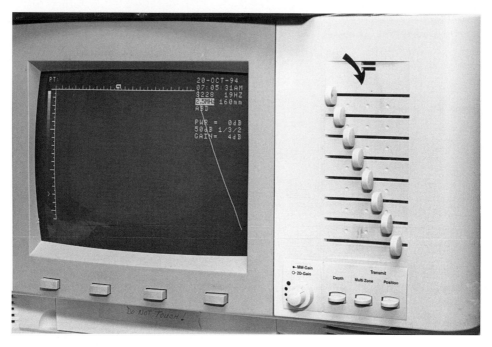

Figure 1–22. Illustration of TGC controls (*curved arrow*). These buttons control amplification in various parts of the image. Each of the eight controls affects the amount of amplification in a part of the image corresponding to the control.

spherical object (such as the gallbladder) can also produce a shadow that is not real (Fig. 1–25).

4. Side lobes and grating lobe artifacts are caused by waves that exit the transducer at an angle, strike a reflector, and then bounce back to the transducer. These appear in the images as though they are straight in front of the transducer when they are actually at an angle to the transducer.

5. Sound passes through a tissue with lower velocity than assumed, such as fat. The sound then takes longer to return than expected and the echoes are depicted on the image at a deeper location (Fig. 1–26).

6. Slice thickness artifacts are caused by a mechanism similar to volume averaging in computed tomography. The sound beam strikes two tissues with different characteristics, such as bladder and adjacent soft tissues. Some of the soft tissue echoes are located in the bladder because of the width of the sound beam (Fig. 1–27).

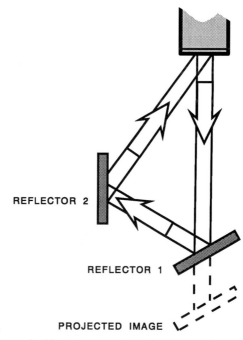

Figure 1–23. *A*, Reflector 1 is falsely depicted as deeper than it truly is because of the long path back to the transducer. *Figure continues on opposite page*

7. Shadows are produced when the ultrasound beam strikes a strong reflector and no or little sound penetrates beyond the reflector. Shadows are described as "clean," meaning there is no sound behind the reflector, and "dirty," meaning the shadow has some echoes within it. A clean shadow results when the sound strikes a rough surface with a small radius of curvature. Dirty shadows are associated with gas. They occur when a smooth surfaced object with a large radius (such as a gas bubble) reflects sound back and forth from reflec-

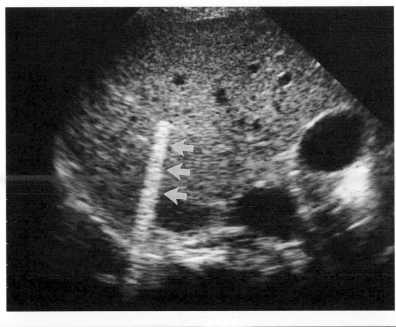

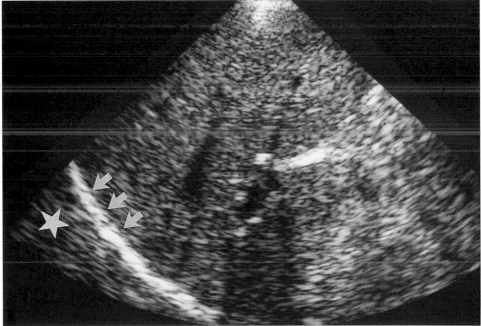

Figure 1–23. *Continued* *B*, Gas bubbles within liver lead to ring down artifact (*arrows*). *C*, Mirror image as a result of multipath. Diaphragm (*arrows*) reflects sound. Sound takes a circuitous route and this results in liver (*star*) being depicted above diaphragm.

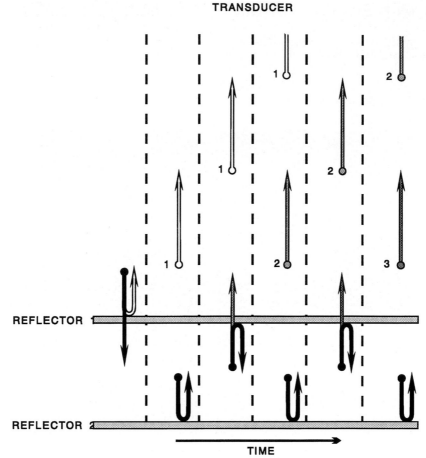

Figure 1–24. Reverberation artifact: sound bounces back and forth between two reflectors. The time spent in this extra travel leads to echoes that are written deeper than either reflector. Pulse 1 reflects off reflector 1 and pulse 2 reflects off reflector 2. Pulse 3 is delayed in returning because it bounces between reflector 1 and reflector 2. Pulse 3 leads to an image with a third reflector depicted deeper than either reflector 1 or 2.

tor to reflector multiple times (reverberation). The echoes are then located deep to the reflector and will partially fill in the shadow.

Doppler Ultrasound

CHARACTERISTICS OF FLOW

Doppler ultrasound uses changes in sound frequency caused by moving blood. Consequently, before discussing Doppler ultrasound and its application to imaging, it is necessary to describe the nature of blood flow. Blood flow is described as laminar or plug (Fig. 1–28). In laminar flow, the velocity of blood varies depending on the distance from the vessel wall. The highest velocities occur in the center of the vessel and the lowest are found at the vessel periphery. This is sometimes called parabolic flow because of a parabolic flow profile. The normal state in most vessels is laminar flow. This type of flow is found in most small arteries. Plug flow occurs in larger vessels. In plug flow, the velocity is the same in the center as at the periphery of the vessel (Fig. 1–28). Average velocity may be estimated to be half of the maximum velocity.

Disturbed flow occurs when flow is disrupted into whirlpools and areas of nonlinear flow. This may occur at a stenosis or bifurcation. For very disturbed flow, the term turbulent is used to imply a very disordered flow pattern in which blood moves

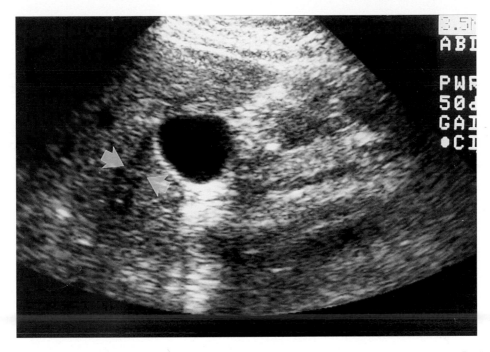

Figure 1–25. Shadow (*arrows*) at edge of gallbladder is due to refraction of the sound.

erratically and randomly. Measuring the average velocity in this situation is difficult and often impossible.

Flow also may be pulsatile or steady. Pulsatile flow occurs in response to periodic ejections of blood from the heart and is most obvious in arteries and arterioles. Steady flow means that the velocity of blood does not vary with time. This type of flow is found in veins.

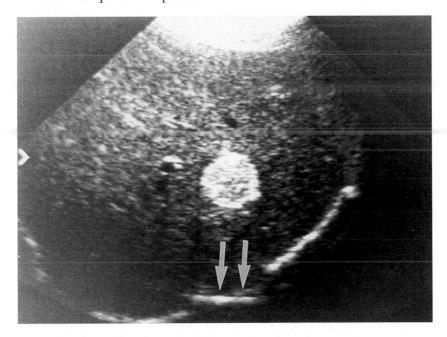

Figure 1–26. Intrahepatic angiomyolipoma with delay of sound, causing diaphragm (*arrows*) to be depicted more distally than it really is. (From Reading CC, Charboneau JW. Ultrasound. Radiographics *10*:511–512, 1990, with permission.)

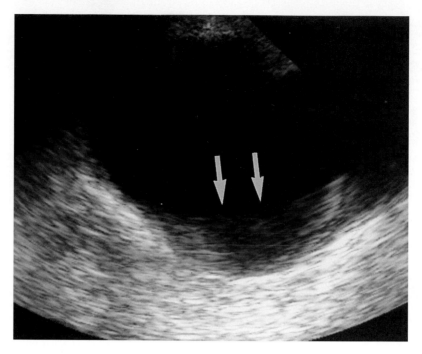

Figure 1–27. Slice thickness artifact causes echoes to be written into bladder (*arrows*).

Other influences on flow include pressure changes during the cardiac cycle. On the arterial side, the ejection of blood causes a typical pattern with a peak corresponding to the "R" wave of the electrocardiogram (Fig. 1–29A). On the venous side, central veins have an "a", "c", and "v" wave (Fig. 1–29B). These waves are usually not seen in peripheral veins except in cases of congestive heart failure or tricuspid valve incompetence. Increased venous flow, which we can see with a Doppler instrument, occurs when central pressure is low: during ventricular systole and when the atrioventricular valves open to fill the ventricles. Respiration influences venous flow. With inspiration, intrathoracic pressure decreases and venous volume increases, resulting in increased venous return to the heart from upper limbs and neck. In the abdomen, inspiration results in increased intra-abdominal pressure and decreased flow into the abdomen from lower extremity veins. These effects are reversed by expiration.

Volume of Flow

The volume of flow may be computed by multiplying the average velocity by πr^2

(cross-sectional area of the vessel):

$$\text{volume} = \text{average velocity} \times \pi \times r^2$$

The velocity of blood is proportional to the radius squared because of Poiseuille's equation:

$$\text{Avg Velocity} = \frac{\text{Pressure Difference} \times r^2}{8 \times \text{Length} \times \text{Viscosity}}$$

The volume of flow is proportional to the radius to the fourth power because the radius is squared in Poiseuille's equation and because the radius is squared in the formula for cross-sectional area. In reality, it is difficult to measure volume of flow accurately because it is difficult to measure the radius (or diameter) of the vessel accurately. Small errors in measurement of the radius may lead to large errors in measurement of the volume of flow.

Stenoses

If volume of flow is to be maintained, velocity must increase through a stenotic area. At the stenosis, laminar flow is usually maintained unless the wall is irregular.

In the poststenotic zone, a 1- or 2-cm

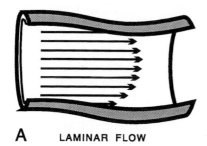

A LAMINAR FLOW

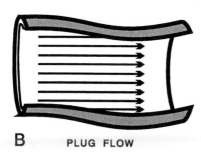

B PLUG FLOW

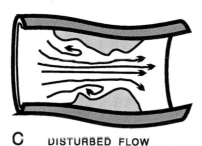

C DISTURBED FLOW

Figure 1–28. *A*, Parabolic or laminar flow. Highest velocities are in center. *B*, Plug flow. All velocities are equal. *C*, Turbulence or disturbed flow due to a stenosis.

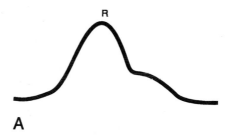

A

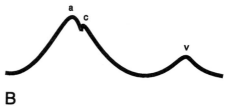

B

Figure 1–29. *A*, Typical arterial pulse wave. *B*, Typical venous wave of jugular vein: ''a'' wave occurs with right atrial systole; ''c'' wave occurs simultaneously with the carotid pulse; ''v'' wave occurs during rise in right atrial pressure during ventricular systole.

length of turbulence may be found. Whirlpools and random flow may give many different velocities by Doppler.

Distal to significant stenoses one may see a damped (decreased maximal velocity) wave form, an increase in the time to peak systole, and broadening of the wave form at half amplitude.

In the region proximal to a severe stenosis, there is a decrease in diastolic flow and an increase in pulsatility, that is, a larger difference between systolic and diastolic velocities.

DOPPLER EFFECT

The Doppler effect occurs when an emitter or reflector of sound is moving relative to a receiver of sound. If emitter and reflector are moving toward each other, the frequency of the sound is increased. If they are moving away from each other, the frequency is decreased. If an ultrasound beam strikes a reflector moving toward it, the reflected sound has a higher frequency than the original beam. If an ultrasound beam strikes a reflector moving away, the frequency of the reflected sound is lower than the original beam. The difference between the original beam frequency and the reflected beam frequency is the Doppler shift:

$$D = \frac{2 f_0 V}{m}$$

D = Doppler frequency shift
f_0 = original frequency
V = velocity of reflector
m = speed of sound in medium (1,540 m/sec)

We can rearrange this equation to get:

$$\frac{Dm}{V} = 2 f_0$$

The factor of ''2'' occurs in the numerator because the sound must make two trips.

One trip goes from transducer to reflector and the second trip from reflector back to transducer. The above equation must be adjusted if the reflector is not moving directly toward or away from the transducer. If the reflector is moving at an angle θ relative to the transducer, then the equation must be multiplied by $\cos \theta$ (Fig. 1–30).

$$D = \frac{2 f_0 V}{m} (\cos \theta)$$

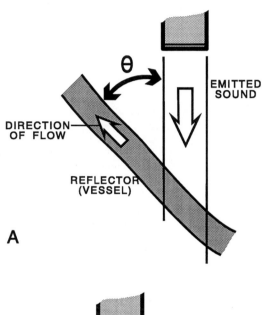

A

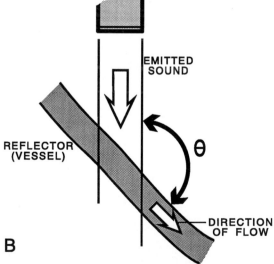

B

Figure 1–30. *A*, Flow is moving toward transducer (θ is less than 90°). Sound will be shifted to a higher frequency and will be depicted above the baseline. *B*, Flow away from transducer (θ greater than 90°). Sound is shifted to a lower frequency and will be depicted below the baseline.

or, rearranging,

$$V = \frac{Dm}{2 f_0 (\cos \theta)}$$

When the angle between transducer and reflector approaches 90°, since the cos 90° = 0, a Doppler shift may not be detected. Between 60° and 90°, small errors in estimation of the angle θ between transducer and reflector may result in huge differences in cos θ with resultant huge errors in Doppler shift calculations (Table 1–2). A 10° error between 75° and 85° makes a difference of .26 vs .09 when cos θ is calculated. A 10° error between 5° and 15° makes a difference of only .99 vs .97 for cos θ. Therefore, the angle between transducer and reflector should be less than 60° whenever possible.

INSTRUMENTATION

Continuous Wave

The most basic Doppler system is the continuous-wave instrument. Sound is emitted continuously. The transducer assembly has both a transmitter element and a receiver element. A demodulator compares the frequency of transmitted waves to the frequency of waves received and computes a difference. Filters eliminate low-frequency Doppler shifts that might be due to the respiratory motion of liver or another organ or due to a pulsating vessel wall. The continuous-wave instrument may not be able to distinguish between several vessels in the same area since any motion within the sample path of the transmit and receive

Table 1–2. ANGLE COSINES

ANGLE A (DEGREES)	COS A
0	1.00
5	.996
15	.98
25	.91
30	.87
35	.82
45	.71
55	.57
60	.50
65	.42
75	.26
85	0.09
90	0.00

transducers will result in a Doppler shift. This sample volume starts near the transducer face and usually extends into the tissues as far as the beam will penetrate. A technique known as phase V quadrature detection determines whether the Doppler shift is higher or lower than the transmitted frequency corresponding to flow toward or away from the transducer. Continuous-wave instruments are good for superficial vessels such as the carotid. They are also very sensitive to weak signals such as might be found in the digital artery of a finger. No depth information is obtained.

Pulsed Doppler

With a pulsed Doppler system, the same transducer element both sends and receives sound, similar to non-Doppler systems. The sound is sent in short bursts and then no sound is sent for a brief interval while the system waits for the returning echo. The depth of tissue that is being examined for flow is determined by varying the length of time after sound is transmitted before the receiver is turned on. The length of inter-

rogated tissue or gate length is determined by the duration of time for which the receiver is on (Fig. 1–31). The length of the emitted pulse also influences the gate length. The effective gate length is one-half pulse length longer than the gate length deduced on the basis of time of reception. The system is repeatedly pulsed. The pulse repetition frequency (PRF) is the frequency at which sound pulses are emitted. The Nyquist theorem states that PRF must be twice the Doppler shift frequency or errors in calculating and reconstructing Doppler curves may result.

An analogy would be a person who is trying to count a train of moving boxcars. This person keeps his eyes closed and opens them periodically for a brief look at the boxcars. He must open his eyes with a high enough frequency so that he sees each boxcar twice according to the Nyquist limit. Otherwise, he cannot be certain he has counted every boxcar and may arrive at a count that is too low. The PRF must be high enough to sample the vessel adequately so that the Doppler information is accurate.

One might think that we could just in-

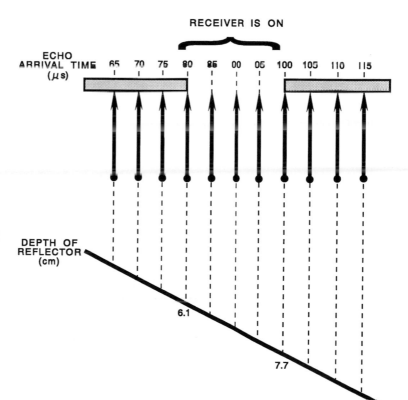

Figure 1–31. Pulsed Doppler. The receiver is "on" only between 80 and 100 seconds after the pulse is emitted. Therefore, only moving objects located at a depth between 6.1 and 7.7 cm will be detected.

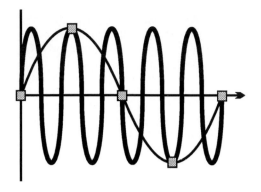

■ **SAMPLE POINTS**

Figure 1–32. Aliasing. If the sampling rate is too low, then the machine cannot accurately calculate the frequency. (Modified from Kremkau F. Diagnostic Ultrasound: Principles, Instruments, and Exercises, 3rd ed. Philadelphia, WB Saunders, 1989, with permission.)

crease the PRF if we encounter rapidly flowing blood. However, if we increase the PRF there is less time between pulses for the sound to return and, therefore, the depth we can examine is decreased. The phenomenon of miscalculating the Doppler shift because the PRF if too low is called aliasing (Fig. 1–32). Aliasing is a commonly encountered error, but it is usually easy to recognize (Fig. 1–33). The high-velocity portions of the Doppler trace are misinterpreted as being of low velocity and in the wrong direction. On most machines, the PRF is decreased when the field of view or depth of examination is increased. The PRF must be decreased to allow more time for the echoes to travel deep into the body and

return when very deep structures are examined. The PRF may be increased by using a smaller field of view or more shallow depth. Another way to effectively increase the PRF is to increase the scale on the Doppler trace. Aliasing occurs more often with high-frequency transducers (because the Doppler shift is greater with high-frequency transducers). One may change to a lower frequency transducer to eliminate aliasing. Another technique is to increase the angle of insonation, which will decrease the Doppler shift. Finally, aliasing may be eliminated by using continuous-wave Doppler instead of pulsed Doppler. Aliasing does not occur with continuous wave. One way to avoid aliasing is to switch to continuous-wave Doppler whenever it may be occurring.

DUPLEX SYSTEM

A duplex system is one in which Doppler and imaging information both can be obtained. In many such systems, the image is frozen and the transducer switched to Doppler mode. Every few seconds Doppler scanning is briefly discontinued and imaging resumed to update the image. Some instruments use the same transducer element and switch between Doppler and imaging modes. Other instruments have two separate transducer elements in the same housing. Usually the Doppler frequency is made lower than the imaging frequency. This minimizes aliasing in the Doppler mode and maximizes resolution. A low-frequency Doppler transducer is not as good as a

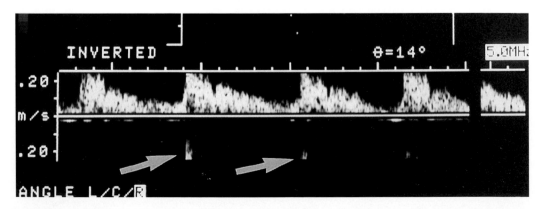

Figure 1–33. Doppler trace showing aliasing. Top of wave (*arrows*) wraps around and is written at bottom of trace.

higher frequency transducer at detecting slow flow, however.

Another way to combine Doppler and imaging in the same instrument is to use an array transducer with multiple elements. Several elements can be assigned to perform Doppler while others do imaging. Rapid switching between modes can make it appear that the image and Doppler data seem to be simultaneously acquired. In addition, the elements that are performing Doppler can be steered or angled to provide a better signal.

COLOR FLOW DOPPLER

Color Doppler ultrasound (CDU) works in a manner similar to pulsed Doppler. Each scan line in an image has multiple gates (Fig. 1–34). Doppler information is sampled from multiple gates from many scan lines in an image and, in effect, the entire image is sampled.

Color is arbitrarily assigned on the basis of flow toward or away from the transducer; e.g., red may mean flow toward and blue flow away from the transducer.

The frequency shift in CDU is determined by using a technique called quadrature detection. In quadrature detection the returning Doppler-shifted signal is compared to the carrier frequency of the original signal and to the carrier frequency, which has been phase shifted 90°. The latter is called the quadrature waveform. Using this method, the direction of flow is determined. Frequency shifts (i.e., Doppler

shifts) are determined by comparing the returning signal to a reference and determining the amount of phase shift of the wave. This is done using a technique called autocorrelation. The amount of frequency shift indicates *average* velocity for each pixel. To calculate these data usually requires 128 pulses for each line. In CDU there is a trade-off between sampling rate for detection of Doppler shifts and pulse rate for image generation. Usually the frame rate of imaging is slowed while CDU is being performed.

SPECTRAL ANALYSIS

Three types of information are available during a Doppler exam: (1) the frequency of returned echoes, which equates to velocity if the angle is known; (2) the amplitude of the returned echoes, which reflects the number of red blood cells in the examined volume; and (3) the time at which each echo returns. Duplex instruments can usually present Doppler information almost instantaneously in graph form with a time versus velocity graph (Fig. 1–35). With this plot, at any point in time we can see what frequencies are present. If angle correction has been made, then this graph is equivalent to time versus velocity. In Figure 1–35, we can see that only a narrow range of velocities is present in this normal patient at any point in time. With a minimal flow disturbance, flow in late systole and early diastole is disturbed first. As the flow becomes more disturbed, the spectral window is "filled in" or "broadened" (Fig. 1–36). This means that at any point in time, a wide range of velocities is present. There may even be forward and reverse flow at the same time. A frequency analyzer can take the frequency and time information, and, using a mathematical technique known as a fast Fourier transform, convert the above graph into a graph of frequency versus amplitude. This is sometimes called a power spectrum and indicates how much blood (amplitude) is present at any velocity (frequency).

INDICES

Indices that reflect the main characteristics of the Doppler waveform have been devised to simplify the analysis of the Doppler trace. These are usually incorporated

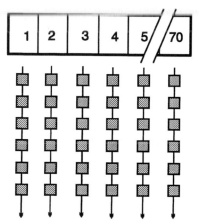

Figure 1–34. Gates from CDU. Each gray box is a Doppler gate. The numbers refer to scan lines of an image.

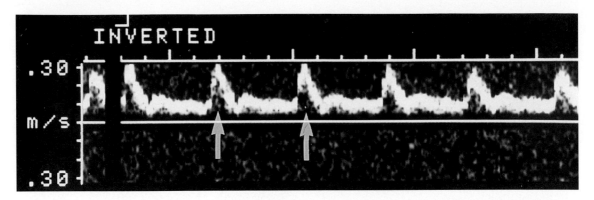

Figure 1-35. Normal Doppler. Area under wave is black (*arrows*).

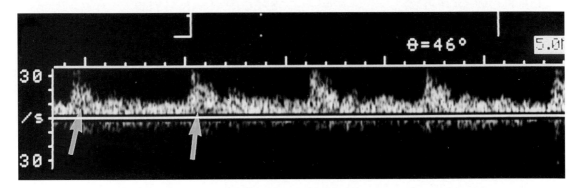

Figure 1-36. Spectral broadening. Area under curve is filled in (*arrows*).

into the software of the ultrasound machine.

Average velocity: indicates the flow rate at any point in time. It can be used with vessel cross-sectional area to calculate flow rates. This requires that the total vessel lumen be included in the Doppler window so that the entire range of velocities from vessel wall to vessel center is included in the calculation. It takes into account the range of velocities and the number of cells moving at each velocity.

A/B ratio: also known as systolic/diastolic ratio. Advantage: simple to use and calculate; disadvantage: cannot account for reverse flow, approaches infinity as diastolic flow becomes small. Commonly used in obstetrics for fetal and umbilical vessel evaluation.

Resistivity index: also known Pourcelot index (see below and Fig. 1–37).

High diastolic flow leads to low values. This does not handle reversed diastolic flow. Commonly used to evaluate renal transplants.

Pulsatility index: (See Fig. 1–38.)

$$PI = \frac{A - B}{\text{mean}}$$

$$= \frac{\text{Peak Systolic} - \text{End-Diastolic}}{\text{Mean Velocity}}$$

Can reflect both reverse diastolic flow and a wide range of velocities because the mean velocity is in the denominator. Commonly used to evaluate the extremities and the carotids.

Normal values for each of these indices will vary depending on the artery being examined. Because the A/B ratio, resistivity index, and pulsatility index are ratios, they

$$\text{Resistivity index} = \frac{\text{Peak Systolic Velocity-End-Diastolic Velocity}}{\text{Peak Systolic Velocity}}$$

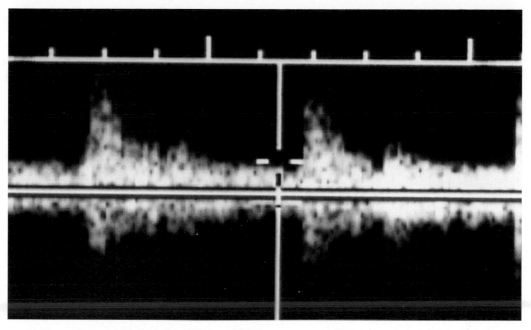

Figure 1–37. Resistivity index is calculated by machine. Peak systolic velocity has been marked and cross hairs are now being used to mark end diastolic velocity.

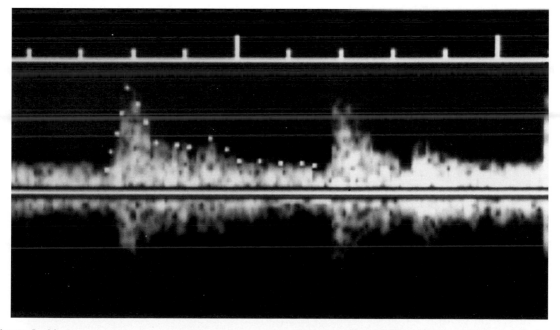

Figure 1–38. To calculate the pulsatility index, the envelope of the Doppler trace must be manually outlined by the operator. This allows the machine to calculate the peak systolic velocity, end diastolic velocity, and the average velocity so that a pulsatility index may be derived.

are not influenced by measurement of the angle of flow.

SOURCES OF ERROR AND DOPPLER ARTIFACTS

One common source of error in velocity measurements is incorrect measurement of the angle of flow. Many vessels are tortuous or curved, and it is difficult to precisely measure an angle. However, errors can usually be kept to less than 5°. As indicated earlier, small errors are not important at angles less than 60° but become more important between 60° and 90°. Estimates of average velocity require that the entire vessel lumen be evaluated so that slowly flowing cells near the vessel wall, as well as rapidly flowing cells at the center, can be counted. To estimate flow, it is necessary to know the average velocity and the cross-sectional area of the vessel. Cross-sectional area is calculated from

$$A = \pi r^2 \text{ or } A = \pi \frac{(d)^2}{(4)}$$

where r = radius and d = diameter.

Because the diameter is squared, 1- or 2-mm errors in diameter measurement can lead to huge errors in calculation of the area. Larger arteries are more elastic and change in diameter during systole. This fluctuation in diameter during the cardiac cycle may lead to large errors.

Movement of vessel walls may lead to large, low-frequency echoes. These are usually removed from the Doppler trace using a "wall thump filter." This filter may also remove signals from slow flow. This is more a problem when the transducer approaches a perpendicular (90°) orientation to the vessel since the expanding vessel may be moving directly toward the transducer in that situation. Aliasing, as described earlier, also can be a problem.

A range ambiguity problem can result from using a high PRF. This means that not all echoes have been received at the transducer before a new pulse is sent out. If an echo returns from pulse number 1 just after pulse number 2 is sent out, the machine infers that the received echo is coming from a superficial location because of the apparently quick transit time.

Mirror image artifacts in Doppler show up as signal, often symmetrical, on both sides of the baseline (Fig. 1–39). This can occur with high receiver gain when high signal confuses the direction-sensing circuitry. It can also occur at angles of 90° or with low-gain signals when the machine has trouble determining the true flow direction. A mirror artifact in color Doppler occurs when a large reflector is posterior to the vessel being examined. This may cause an imaginary extra vessel to appear deep to

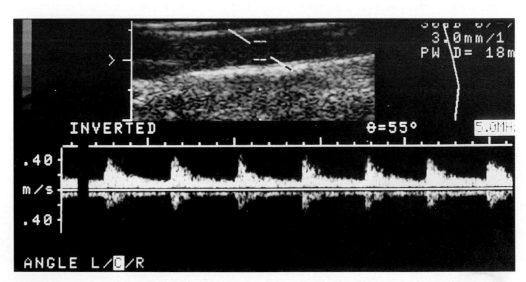

Figure 1–39. Mirror image artifact. This occurs when the machine has trouble telling the direction of flow. In this case the Doppler gate is almost 90° to the vessel.

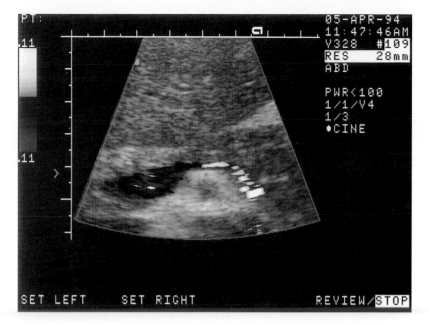

Figure 1–40. Color Doppler. Transverse image of splenic vein. Flow is depicted in two colors with red toward the transducer and green away from the transducer, even though all flow is in the same direction. See color plate 1.

the real vessel. A common error in color Doppler is to assume that all vessels of one color are arteries and all vessels of another color are veins. It is important to remember that color is determined by whether flow is toward or away from the transducer (Fig. 1–40). A vessel with a small bend may have flow depicted as both toward and away from the transducer. In color Doppler, the color of any pixel indicates *average* velocity within that pixel. This is different than pulsed Doppler, where peak velocity is detected.

Aliasing in color flow mimics flow reversal. In true flow reversal there will be a band of nonflowing blood—a no-flow zone—between forward flowing and reverse flowing blood. A no-flow zone may

also be seen when the transducer is perpendicular to the vessel. Aliasing in color flow Doppler may be minimized by changing the color flow scale, by using a lower frequency transducer, or by making the color flow box as small as possible.

Suggested Readings

Kremkau F. Doppler Ultrasound: Principles and Instruments. Philadelphia, WB Saunders, 1990.

Kremkau, F. Diagnostic Ultrasound: Principles, Instruments, and Exercises, 3rd ed. Philadelphia, WB Saunders, 1989.

McDicken, W. Diagnostic Ultrasonics: Principles and Use of Instruments, 3rd ed. New York, Churchill Livingstone, 1991.

CHAPTER 2

Vascular Ultrasound

Technical Aspects

Vascular ultrasound imaging relies heavily on the Doppler effect, which is discussed in detail in Chapter 1. Briefly, the fundamentals of vascular imaging are as follows: sound waves of a known frequency are directed toward moving blood; the sound waves strike the moving blood and are reflected back to the transducer; the frequency of the returning signal is changed depending on the velocity of the blood and the angle at which the sound beam strikes the moving blood. The change in frequency is called the Doppler shift and can be determined by the following formula:

$$D = \frac{2 f_0 V \cos \theta}{M}$$

D = frequency of Doppler shift
f_0 = frequency of sound from transducer
V = velocity of target
θ = angle between transducer and target
M = velocity of sound in tissue
   being examined

In color flow Doppler, the image is best thought of as being divided into pixels. Any flow in a given pixel is detected, but there is no angle correction, and the velocity within the pixel is simply an average velocity of all structures moving within that pixel. Depending upon this velocity, a color is assigned to the pixel that is being interrogated. When performing color Doppler, a box can be placed around the area of interest on most machines. The larger this box, the less time available for gray scale imaging. Therefore, flickers of the gray scale image may be reduced by keeping this box small. Color Doppler aliasing is also reduced with a small box size (i.e., the pulse repetition frequency may be higher).

For carotid Doppler, and for small superficial vessels in general, 7- to 10-MHz transducers are usually ideal. For other vessels such as the aorta or iliac arteries, a 5-MHz or even a 3-MHz transducer may be necessary to get adequate penetration.

The Doppler data are usually displayed as a spectrum adjacent to the ultrasound image. This spectrum is essentially a graph with time on the horizontal axis and velocity on the vertical axis. Shades of gray or different colors indicate how many blood cells are moving at each velocity.

When a stenotic artery is examined, a phenomenon known as spectral broadening may be encountered. Spectral broadening means that the range of velocities seen is much wider than usual and includes high-velocity particles, low velocity particles, and intermediate velocity particles. This is reflected in the Doppler spectrum display by filling in of signal underneath the trace. Spectral broadening may be subjectively quantified. Minimal spectrum broadening occurs mainly in late systole or early diastole (Fig. 2–1). Moderate spectral broadening has the entire window filled in underneath the trace. Severe spectral broadening has reversal of flow during portions of the trace and will show backward and forward flow simultaneously. In color Doppler, a mixture of color and even color adjacent to soft tissues, known as a visible bruit, may be seen. It should be noted that too large a sample volume may give spurious spectral broadening.

Whenever a vessel is stenotic, the following factors affect the significance of the area of narrowing: (1) the length and diameter of a narrowed segment, (2) the roughness of the endothelial surface of the narrowed segment, (3) the irregularity of the narrowed segment, (4) the overall amount of cross-sectional area blocked, (5) the flow

29

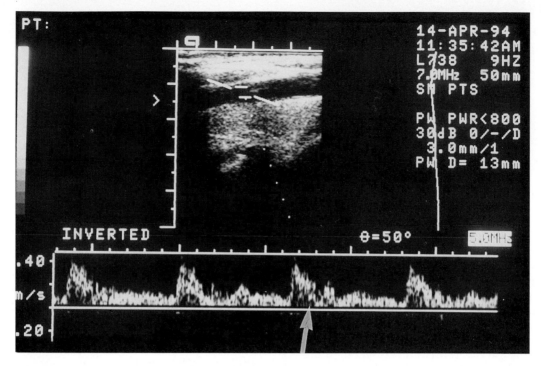

Figure 2–1. Minimal spectral broadening: filling in of area under trace (*arrow*) mainly in late systole and early diastole.

rate, (6) the pressure gradient across the area of stenosis, and (7) the peripheral resistance in the vessel that is being examined.

When there is a stenosis or obstruction in an artery proximal to a site of interrogation, systolic acceleration is slowed, and the maximal velocities are lower than normal during both diastole and systole. This is known as a "damped wave form." A false-positive damped wave form may occur in cases of cardiac dysfunction. Therefore, whenever this situation is encountered, other arteries should be checked to see if the abnormality can be detected in them. If so, a cardiac problem should be suspected.

Whenever there is outflow obstruction, that is, stenosis distal to the site of interrogation, the resistance to flow is increased. In cases of mild stenosis, that is, obstruction that produces only a small increase in resistance, good diastolic flow will be continued. With moderate resistance obstruction (distal to the site of interrogation), there will be little diastolic flow, and with high resistance obstruction, there will be reversal of early diastolic flow.

When the interrogation is within the stenotic zone, the following parameters can be measured: (1) peak systolic velocity, (2) end-diastolic velocity, (3) systolic velocity ratio, (4) diastolic velocity ratio, and (5) poststenotic flow disturbance.

As the degree of stenosis increases (Table 2–1), peak systolic velocity increases until 75 percent of the diameter (95 percent of the area) is occluded. Further increases in the amount of obstruction lead to a decrease in velocity until, at complete occlusion, there is zero velocity. Peak end-diastolic velocity in an area of stenosis increases. This effect is usually only seen after an approximately 50 percent decrease in vessel diameter.

The systolic velocity ratio is obtained by taking the peak velocity in the stenotic zone during systole and comparing it to a peak systolic velocity in a nonstenotic area. The same calculation can be performed with diastolic velocity in the stenotic zone. Usually the peak systolic velocity in the internal carotid stenotic zone is compared to the peak systolic velocity in the common carotid. The velocity in the common carotid is presumed to be normal. A ratio above approximately 1.8 suggests a stenosis of at least 60 percent. The same is true for the diastolic velocity ratio, with the velocity being measured at

Table 2–1. DOPPLER SPECTRUM ANALYSIS

DIAMETER STENOSIS (%)	PEAK SYSTOLIC VELOCITY (CM/SEC)	END-DIASTOLIC VELOCITY (CM/SEC)	SYSTOLIC VELOCITY RATIO (VICA:VCCA)	DIASTOLIC VELOCITY RATIO (VICA:VCCA)	SPECTRAL BROADENING (CM/SEC)
0	<110	<40	<1.8	<2.4	<30
1–39	<110	<40	<1.8	<2.4	<40
40–59	<130	<40	<1.8	<2.4	<40
60–79	>130	>40	>1.8	>2.4	>40
80–99	>250	>100	>3.7	>5.5	>80

end-diastole. One significant caveat is that the effects described above occurring distal or proximal to a stenotic zone may not occur if there is good collateral flow. Table 2–1 summarizes these findings.

Examination of the Carotid Artery

The common carotid artery is examined first. The patient should be positioned supine with the head rotated away from the side being examined. Scanning is usually begun in a posterior lateral position, but it may be worthwhile to move to an anterior position to improve visualization. The velocity spectrum from a typical portion of the common carotid artery is recorded. Since the carotid bifurcation is the area most likely to be involved by disease, this portion of carotid is examined next. The transducer should be placed in the region of the clavicle and should be moved superiorly to the area of the carotid bifurcation. The internal and external carotid artery should be identified and evaluated for patency. One should look for plaque in the region of the bifurcation. The velocity spectrum from both internal and external carotid arteries should be recorded. One must try to find a typical segment. Usually, the external carotid is smaller and has branches, whereas the internal carotid is larger with no branches. The external carotid artery is a high-resistance vessel with very little diastolic flow, while the internal carotid is a low-resistance artery with high diastolic flow. The external carotid usually moves anteriorly toward the face as it branches.

The carotid artery also should be examined in the transverse imaging plane. This allows assessment of the amount of plaque and can also help in estimating the size of residual lumen if a stenosis is present.

At times, it may be difficult to tell which vessel is internal carotid and which vessel is external carotid, in spite of the characteristics mentioned above. If this is the case, then one may tap the superficial temporal artery and look for transmitted pulsations. This procedure may help to identify the external carotid artery.

A normal carotid wall demonstrates a sharp specular reflector at the intimal surface. A hypoechoic layer represents the media of the artery and an outermost white line is the adventitia of the artery (Fig. 2–2). Plaque may be found along the walls of the carotid artery. Early plaque formation may be measured on a transverse image. Intima plus media should not be thicker than 1.2 mm. Fibrofatty plaque is low in echogenicity. More collagen gives more echogenicity. Strongly echogenic plaque may be a result of dystrophic calcifications that occur in the plaque and the adjacent arterial wall. Plaque ulcerations can be a source of emboli that lead to transient ischemic attacks. In general, ultrasound cannot reliably demonstrate ulcerations, however. If the plaque is completely smooth, then it is doubtful if ulcerations are present. If a well-defined crater can clearly be identified in two new imaging planes, then there is a high probability of an ulcer.

Analysis of the common carotid wave form may be quite helpful. If there is a stenosis proximal to the examined area of the common carotid, for example, near where the carotid branches off the aortic arch, then the entire wave form may be of low amplitude and have a damped appearance. On the other hand, if there is an obstruction at

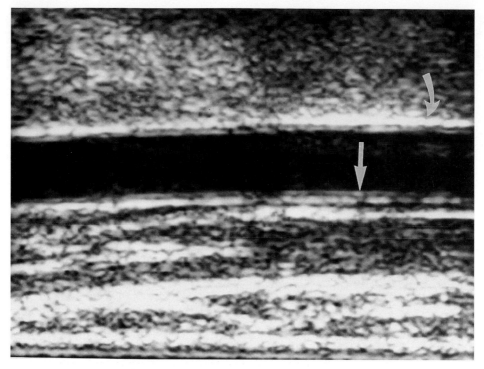

Figure 2–2. Intima (*straight arrow*) and adventitia (*curved arrow*) are seen well in this patient.

the carotid bifurcation (i.e., distal to the common carotid artery), then there may be absence of diastolic flow in the common carotid. It should be noted, however, that the common carotid may have high-resistance characteristics for reasons other than a stenosis at the carotid bifurcation. For instance, hypertension, a rapid heart rate, and severe distal arterial vascular disease leading to decreased arterial compliance may all result in high-resistance common carotid wave forms. However, the abnormality will be present bilaterally in both common carotids in these diseases.

The most commonly used parameter for the evaluation of a stenotic zone is the peak systolic velocity. A peak systolic velocity above approximately 130 cm/sec is abnormal and indicates a stenosis of at least 60 percent of the diameter (Fig. 2–3). Confirmatory evidence may be obtained from the peak end-diastolic velocity, which will be above 40 cm/sec with 60 percent stenosis. High systolic velocities may occur with shunting when there is contralateral disease. Determining the systolic velocity ratio may be useful because it may indicate compensation for changes in heart rate,

blood pressure status, fluid status, and cardiac output. The stenotic zone peak velocity is divided by peak velocity from the common carotid artery. A ratio over 1.8 is considered to be significant and indicates at least a 60 percent diameter decrease. The end-diastolic ratio can be used in a similar fashion. The peak velocity at end diastole in the area of stenosis is divided by the peak velocity at the end of diastole in the normal common carotid. A ratio greater than 5.5 may predict an 80 percent reduction in diameter. The examiner should also look for spectral broadening in the post-stenotic zone. Spectral broadening will be most severe in the 1 cm beyond the stenosis because this is where turbulence is the worst. Artifactual spectral broadening may occur when the gain is too high or when the sample volume is too near the wall.

Higher peak systolic velocities indicate greater degrees of stenosis (Fig. 2–4).

Care must be taken not to miss a totally occluded or near-totally occluded internal carotid artery. In this situation, the external carotid artery may be mistaken for the non-visible internal carotid.

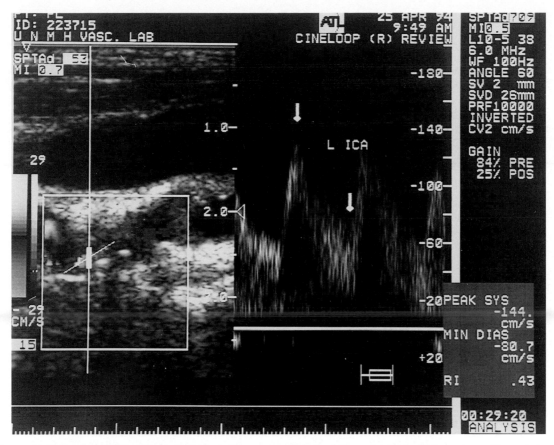

Figure 2–3. Peak systolic velocity is 144 cm/sec and end-diastolic velocity is 80.7 cm/sec. Stenosis is at least 60 percent of the diameter.

Examination of the Vertebral Artery

The vertebral arteries are examined after the carotids. Vertebral basilar insufficiency is a poorly defined and poorly understood syndrome. Symptoms may include dizziness or fainting. Visual field problems may occur, as well as problems with multiple cranial nerves. However, the therapeutic options in regard to the vertebral and basilar arterial systems are limited.

It should be noted that approximately three-quarters of patients have asymmetric vertebral arteries, and about four-fifths of these have a larger left vertebral artery. A vertebral artery smaller than 2 mm in diameter is probably abnormal.

The vertebral arteries originate from the subclavian arteries, but they may be difficult to see on ultrasound. The vertebral artery is commonly tortuous at its origin. The vertebral arteries pass through the foramen transversarium of the cervical vertebrae, a small series of rings along the lateral side of each vertebral body. Normally, there are foramen transversaria of C1 through C6. Not uncommonly, however, C7 will also have a foramen.

In general, the vertebral arteries are found by angling the transducer more posteriorly until the vertebral bodies are identified and then the vertebral arteries can be examined between the vertebral bodies. Only small portions of the vertebral artery will be outside of the foramen transversarium. Color flow Doppler is used to make certain that the direction of flow is correct. The velocity wave form of each vertebral artery should be recorded and each should be followed as far proximally and distally as possible.

Frequently, veins will be seen in the region of the vertebral artery, and one must

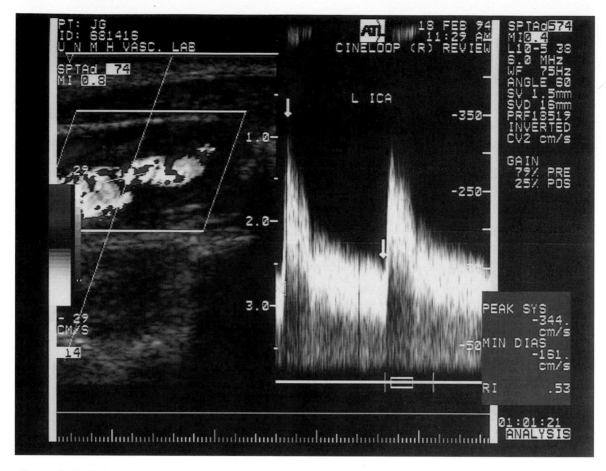

Figure 2–4. Color Doppler image of internal carotid artery shows obvious stenosis. Doppler spectrum shows peak systolic velocity of 344 cm/sec and end-diastolic velocity of 161 cm/sec, indicating stenosis should be at least 80 percent. See color plate 2.

take care to make certain that one has arterial pulsations and not venous pulsations in the spectral display. The vertebral system is low resistance, so there should be flow throughout diastole and flow reversal should not occur. The wave form should be symmetric.

The examiner must watch for either increased or decreased velocity, abnormal direction of flow, and lack of flow. Failure to identify the vertebral artery may mean that it is totally occluded, but it may also be invisible due to poor visualization. It may be useful to make certain that the duplex instrument is set for a low flow state if the vertebral artery cannot readily be identified. Usually, the flow rate in the vertebral artery will be less than 40 cm/sec at peak systole. If increased velocity is seen, then turbulence should be looked for as an indicator that there is a stenosis causing the

increase in velocity. With severe stenosis, the velocity may decrease. The sensitivity of duplex Doppler in vertebral artery stenosis is approximately 75 percent and specificity approximately 95 percent. However, these values may be inaccurate because they are based on studies in which only about 80 percent of patients are examined successfully.

TRANSCRANIAL DOPPLER

Transcranial Doppler is a relatively new technique. It is used to detect intracranial stenosis in major arteries at the base of the brain and can also be used to evaluate the effects of extracranial occlusive disease, such as subclavian steal or intracranial blood flow. It has been used to evaluate arteriovenous malformations, to monitor patients with vasospasm after subarachnoid hemorrhage, and to monitor patients during balloon occlusion and balloon embolization procedures.

Before performing transcranial Doppler, the extracranial vessels must be completely evaluated. The patient must be calm, comfortable and quiet so that changes in pCO_2, which may affect dilatation and contraction of intracranial vessels, do not occur. In general, 2-MHz duplex Doppler systems are used. Focusing is performed at a distance farther from the transducer than usual, about 5 cm. Scanning can be performed from the transtemporal, transorbital, suboccipital, and submandibular approaches. Usually, the transtemporal approach is the most useful and is performed through the temporal bone just anterior to the ear. M1 and M2 segments of the middle cerebral arteries, the C1 segment of the siphon, as well as the A1 segment of the anterior cerebral artery can be evaluated.

Sometimes the anterior communicating artery can be evaluated. By angling posteriorly, the P1 and P2 segments of the posterior cerebral artery and most distal basilar artery can be identified. Usually, the posterior communicating arteries are visible. By scanning through the orbit with the transducer against a closed eyelid, the anterior portion of the carotid siphon can sometimes be examined. The suboccipital approach may be useful for screening the vertebral and basilar arteries. The transducer is placed between the foramen magnum and the spinous process of the first cervical vertebral body with the beam aimed toward the eyes. The submandibular approach may be useful for examining the distal parts of the internal carotid artery. When stenosis is present, increased velocity of peak systolic flow may be detected as well as disturbed flow. Little information is available regarding the accuracy of transcranial Doppler and the detection of intracranial lesions, however.

Examination of the Upper Extremities

Usually a 3- or 5-MHz transducer is needed to examine the origins of the subclavian artery. As one moves more peripherally in the upper extremity, a higher frequency transducer (either 5.0 or 7.0 MHz)

will be needed. Standoff pads also may be necessary. Arteries of the upper extremity show higher resistance and a triphasic pattern. Early in diastole there is reversal of flow, with forward flow in late diastole. A biphasic pattern may also be normal but a monophasic pattern is abnormal and occurs with high distal metabolic demand, such as distal infection or after exercise; insufficient arterial inflow; or distal arteriovenous shunting. Normal peak systolic velocities will vary widely but generally have values between 60 and 100 cm/sec. If there is stenosis, the velocity will be increased within the stenotic zone and there will be turbulent flow in the poststenotic region. When sites of suspected stenosis have been identified, it is worthwhile to measure the peak systolic velocity in the stenotic zone and then to measure peak systolic velocity several centimeters proximal to the systolic zone in an area of normal artery. If this peak systolic velocity ratio is greater than 2, then stenosis of the artery is likely. Generally, a 50 percent decrease in diameter leads to doubling of peak velocity and a quadrupling indicates a 75 percent diameter reduction.

Any bypass grafts should be examined for patency as stenosis can occur in them also. An entire bypass graft can be scanned using color Doppler. Again, the peak systolic velocity ratio can be used to identify areas of possible stenosis. A doubling of peak systolic velocity along the length of a graft usually indicates stenosis. A velocity of greater than 200 cm/sec also indicates stenosis. Low velocity flow in a graft (less than 45 cm/sec) indicates probable near term graft failure. Monophasic flow in a graft may be normal.

Dialysis fistulas may develop infection, aneurysms, or stenosis. A fistula can be examined for infection by looking for fluid collections around the region of the anastomosis. Stenosis can be evaluated by using the peak systolic velocity ratio with the feeding artery being used as a reference. Aneurysms present as a mass adjacent to the fistula and should demonstrate turbulent or to-and-fro flow.

Pseudoaneurysms may develop in either bypass grafts or dialysis fistulas. These will also have to-and-fro flow. They appear as a mass adjacent to the vessel. Pseudoaneurysms have a differential diagnosis that includes a saccular true aneurysm and hematoma. A pseudoaneurysm may also develop in a native artery after trauma or puncture. A pseudoaneurysm is nothing more than a contained leak. Treatment is surgical ligation or ultrasound-guided compression. Ultrasound-guided compression is performed by putting steady pressure on the neck of the pseudoaneurysm for 10 to 20 minutes. Compression is repeated multiple times for a total of 1 hour. Compression is contraindicated if the pseudoaneurysm is the result of infection or if it is near the inguinal ligament so that intraperitoneal rupture is a possibility. The arterial lumen should be maintained in a patent state during compression. If the pseudoaneurysm is at a graft anastomosis, then repair should be surgical.

EVALUATION OF PERIPHERAL VEINS

Doppler has now become the preferred method to screen for peripheral venous thrombosis. Veins should have constant forward velocity with respiratory variation. In the lower extremity, inspiration should produce decreased flow because of an increase in intra-abdominal pressure. In the upper extremity, inspiration should produce increased flow. Obstructed veins lose this respiratory variation.

When thrombus forms in a peripheral leg vein, it is usually sonolucent initially and becomes more echogenic over a period of days. In acute deep venous thrombosis, the vein will usually be distended and larger than the adjacent artery. In chronic thrombosis, the vein will usually be echogenic and be either equal in size or smaller in size than the adjacent artery. Collateral veins may also be seen. Color Doppler for acute deep venous thrombosis above the knee is 95 to 98 percent accurate when performed by an experienced examiner. In the calf, accuracy is lower but may be up to 80 percent.

Five criteria are used to determine whether or not a vein is thrombosed (Table 2–2): compressibility, augmentation, spontaneity, respiratory variation, and presence of intraluminal thrombus. Compressibility means that when the transducer is placed over a peripheral vein and pressure is applied, the two walls collapse and the lumen is obliterated. A caveat: The vein may not

Table 2–2. CRITERIA FOR DIAGNOSIS OF DEEP VENOUS THROMBOSIS

1. Compressibility	Walls of vein should collapse together when transducer used to apply pressure
2. Spontaneity	Doppler signal easily detected
3. Augmentation	Contraction of calf muscles should increase flow
4. Respiratory variation	Expiration should increase flow in lower leg veins
5. Thrombus in lumen	May occasionally see thrombus in lumen

easily be compressed in Hunter's canal. Compressibility is one of the most important signs that no thrombus is present. Spontaneity occurs when a Doppler signal is detected within the lumen of the vessel spontaneously or instantaneously upon sampling of that vessel. Augmentation is an increase in the flow through the vessel when the calf is squeezed or when the patient contracts the calf muscles, resulting in an increase in flow through the lower extremity venous system. Augmentation implies unimpeded flow between the point of compression and point of examination. Respiratory variation occurs when there are spontaneous changes in the velocity of flow as the patient breaths. Finally, the visualization of clot within the vein is evidence of thrombosis (Fig. 2–5). It should be noted that extrinsic masses may obstruct a vein and may lead to abnormalities in many of these signs.

The leg should normally be examined with the patient supine. The knee may be bent for greater accessibility to the calf veins. One should begin the examination in the femoral region and work distally. The detection of thrombosis between inferior vena cava and knee is felt to be more important than the detection of thrombosis in the calf veins since embolization of calf thrombus is debatable. The examiner should continue below the knee remembering that, usually, the deep veins are paired below the knee.

Also keep in mind that congestive heart failure can change the respiratory phasicity of a normal vein. We image only the symptomatic limb, although there are advocates of imaging both limbs as there may be

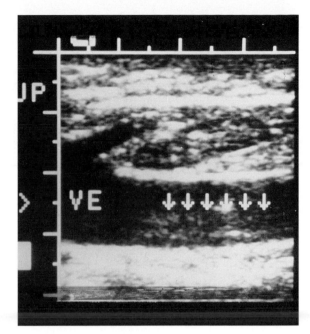

Figure 2–5. Superficial femoral vein has visible clot within it.

thrombosis in an asymptomatic limb in a high-risk patient. If it is difficult to demonstrate spontaneous venous flow, then the amount of reverse Trendelenburg should be increased. In pregnant patients, a lateral decubitus position may be useful. The fetus and enlarged uterus may result in extrinsic compression and cause abnormal signs of thrombus when none are present. For venous studies, the color Doppler flow settings must be at their lowest so that low flow states may be detected. If no flow is detected, it may be useful to switch to a higher frequency transducer since the Doppler shift will be greater, and slow flow is detected better. If flow still cannot be detected, a switch to a lower frequency transducer may give more power and penetration.

CHRONIC DEEP VENOUS THROMBOSIS

Chronic thrombosis is manifest by focal wall thickening; residual thrombus, especially along the wall; and valve thickening, calcification, or incompetence. Doppler of these veins may range from normal to a dampened monotonous wave form. If clot is seen within a vein, there are no criteria to determine clot age based on echogenicity. Acute clot is more likely to expand the vein and be tender to direct compression. The differentiation of chronic venous thrombus from acute disease may not be possible.

VENOUS INSUFFICIENCY

Incompetent valves may be a result of chronic deep venous thrombosis, or episodes of acute thrombosis. Primary incompetence may also occur without antecedent history. Patients may present with swelling, pain, induration, and ulceration. Descending venography has been the gold standard for this diagnosis. Color Doppler has been used to make this diagnosis but the accuracy is uncertain. Reversal of flow with the Valsalva maneuver or with compression of the vein proximal to the valve or reversal following the release of distal compression all suggest the diagnosis.

ARTERIOVENOUS FISTULAS

These occur because of puncture or trauma of adjacent arteries and veins. Symptoms may include distal ischemia, venous stasis, deep venous thrombosis, and infection. These lesions have high diastolic flow on the arterial side due to low resistance. There is "arterialization" of the wave form on the venous side with high velocity flow. A color Doppler bruit may be present where color is seen in the soft tissues adjacent to the vessels. In situ grafts where native veins are used for arterial bypass grafts may develop fistulas if there is incomplete ligation of feeding veins. Diagnosis depends on color visualization of abnormal flow away from the graft.

EXAMINATION OF THE AORTA

The aorta should be examined from diaphragm to bifurcation into iliac arteries. The diagnosis of abdominal aortic aneurysm (AAA) depends on identifying a segment of aorta that is greater than 3 cm in diameter. We measure the lumen from inner wall to inner wall in both the anteroposterior and transverse planes. Measurements are made in the epigastric region, at the level of the take-off of the superior mesenteric artery (about 1 to 2 cm above the renal artery origins), at the level of the renal arteries (if not obscured by bowel gas), and then at 3- to 4-cm intervals inferiorly to the level of the bifurcation into iliac arteries. Care must be taken to make measurements perpendicular to the long axis of the aorta since oblique measurements exaggerate the size of the aorta. If measurements greater than 3 cm are found, a diagnosis of AAA is made. Measurements greater than 5 cm are an indication for surgery. It is important to determine the length of the aneurysm if one is found. It is also important to determine if the aneurysm extends proximally to the level of the renal arteries, making surgery more difficult, and if it extends distally to involve the common iliac arteries. Common iliac arteries greater than 1.5 cm are abnormal.

It is very common for AAAs to have extensive circumferential clot. Color Doppler can be used to separate clots from lumen. This clot does not often embolize distally and is not a bad prognostic factor.

Some have advocated scanning the popliteal arteries whenever a AAA is found since a small percentage of AAA patients will also have popliteal artery aneurysms. We have not found this to be useful or productive, however.

Suggested Readings

Brown LK, Carroll BA. The extracranial cerebral vessels. *In* Rumack CM, Wilson SR, Charboneau WJ (eds): Diagnostic Ultrasound, vol 1. St. Louis, Mosby-Year Book, 1991.

Merritt C. Doppler Color Imaging. New York, Churchill Livingstone, 1992.

Zweibel WJ. Introduction to Vascular Ultrasonography, 3rd ed. Philadelphia, WB Saunders, 1992.

CHAPTER 3

Thyroid and Parathyroid Glands in Ultrasound

Thyroid

EXAMINATION TECHNIQUE

Ultrasonography of the thyroid gland should be performed using high-resolution equipment, preferably a 7.5-MHz transducer. Some sonographers advocate the use of a 10.0-MHz transducer, although even a 5.0-MHz transducer can be used in most cases, if it is properly focused. When possible, one should use a linear array to obtain a wider field of view. The patient should be in a supine position with the neck hyperextended. It may be useful to put a small pillow or towel under the patient's shoulder blades to assist hyperextension. Having the patient swallow aids in visualizing the most inferior portions of the thyroid, especially those parts that are behind the upper sternum. The gland should be examined longitudinally and transversely.

INTERPRETATION

The precise role of ultrasound in the examination of the thyroid is unclear. It is not possible, for instance, to distinguish malignant from benign diseases using ultrasound. True epithelial-lined cysts that meet all the criteria of a simple cyst are exceedingly rare.

In an examination of the thyroid glands of 1,060 people living near Chernobyl (both persons exposed to radiation and a control population), only one simple cyst was found. Nineteen complex cysts and 61 nodules were found. These findings show that ultrasound has limited utility in detecting a simple cyst in the thyroid gland because true simple cysts are rare.

Most of the cystic lesions in the thyroid gland are degenerated thyroid adenomas. These degenerated tumors frequently have small amounts of debris in them and, therefore, do not meet the criteria for a simple cyst. A simple cyst should have no internal echoes, be spherical in shape, have good through transmission, and have thin walls. A study by Hayashi found that as many as 20 percent of malignant lesions have some area of cyst formation. Therefore, the identification of a cyst in the thyroid gland does not exclude malignancy, unless it is a simple cyst. In the same study, cystic areas were also identified in 64 percent of benign lesions.

Previously, a sonolucent band surrounding a lesion (the "halo" sign) was thought to indicate a benign lesion. It is possible that this appearance is caused by vessels around the lesion. However, this "halo" sign has been noted in 29 percent of carcinomas and 42 percent of benign lesions and consequently is of limited use.

Some clinicians recommend using ultrasound when a single nodule is palpated on the thyroid gland. They theorize that if more than one nodule is identified by ultrasound, then a diagnosis of multinodular goiter is possible. They presume that if a multinodular goiter is present, the risk of malignancy is very small. In fact this is not true. Patients who have multinodular goiter may also have malignant nodules. When multiple nodules are identified (Table 3–1), the risk of malignancy is decreased but is not negligible.

Table 3-1. MULTIPLE NODULES (HYPOECHOIC OR HYPERECHOIC)

COMMON
Multinodular goiter
Subacute thyroiditis
Chronic thyroiditis
Multiple adenomas

UNCOMMON
Lymphoma
Anaplastic carcinoma
Acute thyroiditis
Carcinoma plus benign nodules

We have used ultrasound in the situation where a patient is known to have multinodular goiter. Periodic ultrasound examinations have been used to measure the size of specific nodules. If a nodule has been shown to increase in size over time, then ultrasound has been used to guide fine-needle aspiration.

Another fallacy is that the presence or absence of calcification on ultrasound helps in differentiating malignant from benign lesions (Table 3-2). Although the most common cause of small calcifications seen within the thyroid is an adenoma, carcinomas can also show calcification. If the calcifications are peripheral (sometimes called eggshell), then there is a high probability the lesion is benign. This pattern is rarely seen.

The only definite sign of malignancy that is visible in a sonogram is a very irregular appearance indicating invasion of the adjacent thyroid or surrounding soft tissue. This sign is found in a minority of malignant lesions.

The main uses of ultrasound in thyroid disease, therefore, are to confirm a lesion as

Table 3-2. ULTRASONOGRAPHIC (US) APPEARANCE OF THYROID PATHOLOGY

DISEASE PROCESS	US APPEARANCE	COMMENTS
Graves' disease	Enlarged, ± hypoechoic; "thyroid inferno" with color Doppler	
Multinodular goiter	Multiple hypoechoic lesions	
Colloid nodule	Hypoechoic, some are complex cystic	Area of glandular hyperplasia AKA "adenomatous hyperplasia"
Adenoma	Hypoechoic	
Carcinoma, follicular or papillary	Hypoechoic	Follicular is more aggressive than papillary
Anaplastic carcinoma	Large heterogeneous mass	Older female, bad prognosis
Medullary carcinoma	Hypoechoic, may have bright echogenic foci or calcification	
Acute thyroiditis	May see abscess collection, heterogeneous gland	Bacterial, patient very ill
Subacute thyroiditis	Variable from normal to heterogeneous US appearance that may simulate nodule	Postviral
Chronic thyroiditis	Variable; small to large gland, normal to heterogeneous appearance that may simulate nodule	AKA Hashimoto's autoimmune thyroiditis

intrathyroidal or extrathyroidal, to detect adenopathy, to assist in biopsy of palpable abnormalities, to follow the size of known lesions, and to evaluate the extent of disease. Normal thyroid anatomy is shown in Figure 3–1. Differential diagnoses for an enlarged thyroid, for solitary nodules, and for hypoechoic areas are given in Table 3–3, Table 3–4, and Table 3–5, respectively.

ULTRASOUND APPEARANCE OF THYROID PATHOLOGY

Table 3–2 gives a list of various forms of thyroid pathology and their ultrasonographic appearance.

Graves' Disease

Graves' disease usually affects young to middle-aged females. The thyroid gland is diffusely enlarged and sometimes is hypoechoic. Usually no focal lesions are visible. The gland is extremely vascular and the pattern known as "thyroid inferno" may be seen by using color Doppler ultrasound. Areas of color consistent with high flow will be visible throughout the gland during both systole and diastole.

Multinodular Goiter

Multinodular goiter (Fig. 3–2) is an enlarged thyroid gland with multiple hypoechoic nodules throughout both lobes. Unfortunately, the multiple nodules in multinodular goiter are not distinguishable from cancer. At one time it was thought that patients with multinodular goiter had a lower risk of cancer, but it is now known that cancer may occur in a multinodular gland and that the risk is not negligible. Ultrasound may be used to follow nodules to look for an increase in size and to direct aspiration.

Colloid Nodules

Colloid nodules are not true adenomas but are simply areas of glandular hyperplasia. They also are hypoechoic in appearance. Hemorrhage or necrosis of these nodules may result in a complex cystic appearance.

Adenoma

Adenomatous hyperplasia differs from an adenoma of the thyroid in that an ade-

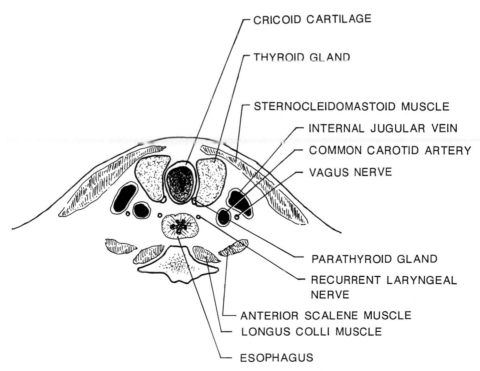

CRICOID CARTILAGE

THYROID GLAND

STERNOCLEIDOMASTOID MUSCLE

INTERNAL JUGULAR VEIN

COMMON CAROTID ARTERY

VAGUS NERVE

PARATHYROID GLAND

RECURRENT LARYNGEAL NERVE

ANTERIOR SCALENE MUSCLE

LONGUS COLLI MUSCLE

ESOPHAGUS

Figure 3–1. Normal cross-sectional thyroid anatomy.

Table 3–3. ENLARGED THYROID

COMMON
Graves' disease
Subacute thyroiditis (de Quervain's)
Chronic thyroiditis (Hashimoto's)

UNCOMMON
Acute thyroiditis
Lymphadenoid goiter
Riedel's struma or thyroiditis
Lymphoma
Anaplastic carcinoma

Table 3–4. SOLITARY NODULES (HYPOECHOIC OR HYPERECHOIC)

COMMON
Adenoma

UNCOMMON	COMMENT
Papillary thyroid cancer	Usually solid, hypoechoic; occasionally cystic
Follicular thyroid cancer	
Metastases	
Parathyroid adenoma	May be intrathyroidal
Colloid nodule	Area of glandular hyperplasia

Table 3–5. HYPOECHOIC AREAS

COMMON	COMMENT
Subacute thyroiditis	Also known as de Quervain's thyroiditis
Hashimoto's thyroiditis	Also known as chronic thyroiditis
Multinodular goiter	
Multiple adenomas	

UNCOMMON
Acute thyroiditis

noma has a collagen capsule. Cells in adenomatous hyperplasia often resemble, microscopically, the cells in the adjacent thyroid.

The cells in an adenoma may have a totally different microscopic appearance than the cells of the adjacent thyroid. A thyroid adenoma and adenomatous hyperplasia appear hypoechoic on ultrasound. There are no specific characteristics to reliably distin-guish a thyroid adenoma from a thyroid carcinoma.

Thyroid Cancer

Papillary cancer is the most common type of thyroid cancer. It affects women more than men. It is less aggressive than other types of thyroid cancer and usually metastasizes locally to lymph nodes in the neck. The ultrasound appearance is of a hypoechoic nodule that may have tiny calcifications (psammoma bodies).

Follicular carcinoma is a second type of well-differentiated cancer. Follicular carcinoma is more aggressive than papillary carcinoma and is more likely to produce distant metastases. It is also seen more often in females than males and has a hypoechoic appearance. A Hürthle cell tumor of the thyroid is a type of follicular cell carcinoma. Hürthle cell tumors have the same prognosis as follicular cell carcinomas and the same ultrasonographic appearance.

Anaplastic thyroid carcinoma usually occurs in women over age 65. These patients frequently present with difficulties swallowing or breathing because the cancer has invaded the adjacent trachea and esophagus. Patients with this tumor have a very poor prognosis. On ultrasound, there is usually a large mass in the neck with a very heterogeneous echo appearance. The tissue is very disorganized.

Medullary carcinoma is derived from parafollicular or C cells and typically these secrete calcitonin. Medullary carcinoma may occur as part of the multiple endocrine neoplasia syndromes, types II and III. This lesion is frequently hypoechoic, but it may contain bright echogenic foci also. There may even be calcifications visible that demonstrate shadowing. If large calcifications with shadowing are seen, medullary cancer should be considered. The metastases to nodes from this disease may also calcify and shadow.

It should be noted that hyperechoic nodules in the thyroid are more likely to be benign than malignant.

Thyroiditis

Acute thyroiditis is a bacterial process. These patients are usually quite ill. They may develop an abscess in the thyroid

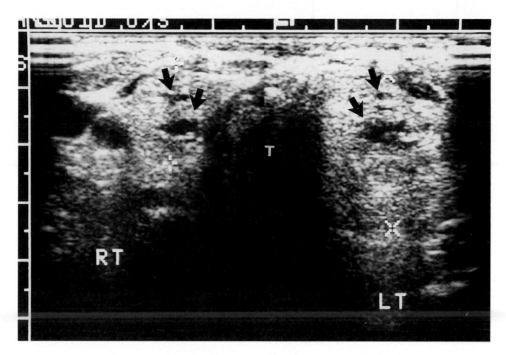

Figure 3–2. Multiple hypoechoic nodules (*arrows*) are visible in this patient with multinodular goiter. T = trachea.

gland that usually makes the gland tender to palpation. Ultrasonography may reveal an abscess consisting of a complex hypoechoic fluid-like area within the gland or it may be very disorganized in appearance.

Subacute thyroiditis usually occurs as a postviral phenomenon. The thyroid gland is temporarily damaged as a result of the effects of a viral upper respiratory infection or virus somewhere else in the body. Prognosis is quite good. Typically, complete recovery is seen over a period of weeks to months. These patients may present with hyperthyroidism very early due to the liberation of large amounts of thyroid hormones but usually will present with hypothyroidism of relatively acute onset due to a temporarily nonfunctioning gland. The ultrasonographic appearance of subacute thyroiditis varies. The gland may be enlarged and show areas of increased and decreased echogenicity, or it may appear similar to a gland with multiple nodules throughout. This disease is also known as de Quervain's thyroiditis.

Chronic thyroiditis is an autoimmune disease caused by lymphocytic infiltration of the thyroid gland. These patients usually present with hypothyroidism. About one third of them may retain the ability to trap iodine but are unable to use the iodine in the organification process to create thyroid hormone. Therefore, they may have a normal or increased radioiodine uptake when measured at 4 or 6 hours with a low uptake when measured at 24 hours but low serum thyroid hormone levels. The appearance of this condition on sonograms varies. The gland may show increased and decreased echogenicity, or it may show areas simulating multiple nodules. The gland may be enlarged, normal size, or small. This disease is also known as Hashimoto's thyroiditis.

Parathyroid Glands

Ultrasonography of the parathyroid glands is performed with the patient in the same position used to image the thyroid. An autopsy series found an average parathyroid gland to measure 5×3×1 mm, with the largest being 12×2×1 mm, and the smallest being 2×2×1 mm. Five percent were located in ectopic locations and the other 95 percent were located in areas around the thyroid. The average parathyroid adenoma is approximately 15×10×9 mm. A typical parathyroid adenoma is oval, solid, and of low echogenicity and lies along the posterior surface of the thyroid gland. An adenoma may become tubular as it enlarges. Usually the parathyroid glands are not more lateral than the carotid artery and they will usually lie anterior to the longus colli muscle.

A single enlarged parathyroid gland suggests an adenoma. Multiple enlarged glands suggest hyperplasia. Hyperplastic glands are still responsive to physiologic feedback mechanisms, while adenomas no longer respond to feedback but function autonomously. An experienced neck surgeon can find over 90 percent of adenomas without imaging guidance. After a failed neck exploration, scar tissue and anatomic distortion make reoperation more difficult. Ultrasound, computed tomography, magnetic resonance imaging, and dual isotope nuclear medicine examinations all have their advocates. These tests generally have 60 to 70 percent success rates in finding diseased glands after failed surgical exploration. We recommend that the radiologist use the test with which he or she is most experienced.

A normal parathyroid gland is usually not visible on ultrasound. Most patients have four parathyroid glands. About 6 percent of patients may have three glands and about 6 percent may have five glands. Eleven percent of all parathyroid glands have been found to be 1 to 4 cm below the lower pole of the thyroid. Therefore, it is important to ask the patient to swallow so that the inferior portion of the thyroid can be well examined.

The superior parathyroids derive from the fourth brachial cleft pouch, as does the thyroid. These glands are usually close to the thyroid, usually near the posterior surface of the middle to upper thyroid gland. Inferior parathyroids arise from the third brachial cleft pouch and migrate with the thymus. These may be located anywhere from the thyroid gland to the superior mediastinum. Ectopic glands may occasionally be found in distant locations such as the inferior mediastinum, but usually parathyroid glands are located medial to the carotid arteries and between the thyroid gland and the superior mediastinum. Parathyroid glands may be intrathyroidal in location. If so, they will usually have a thin fat plane around them.

Hyperplastic glands cannot be reliably differentiated from adenomatous glands using ultrasound. The appearance of more than one enlarged parathyroid gland suggests hyperplasia. A characteristic highly suggestive of parathyroid adenoma is a hypoechoic, teardrop-shaped mass, aligned in a craniocaudad direction (Fig. 3–3). One potential indicator of the presence of a parathyroid adenoma is an asymmetric neurovascular bundle lying anterior to the longus colli muscle. This asymmetry may result from hypertrophy of the inferior thyroidal artery. Parathyroid carcinomas have an appearance that is identical to parathyroid adenomas, except they may have invaded adjacent tissues. Some adenomas have areas of varying echo intensity, whereas hyperplastic glands are usually homogeneous. Hyperplastic glands also are usually smaller than adenomatous glands, but this is not a reliable distinguishing characteristic.

False-negative diagnoses of adenomas of the parathyroid glands are made because of ectopic parathyroids and sometimes due to glands that are only minimally enlarged. False-positive diagnoses are the result of thyroid nodules or lymphadenopathy.

Occasionally, parathyroid glands have a cystic appearance. This may make them difficult to distinguish from thyroid lesions.

Calcification of a parathyroid adenoma is rare, but a single case was seen in a series of 63 patients.

Ultrasound-Guided Biopsy

Ultrasound-guided biopsy of a thyroid or parathyroid lesion can be done. Usually a very small needle is used. When a parathyroid gland is aspirated, the aspirate is usually checked for high levels of parathormone. When the thyroid is aspirated, cytology is used to look for indications of malignancy. Percutaneous ethanol injection of parathyroid tumors under ultrasound guidance has also been used as a treatment for hyperparathyroidism.

Other Neck Pathology

Ultrasound is used to examine the neck for other pathology (Table 3–6). A thyro-

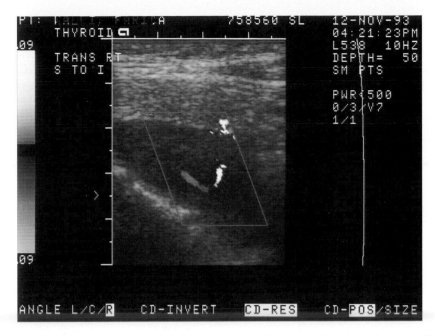

Figure 3–3. Transverse image of a teardrop-shaped hypoechoic parathyroid adenoma. This color Doppler image shows a small amount of flow. See color plate 3.

glossal duct cyst may occur anywhere from the base of the tongue to the thyroid gland. These are frequently seen in the midline and should have the ultrasound characteristic of a cyst, but they may have debris within them and therefore have a complex appearance.

Brachial cleft cysts or sinuses are lateral neck masses usually seen in children. Most of these masses arise from the second brachial cleft and lie just anterior to the upper portion of the sternocleidomastoid muscle. They are usually anterior and lateral to the carotid artery. These may be infected and symptomatic. On sonograms, they usually have a complex appearance.

Table 3–6. NECK MASSES

COMMON
Nodal metastases
Inflammatory adenopathy

UNCOMMON
Thyroglossal duct cyst
Brachial cleft cysts
Neck abscesses
Parathyroid adenoma
Lateral pharyngoesophageal diverticulum

Suggested Readings

Brander A, Viikinkoski P, Nickels J, et al. Thyroid gland: ultrasonography screening in middle-aged women with no previous thyroid disease. Radiology 173:507–510, 1989.

Hammer M, Worstman J, Folse R. Cancer in cystic lesions of the thyroid. Arch Surg 117:1020–1023, 1982.

Hay ID. Thyroiditis: a clinical update. Mayo Clin Proc 60:836–843, 1985.

Hayashi N, Tamaki N, Yamamoto K, et al. Real-time ultrasonography of thyroid nodules. Acta Radiol [Diagn] (Stockh) 27:403–408, 1986.

James EM, Charboneau JW. High frequency (10 MHz) thyroid ultrasonography. Semin Ultrasound, CT, MR 6:294–309, 1985.

Katz JF, Kane RA, Reyes J, et al. Thyroid nodules: sonographic-pathologic correlation. Radiology 151:741–745, 1984.

Mettler FA Jr, Williamson MR, Royal HD, et al. Thyroid nodules in the population living around Chernobyl. JAMA 265:616–619, 1992.

Ralls PW, Mayekawa DS, Lee KP, et al. Color-flow Doppler sonography in Graves' disease: "thyroid inferno." AJR 150:781–784, 1988.

Rojeski MT, Gharib H. Nodular thyroid disease: evaluation and management. N Engl J Med 313:428–436, 1985.

CHAPTER 4

Breast Ultrasound

Equipment

It is important that breast ultrasound be performed only with specific types of equipment. Real-time scanning can be performed using transducers with a frequency between 5.0 and 10.0 MHz. A 10.0-MHz transducer may not adequately penetrate large breasts, however. Either linear or sector-type transducers may be used. The transducer should have a small dead zone so that superficial lesions can be seen. An alternative is to use a stand-off pad. In general, a focal zone of less than 3 cm is ideal.

Automated scanning equipment also is available for breast examination. There are two basic methods for using these machines. Either the patient lies supine with a water bath over the breasts or she lies prone with the breasts immersed in a water bath. However, standard real-time equipment is used in most institutions.

Who Should Have Breast Ultrasound

In the past, ultrasound was advocated as a method of screening for breast cancer. However, ultrasound is now considered inadequate for breast cancer screening and should not be used. Nor is it adequate for screening women with breast implants. Research has shown that ultrasound may detect fewer than 50 percent of nonpalpable breast cancers. Although there are rare cancers that are missed by mammography and seen by ultrasound, most abnormalities detected by ultrasound only are benign. Evidence to support this comes from Kopans, who studied 94 women with normal mammograms and physical findings but suspi-

cious lesions on ultrasound. After 3 years of follow-up, no cancers had occurred.

The primary utility of ultrasound is to separate simple cysts from solid lesions and complex cysts (Tables 4–1 and 4–2). In making this distinction, strict criteria must be followed. Simple cysts must be round or oval, have no internal echoes, be sharply marginated, and demonstrate posterior acoustic enhancement (or through-transmission) (Fig. 4–1). Lesions that do not meet these criteria should be classified as complex-cystic or solid. The most common error that we see is to misclassify a solid lesion as a cyst. Many solid lesions have low-level internal echoes and posterior enhancement. Therefore, care should be taken before concluding that a lesion is a cyst. Attention must be paid to the machine settings when deciding whether a lesion is cystic or solid. If the gain is too high, the lesion may have artifactual internal echoes. The gain should be just high enough to produce posterior enhancement. When the gain is turned higher, the anterior part or the perimeter of a cystic lesion will fill in first. A solid lesion will fill in homogeneously. The cyst must be imaged within the focal zone or artifactual internal echoes may be produced. Small cysts may have internal echoes because of a beam width artifact. It may not be possible to demonstrate posterior enhancement in deep lesions or lesions against the chest wall. These lesions should be considered indeterminate. If a lesion has no internal echoes but has septa, debris, or irregular walls, then it is complex-cystic. These lesions can be aspirated for confirmation of benignity or ultrasound-guided core biopsy may be performed. If no lesion is seen with ultrasound and a lesion has been detected with mammography or by palpation, then management should be the

Table 4–1. CYSTIC LESIONS

COMMON
Benign simple cysts
Breast carcinoma
Abscesses

UNCOMMON
Galactocele
Hematoma
Metastases

Table 4–2. MASSES

COMMON
Fibroadenoma
Ductal carcinoma
Lymph node

UNCOMMON
Cystosarcoma phyllodes
Hematoma
Abscess
Metastases
Lobular carcinoma of breast
Giant fibroadenoma
Hamartoma
Cysts

same as for a solid mass. Simple cysts are benign and require no further action.

Women over 35 should have mammography before ultrasound. Ultrasound usually is performed only to make the cyst versus solid distinction. For women under age 30 who have a palpable mass, ultrasound should be performed before mammography. This prevents some exposure to ionizing radiation in young women. If a simple cyst is detected by ultrasound, no mammogram or further action is needed. If a complex cystic or solid mass is seen, mammography should be performed. For women between the ages of 30 and 35, ultrasound should be performed first, unless there is a strong family history of breast cancer. In these cases, mammography may be justified. A list of breast ultrasound indications is shown in Table 4–3.

Technique and Normal Anatomy

Scanning is normally performed with the patient supine. The patient's hand is placed over her head to examine axillary lesions and at her side for other lesions. All lesions should be examined in two orthogonal planes. Scanning also can be done with the

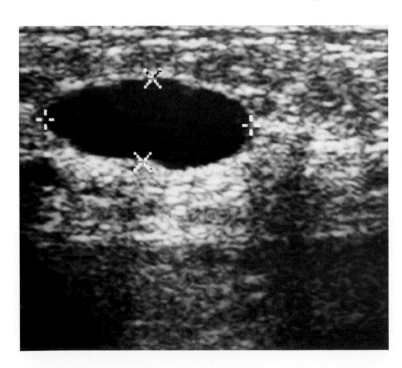

Figure 4–1. Breast cysts. This lesion meets all criteria for a benign cyst: good through transmission, no internal echoes, indiscernible walls, round or oval shape.

Table 4–3. INDICATIONS FOR BREAST ULTRASOUND

1. Mass detected by mammography or palpation (to determine if it is cystic or solid)
2. Asymmetric breast density on mammogram (to further evaluate the breasts and exclude underlying lesion)
3. Mass palpated but mammogram is negative
4. Localized breast pain and tenderness prevents mammography
5. Guidance for cyst aspiration
6. Lesion seen on only one mammographic view of breast or is in a difficult location for mammographic localization guidance
7. Women under age 30 with a palpable mass and most women under age 35 with a palpable mass (to avoid ionizing radiation exposure). Mammography may be needed after ultrasound
8. Suspected breast implant rupture
9. Guidance for core biopsy or cyst aspiration

patient seated, especially if the lesion is more easily palpated in that position.

The retroareolar area can be difficult to scan as the protruding nipple may create an artifact. The application of additional gel and angling the beam from the edge of the areola may help. A stand-off pad may also be useful. In general, superficial abnormalities should be examined with a stand-off pad.

Normal deep structures include the ribs and pectoralis muscles. Breast parenchyma is usually echogenic, especially in younger women. Masses within the breast are usually hypoechoic. Fat is hypoechoic when compared to fibroglandular elements. Cooper's ligaments are fibrous and echogenic (Fig. 4–2). A breast lobule surrounded by Cooper's ligaments may simulate a mass.

It is not abnormal to be able to see ducts in the retroareolar area. These may measure up to 8 mm in size. In the periphery of the breast, the ducts are less visible. Lymph nodes may not be distinguishable from fat lobules, cysts, or hypoechoic masses.

Pathology

The ultrasonographic and mammographic appearances for benign and malignant breast pathology are given in Tables 4–4A and 4–4B. Comments about each entity follow. In general, breast carcinoma will be hypoechoic and poorly defined. It may be sound attenuating (Fig. 4–3 and Tables 4–4A and B and 4–5). The malignant-type

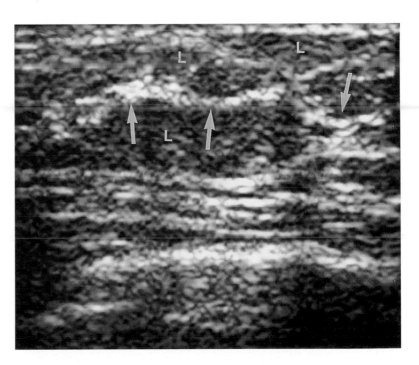

Figure 4–2. Normal breast lobules. Note that Cooper's ligaments are echogenic (*arrows*). L = lobule.

Table 4–4A. BENIGN BREAST LESIONS

	MAMMOGRAPHIC APPEARANCE	ULTRASOUND APPEARANCE	COMMENTS
Adenosis	Calcifications; patchy densities	Nothing seen	Benign proliferation of stromal and epithelial tissue. Increase in acini
Cysts	Round density	Well marginated, no internal echoes, through transmission, round or oval	Dilated acini
Fibroadenoma	Well-defined large calcifications	Variable: hypoechoic, through transmission	
Papillomatosis	Clustered calcifications	Not seen	Distal ducts, multiple
Hamartoma (fibroadenolipoma)	Well-defined, mixed density with some fat lucency	Well-defined, echogenic and echo-poor zones, may attenuate	
Cystosarcoma phyllodes	Well-defined, large mass, no calcification	Hypoechoic, large mass	Rapidly enlarging
Nodes	Small mass with cleft	Hypoechoic mass	Usually upper, outer breast
Lipoma	Lucent, smooth	Hypoechoic, well-defined	
Galactoceles	Lucent	Mass or cyst with low level echoes well-defined	Occur after lactation
Fat necrosis	May look like cancer; may form oil cyst; may calcify	May not through transmit; oil cysts look like cysts; others look like solid ill-defined masses	
Oil cysts	Rim calcification of a spherical lesion	Cysts. If calcified, may block sound	
Intraductal papilloma	Most not seen; occasionally lobulated mass; rarely calcify	Solid, hypoechoic, lobulated; may be within cyst	Filling defect on galactogram
Hematoma	Variable: vague density to well-circumscribed mass	Variable: early may see echogenic; later, becomes cyst-like	
Radial scar (elastosis)	Spiculated; no central mass; lucent center	No reports	
Abscess	Increased density with amorphous shape, poorly defined	Complex cystic	
Duct ectasia	Tubular, serpiginous densities; often have calcification	Tubular lucency; may be solid	

of microcalcifications seen at mammography will often not be seen by ultrasound.

SKIN LESIONS

Occasionally, skin lesions from acne or sebaceous cysts may be confused with breast pathology. At ultrasound, skin lesions will be seen to lie between two echo-genic lines of skin (Fig. 4–4). Breast lesions will lie deep to these two lines.

Interventional Breast Ultrasound

Ultrasound guided interventions are useful in four situations: (1) cyst aspiration, (2)

Table 4–4B. MALIGNANT BREAST LESIONS

	MAMMOGRAPHIC APPEARANCE	ULTRASOUND APPEARANCE	COMMENTS
Carcinoma in situ			
Ductal	Not seen	Not seen	
Comedo	Not seen	Not seen	
Noncomedo	Not seen	Not seen	
Cribriform	Not seen	Not seen	
Micropapillary	Not seen	Not seen	
Lobular	Not seen; histologic diagnosis	Hypoechoic, may be due to tissue rx, not tumor itself	
Infiltrating ductal cancer			
Usual–not otherwise specified	Irregular, spiculated, poorly defined masses	Irregular, poorly defined border, hypoechoic, sound attenuating	80–90% of all cancers
Medullary	May be well circumscribed	Well defined, hypoechoic may simulate cysts	5% of breast cancer
Colloid (mucinous)	Spiculated mass but may be better defined than many cancers	Hypoechoic, may have through transmission	1–2% of cancers; better prognosis older women
Paget's	May have no mammogram abnormality or may see mass	Not usually seen but may see mass	Ductal cancer with spread to nipple
Tubular	Small mass	Well-defined mass	Good prognosis, rare
Papillary	May be well circumscribed	Cystic mass with solid projection	Bloody discharge
Comedo	Exuberant calcification oriented parallel to ducts	May see hypoechoic mass; will not see calcification	Much necrotic cellular debris
Inflammatory cancer	Skin thickening, may see underlying mass	Skin thickening	A clinical diagnosis
Lobular	Spiculated mass	Looks like mass of ductal cancer	
Sarcomas			
Phylloides	Well circumscribed mass, looks like fibroadenoma	Looks like fibroadenoma	
Lymphoma	Range from nodules to diffuse density increase	Hypoechoic mass, may have through transmission	
Metastases	Multiple masses	Multiple masses, variable appearance	

fine-needle aspiration biopsy (FNAB), (3) needle/hook wire placement prior to surgical biopsy, and (4) core biopsy.

TECHNIQUE

A 5.0- or 7.5-MHz transducer is used as in routine ultrasound imaging of the breast. Either a needle guide or a freehand technique may be used. The patient is draped and cleansed with Betadine. The transducer should be placed in a sterile glove or sheath and the operators should wear sterile gloves.

The lesion should first be located and the shortest path from skin surface to lesion identified. The depth of the lesion should be determined. For FNAB, a 21-gauge needle is then inserted through a biopsy guide or the freehand technique may be used. If a freehand technique is used, the needle may be inserted alongside and parallel to

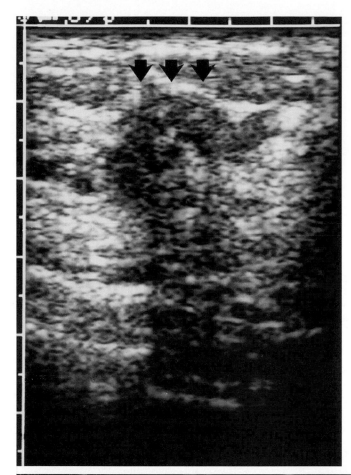

Figure 4–3. Two lesions from different patients (*arrows*). Both are hypoe-choic, sound attenuating, and poorly defined. Both proved to be carcinomas.

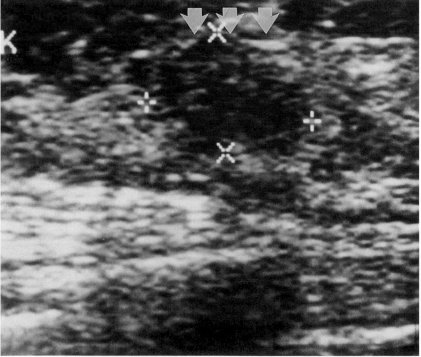

Table 4-5. SHADOWING FROM BREAST LESION

Carcinoma
Fat necrosis
Foreign body
Lipoma
Galactocele
Fibrocystic disease
Granular cell tumor (myoblastoma)
Hamartoma

the transducer. This requires some experience as the needle will not be seen as it is inserted and will be seen only when it reaches the lesion. An alternative method is to insert the needle perpendicular to the transducer. The needle may be followed along its entire course and seen as it enters the lesion. We prefer this method but a disadvantage is that it may not always provide the shortest route to the lesion. Some prefer a compromise of the above two approaches in which the needle is inserted obliquely. Usually, the tip can be followed into the lesion and seen on the ultrasound image. Sometimes the needle is difficult to identify. This problem is worse with smaller gauge

needles such as 21s. Some manufacturers have attempted to roughen or coat the needle tips to make them more visible. In our experience, these needles are only slightly more visible than standard needles. It is important to determine that the tip of the needle has reached and is in the target lesion. At times, the needle is visible but the tip is not. Injecting a few air bubbles can help locate the needle tip in these situations. When core biopsy with a larger needle is performed, visualization is less of a problem.

When the goal is to aspirate a cyst, a 21-gauge needle is usually used. Fluid should be sent for cytologic examination. After aspiration, imaging is performed to make certain the lesion is smaller or gone. Tabar advocates injecting a few milliliters of air into the cyst after aspiration as a therapeutic procedure. The air may cause infarction of the cyst so it will not reaccumulate fluid. When FNAB of a mass is the goal, it is imperative that the needle reach and be seen within the lesion. Otherwise, a negative biopsy result is meaningless. After the needle is in the lesion, suction is applied and the needle is moved rapidly back and forth to sample the lesion. Suction is then released

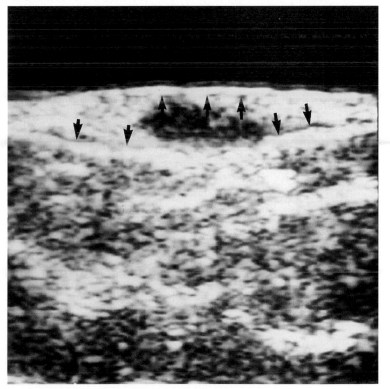

Figure 4-4. Sebaceous cyst. This lesion lies in the skin, not the breast. When a lesion is seen between the two echogenic lines (*arrows*) then a certain diagnosis of skin lesion may be made.

and, ideally, the syringe and needle are passed to a cytopathologist who is present. Usually several samples are taken once the lesion is pierced. A positive biopsy prevents a surgical biopsy. A negative biopsy result must be evaluated with care because of the possibility that the lesion was not adequately sampled. Negative biopsies should be followed up at 6-month intervals by mammography and/or ultrasound to look for changes that would signal a malignancy has been missed. This follow-up should be continued for 2 to 3 years.

Ultrasound guidance can be used for needle/hook wire localization prior to surgical biopsy. The procedure is the same as for cyst aspiration except a hook wire is placed into the lesion as a road map for the surgeon. It is important to pick the shortest path to the lesion to simplify the surgical biopsy. Ultrasound is used to guide the needle into the lesion. When the needle is in or beside the lesion, mammography can be done (if the lesion was previously seen on at least one mammographic view). If the mammogram confirms correct needle placement, a wire with a hook on the end is placed through the lumen of the needle and hooked into the breast tissue near the lesion. The patient may then be sent to surgery. A mammogram and/or sonograms should be obtained to be certain the lesion was truly located.

There is a trend toward the use of ultrasound as guidance for core biopsies of breast lesions. Large needles ranging in size from 14 to 18 gauge are used for these procedures. Multiple passes are made, with the average number being 5. Patient acceptance is high when the alternative is surgical breast biopsy. Negative results require close imaging follow-up just as with FNAB negatives.

Doppler of Breast Lesions

Doppler has been advocated as a means of separating benign breast lesions from those that are malignant. High flow suggests arteriovenous shunting as occurs in neovascularity of tumors. Most benign tumors have little flow. This technique currently is not widely accepted and should be considered investigational.

Characterization of Breast Lesions by Ultrasound

Currently, between three and five breast biopsies must be performed to detect one

Table 4–6. MALIGNANT SONOGRAPHIC CHARACTERISTICS VERSUS MALIGNANT PATHOLOGIC DIAGNOSIS

CHARACTERISTIC	SENS	SPEC	PPV	NPV	ACC	ADJ RISK
Spiculation	36.0	99.4	91.8	88.6	88.8	5.5
Taller-than-wide	41.6	98.1	81.2	89.4	88.7	4.9
Angular margins	83.2	92.0	67.5	96.5	90.5	4.0
Shadowing	48.8	94.7	64.9	90.2	87.1	3.9
Branch pattern	29.6	96.6	64.0	87.3	85.5	3.8
Hypoechoic	68.8	90.1	60.1	93.6	87.2	3.6
Calcifications	27.2	96.3	59.6	86.9	84.8	3.6
Duct extension	24.8	95.2	50.8	86.4	79.3	3.0
Microlobulation	75.2	83.8	48.2	94.4	82.4	2.9

In order of positive predictive value; prevalence = pretest probability = 16.7%; positive predictive value (PPV) = posttest probability; adjusted risk = odds ratio = PPV/prevalence.

Sens = sensitivity; spec = specificity; PPV = positive predictive value; NPV = negative predictive value; ACC = accuracy; Adj risk = adjusted risk.

From Stavros AT, Rapp CL, Thickman D, et al. Sonography of Solid Breast Nodules— Benign or Malignant? Presented at Advances in Sonography, Chicago, October 14–16, 1994, with permission.

**Table 4–7. BENIGN SONOGRAPHIC
CHARACTERISTICS VERSUS BENIGN
PATHOLOGIC DIAGNOSIS**

CHARACTERISTIC	SENS	SPEC	PPV	NPV	ACC	ADJ RISK
Hyperechoic	100.0	7.4	17.8	100.0	22.8	0.00
Two or 3 lobulations	99.2	19.4	19.7	99.2	32.7	0.05
Ellipsoid shape	97.6	51.2	28.6	99.1	59.2	0.05
Thin capsule	95.2	76.0	44.2	98.8	79.2	0.07

In order of negative predictive value; prevalence = pretest probability = 16.7%; (1 − negative predictive value {NPV}) = posttest probability; adjusted risk = odds ratio = posttest probability/prevalence.
From Stavros AT, Rapp CL, Thickman D, et al. Sonography of Solid Breast Nodules— Benign or Malignant? Presented at Advances in Sonography, Chicago, October 14– 16, 1994, with permission.

breast cancer. Another way to say this is that a large number of breast lesions detected by mammography are benign but we have no way of distinguishing malignant from benign by mammographic criteria. Stavros et al. have evaluated the ultrasound characteristics of 750 solid breast nodules and have obtained biopsy data on these nodules. They have been successful in classifying breast lesions as probably malignant versus probably benign. The sonographic characteristics that suggest malignancy are as follows:

1. Spiculation—either hypoechoic and hyperechoic (not both) straight lines radiating from the lesion.
2. Taller than wide—with patients supine, normal tissue planes are horizontal. Some malignant lesions grow vertically (craniocaudad direction). Taller than wide also suggests that the lesion is relatively incompressible.
3. Angular margins—sharp angles as opposed to a gently curving contour suggest malignancy.
4. Shadowing—a malignant characteristic
5. Calcifications—sonography is better at detecting malignant calcifications than benign calcifications because breast cancers are hypoechoic and the calcifications sometimes are conspicuous on a hypoechoic background. Mammography is better at detecting and characterizing calcifications. However, if calcifications are seen in a nodule, it should raise concern for malignancy.

6. Duct extension—malignancies will sometimes have projections that extend radially within a duct toward the nipple.
7. Microlobulation—many small lobulations on the surface of a nodule suggest malignancy.

The sonographic findings that suggest benignancy are:

1. Hyperechogenicity—most women have some hyperechoic tissue and care must be taken that the mammographic abnormality is the same as what is being seen on the ultrasound exam.
2. Ellipsoid shape—cancers rarely have this shape.
3. Two or three gentle lobulations—should be smooth and gently undulating.
4. Thin, echogenic capsule—this suggests slow growth and lack of infiltration.

Each of these characteristics is listed in Tables 4–6 and 4–7, compiled by Stavros. This detailed information is fascinating. It is not yet in widespread use and has not been confirmed by other investigators. It therefore may be considered investigational at this time.

Suggested Readings

Feig SA. Breast masses: Mammographic and sonographic evaluation. Radiol Clin North Am 30:67– 92, 1992.
Mendelson EB. Ultrasound of the breast. Semin Ultrasound, CT, MR. Vol 10, no. 2, 1989.

CHAPTER 5

Abdominal Ultrasound

Anatomy

Anatomy of the upper abdomen can be complex. It is more easily understood after referring to an overall diagram (Fig. 5–1) and then focusing on subsections. Patients should fast for 4 to 6 hours before undergoing abdominal ultrasound. Ultrasound examination of the abdomen begins in the right upper quadrant where the liver, biliary tree, gallbladder, pancreas, and right kidney are examined.

The splenic vein is a marker for the *pancreas* (Fig. 5–2). One should identify the splenic vein first, and then look anteriorly to find the pancreas. The head and body of the pancreas have a relatively transverse orientation but the tail may angle either superiorly or inferiorly. In many patients, the tail cannot be identified. The superior mesenteric vein separates the pancreatic head from the body. The left margin of the lumbar vertebral body separates body from tail. In very thin patients, the left lobe of the liver may provide a sonographic window for visualizing the pancreas. In heavy patients, the pancreas sits inferiorly to the left lobe of the liver, making it more difficult to find. The pancreatic duct passes through the center of the pancreas and should be no larger than 2 mm in diameter. It is usually not seen in normal patients. We sometimes have the patient drink water to fill the stomach and thereby create a window for scanning the pancreas.

Several schemes for measuring the pancreas have been developed. The most reliable is to measure the pancreas in a direct anteroposterior plane perpendicular to the long axis of the gland and measure the head, body, and tail individually (Fig. 5–2).

Using this method, the head should be no greater than 3.0 cm and the body no greater than 2.6 cm in diameter. The tail should show nice tapering and be no greater than 2.0 cm thick. Exact measurements are less important for the tail.

The *common bile duct* is sometimes seen in the posterior portion of the head of the pancreas. There are no standard measurements for the common bile duct at this level, but, if it is easily seen and prominent, then one may conclude that there is a possibility it is enlarged. The gastroduodenal artery may be seen anterior to the head of the pancreas.

By keeping the field of view in the transverse plane and looking posterior to the splenic vein, the origin of the superior mesenteric artery should become visible (Fig. 5–3). This artery is surrounded by echogenic fat, has a very characteristic appearance, and should be easily recognizable. The left renal vein also should be visible between the superior mesenteric artery and the aorta (Fig. 5–4).

The superior mesenteric vein is just to the right side of the superior mesenteric artery. The point where the superior mesenteric vein and splenic vein join is called the portal confluence, and from this point this vessel is called the portal vein.

The portal vein runs in an oblique direction toward the porta hepatis. The long axis of the portal vein may be viewed by following a line from the umbilicus to the patient's right shoulder. This portion of the portal vein is located in the hepatoduodenal ligament. The other two portions of the portal triad, the hepatic artery and the common bile duct, are anterior to the portal vein. The common bile duct is identified by turning the patient to a left lateral decubitus posi-

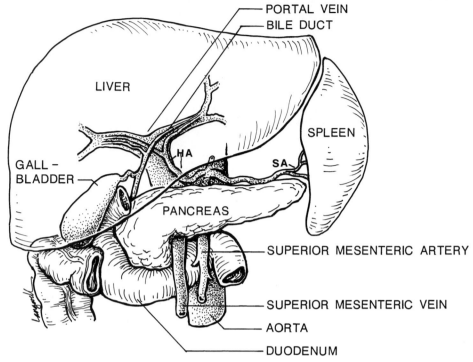

Figure 5–1. Upper abdominal anatomy. HA = Hepatic artery, SA = splenic artery.

tion, identifying the long axis of the portal vein as just described, and then looking anterior to the portal vein (Fig. 5–5). The common bile duct is the structure located anterior to the portal vein. This can sometimes be found with the patient in the supine position, but it is easier to find it with the pa-

tient in the left lateral decubitus or left posterior oblique position.

If imaging is continued in the transverse plane and superiorly from the splenic vein and pancreas, a structure resembling a set of gull wings may be seen coming off the aorta (Fig. 5–6). These gull wings are two

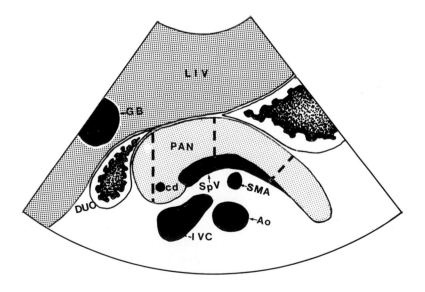

Figure 5–2. Transverse image of the pancreas (PAN). Find the transversely oriented splenic vein (SpV) and look anteriorly. Dotted lines are locations for measurement of the pancreatic head, body, and tail. LIV = liver, GB = gallbladder, DUO = duodenum, cd = common bile duct, SMA = superior mesenteric artery, IVC = inferior vena cava, Ao = aorta.

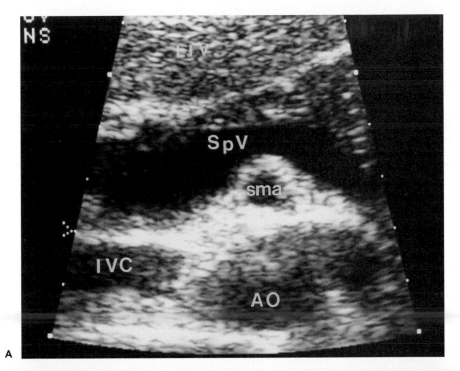

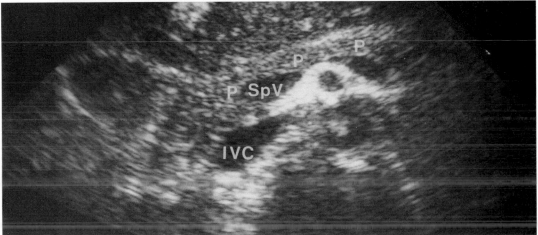

Figure 5–3. *A*, Transverse image at the level of Figure 5–2 near origin of superior mesenteric artery (sma). AO = aorta, IVC = inferior vena cava, SpV = splenic vein, LIV = left lobe of liver. *B*, Different patient showing entire pancreas (P) sitting anterior to splenic vein (SpV). IVC is seen.

of the vessels of the celiac axis, the splenic artery and the hepatic artery. The left gastric artery, which is the third portion of the celiac axis, is usually not seen on ultrasound as it is very short and runs cephalad.

The intrahepatic biliary radicals should not be larger than 2 mm. These ducts are frequently difficult to identify, although they can sometimes be seen with a 5.0-MHz or higher frequency transducer. They are smaller than the portal venous radicals that they accompany. In an intrahepatic location, the relationship between portal venous radicals and biliary radicals is variable. Sometimes the biliary structure will be anterior and sometimes it will be posterior to the portal venous structure. Intrahepatic biliary dilatation is present when two parallel channels are seen, since normally only one channel should be seen. This is sometimes

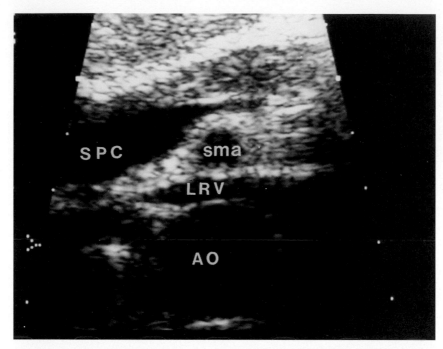

Figure 5–4. Transverse image 1 cm inferior to Figure 5–3 showing left renal vein (LRV) passing between the superior mesenteric artery (sma) and the aorta (AO). SPC is the splenoportal confluence, the point where the superior mesenteric vein and the splenic vein meet to form the portal vein.

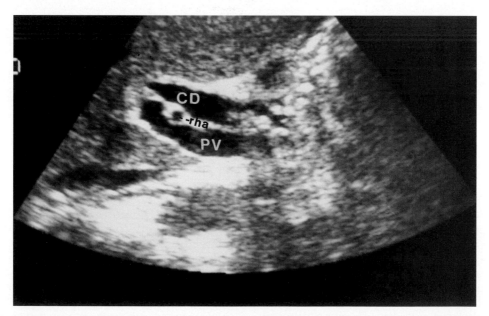

Figure 5–5. Oblique image along the long axis of the portal vein (PV) at the porta hepatis. CD = common duct, rha = right hepatic artery. Patient is in left posterior oblique position. The right hepatic artery should not be mistaken for a lesion in the common duct.

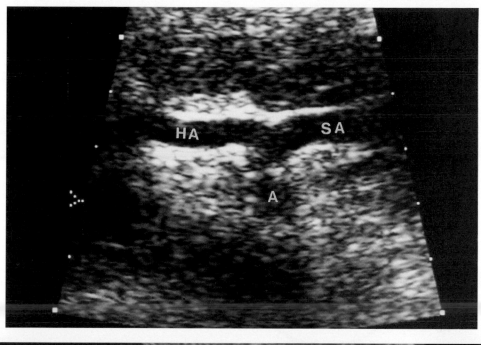

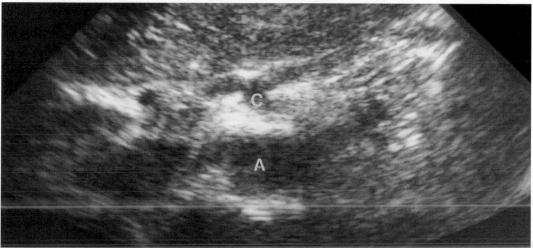

Figure 5–6. *A*, Gullwings. The celiac trunk divides into the hepatic artery (HA) and splenic artery (SA). A = aorta. *B*, Gullwings. Origin of celiac axis (C) from the aorta (A).

called "train tracks" or the "shotgun sign." The biliary structures should be more irregular and serpiginous than the venous structures. In addition, there sometimes is through transmission posterior to dilated bile ducts. The portal venous structures have blood within them that will attenuate the sound so they will not show through transmission. Color Doppler may help distinguish biliary ducts from blood vessels. Doppler settings should be set to detect slow flow.

The portal vein runs into the *liver* at the porta hepatis, supplying most of the blood to the liver. The liver has four lobes. Each of these lobes has a major branch of the portal vein supplying it (Fig. 5–7). The portal venous branches flow into the central portion of each of these lobes. The hepatic vein drains each lobe and lies at the periphery of the lobe.

The hepatic veins provide demarcation of the lobes. The right hepatic vein divides the anterior and posterior segments of the right

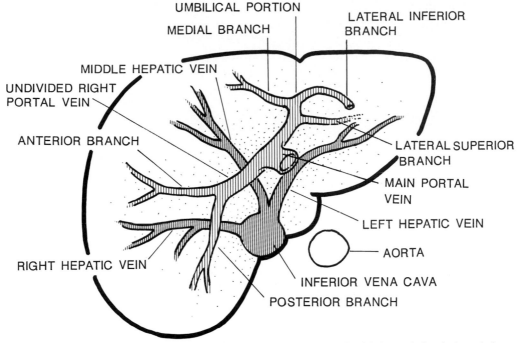

UMBILICAL PORTION

MEDIAL BRANCH

LATERAL INFERIOR BRANCH

MIDDLE HEPATIC VEIN

UNDIVIDED RIGHT PORTAL VEIN

ANTERIOR BRANCH

LATERAL SUPERIOR BRANCH

MAIN PORTAL VEIN

LEFT HEPATIC VEIN

AORTA

RIGHT HEPATIC VEIN

INFERIOR VENA CAVA

POSTERIOR BRANCH

Figure 5–7. Transverse anatomy of hepatic veins and portal vein. Main portal vein is not shown.

lobe. The middle hepatic vein divides the right lobe from the left lobe, and the left hepatic vein separates the lateral and medial segments of the left lobe. A line from the inferior vena cava through the middle hepatic vein and through to the gallbladder fossa demarcates the right lobe from the left lobe. This is the location of the main interlobar fissure. Sometimes, this fissure is seen running between the right portal vein and the gallbladder on a sagittal ultrasound image (Fig. 5–8). The Chewnard system has

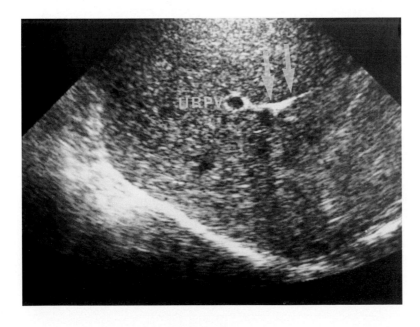

URPV

Figure 5–8. Sagittal image through right lobe of liver. URPV = undivided right portal vein. Caudal to this portion of the right portal vein is the main interlobar fissure (*arrows*). This echogenic line runs to the gallbladder, which is located more caudad out of the image.

recently come into widespread use. This further divides each lobe of the liver into a lobule (Fig. 5–9).

The lateral and medial segments of the left lobe are divided by the falciform ligament (Fig. 5–10). The falciform ligament consists of two layers of parietal peritoneum that, in fetal life, contain the umbilical vein. The umbilical vein becomes the ligamentum teres and this ligamentum teres runs in the free edge of the falciform ligament. In fetal life, the umbilical vein carries blood to the left portal vein. Blood is shunted into the left portal vein and then out the ductus venosus. The ductus venosus wraps around the caudate lobe and empties into the inferior vena cava. After birth, this becomes the fissure for ligamentum venosum. On a transverse image, this fissure for the ligamentum venosum can frequently be identified as it goes around the caudate lobe (Fig. 5–11).

Portal veins can be distinguished from hepatic veins by the fact that portal veins

have a bright echogenic wall, probably as a result of more fibrous tissue in the wall.

ABSCESS OR ASCITES

The radiologist is frequently asked to use ultrasound to rule out an abdominal abscess or ascites. This amounts to a search for collections of either complex or simple fluid. It is important to examine all the areas of the abdomen that are potential hiding places for a fluid collection. There are at least seven of these: (1) right subphrenic area, (2) left subphrenic area, (3) lesser sac (anterior to pancreas), (4) Morison's pouch (Fig. 5–12), (5) left paracolic gutter, (6) right paracolic gutter, and (7) retrovesicle space. The area around both kidneys also should be examined to make certain there are no retroperitoneal fluid collections, and it is important to compare the size of the psoas muscles to make sure a psoas abscess is not present. If fluid is detected, then the differential diagnosis is listed in Table 5–1.

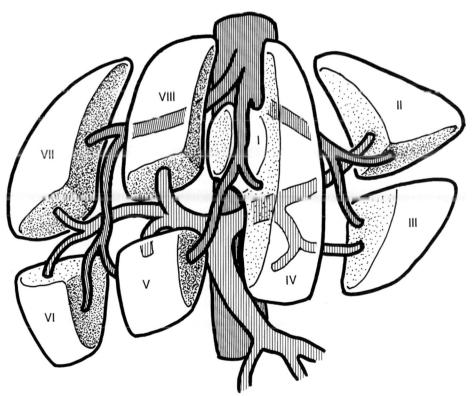

Figure 5–9. Chewnard system: caudate lobe is segment I. Lateral segment left lobe has segments II and III. Medial segment left lobe is IV. The right lobe is divided into four segments: V through VIII. This system is based on the vascular supply to the segments. Segments V and VIII are anterior while segments VI and VII are posterior.

RIGHT LOBE   LEFT LOBE

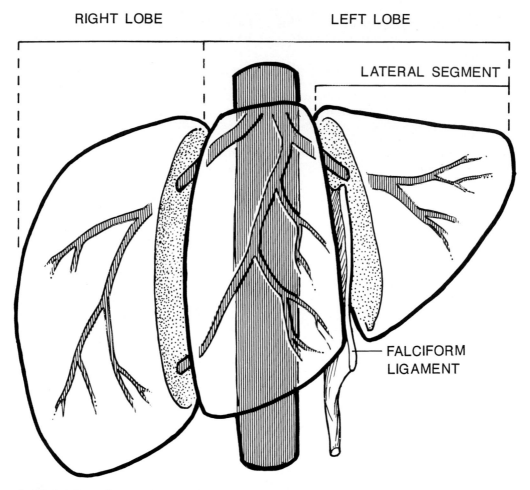

Figure 5–10. Falciform ligament separates the lateral and medial segments of the left lobe. The terms fissure for ligamentum teres and falciform ligament are often used interchangeably.

LYMPHADENOPATHY AND MASSES

Lymphadenopathy in the abdomen is usually seen as a hypoechoic mass; it may be so hypoechoic as to resemble a cyst (Fig. 5–13). Most lymph nodes will not have through transmission and, therefore, the distinction between cyst and enlarged lymph node can be made on the basis of through transmission. Careful examination may reveal internal echoes in lymph nodes. When looking for lymphadenopathy, one should look around the portal vein and common duct in the porta hepatis and in the para-aortic area along the aorta. Scanning of this area is frequently limited by overlying bowel gas, but sometimes in a child or a thin adult, a good view of the para-aortic area is possible. Retrocrural lymph nodes are sometimes seen in the up-

per abdomen. In the pelvis, the pelvic side walls should be examined by using the bladder as a window.

Masses that are identified in the abdomen and pelvis may have an extensive differential diagnosis that is listed in Table 5–2.

HEMATOMAS IN THE ABDOMEN

The best rule of thumb for the ultrasonographic appearance of a hematoma is that it is variable. Investigators have attempted to characterize hematomas by various means: time since the bleed, frequency of the transducer being used, and other factors. In our experience, the hematoma is usually a complex fluid collection with much material in it that simply appears as debris. Certainly as the clot ages, it becomes

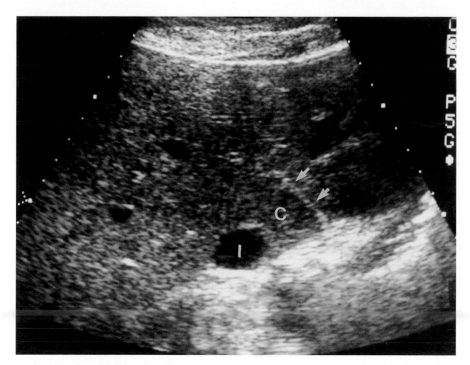

Figure 5-11. Transverse image of liver. Fissure for ligamentum venosum wraps around caudate lobe (C). I = inferior vena cava.

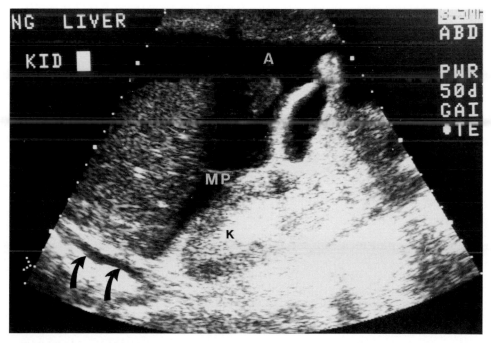

Figure 5-12. Sagittal image. MP = fluid in Morison's pouch, an intraperitoneal space between liver and kidney (K). Note right pleural effusion (*curved arrows*). A = ascites around liver.

Table 5–1. PERITONEAL FLUID COLLECTIONS

COMMON
Ascites
Mesenteric metastases
Peritoneal carcinomatosis
Hematoma
Abscess
After surgery
After peritoneal lavage
Pelvic inflammatory disease
Ectopic pregnancy

UNCOMMON
Peritoneal infection
After renal stone removal percutaneously
Hepatic tuberculosis
Hepatic dysfunction
Inferior vena cava thrombosis
After trauma

more echolucent. At least one study has indicated that higher frequency transducers cause a clot to have a more echogenic appearance. The presence of debris and septations does not necessarily indicate infection and, in general, has no significance.

ABDOMINAL WALL

Ultrasound may be used to evaluate abdominal wall masses and lumps. These usually occur after surgery and represent either abscesses or hematomas. We are often asked to look for ventral hernias. The patient should be examined supine, standing, and sometimes, resting on all four extremities on the examining table. Scanning during a Valsalva maneuver may also be useful. The differential diagnosis for abdominal wall masses is listed in Table 5–3.

Pancreas

PANCREATITIS

Ultrasound of the pancreas (Fig. 5–14A) is frequently performed to look for acute pancreatitis, pancreatic pseudocysts, or pancreatic neoplasms. The classic appearance of acute pancreatitis is that of an enlarged irregular pancreas that is of lower echogenicity than expected (lower than adjacent liver) (Fig. 5–14B). This is best thought of as being an edematous pancreas.

About two-thirds of the patients with acute pancreatitis will have a normal-appearing pancreas. Therefore, ultrasound is not a sensitive detector of acute pancreatitis. Occasionally acute pancreatitis will involve not the entire gland but only a small area of it. This small area may be somewhat enlarged and of lower echogenicity than the remainder of the pancreas. This is called focal pancreatitis.

If the pancreatitis is of the hemorrhagic type, then an echogenic, relatively homogeneous mass may be seen in the region of the pancreatic bed. The differential diagnosis for an echogenic pancreas is listed in Table 5–4. Over time, this hemorrhage may become more echolucent. Phlegmonous pancreatitis is an inflammatory mass that extends outward from the pancreas to involve adjacent tissues and to blur the tissue planes with ultimate necrosis. A phlegmon has the appearance of a complex, usually hypoechoic, mass. It will be located in the pancreatic bed or in the adjacent lesser sac or splenic hilum. The pancreatic duct may be dilated in acute pancreatitis due to obstruction by the pancreatic inflammation.

When searching for pancreatic pseudocysts (Fig. 5–15), one should examine the entire abdomen and pelvis since a pseudocyst may occur in a location far removed from the pancreas. When a cystic structure is found, it is wise to use Doppler sonography because, occasionally, pancreatitis can cause aneurysms in adjacent vessels, most often the splenic artery. Other causes of pancreatic cysts are listed in Table 5–5. Pancreatitis can also cause thrombosis of either the portal vein or the superior mesenteric vein. It is nearly impossible, using ultrasound, to distinguish between a pancreatic pseudocyst and an infected pseudocyst. If gas is identified within the lesion, then a presumptive diagnosis of infection can be made.

Once the pancreatic pseudocyst is identified, ultrasound can be used to monitor its progress. A pseudocyst that remains stable or regresses probably can be treated conservatively, but a pseudocyst that continues to increase in size or does not regress may need either percutaneous drainage with ultrasound or computed tomography (CT) guidance, or definitive surgical treatment.

Chronic pancreatitis classically appears as a small, relatively atrophic pancreas with

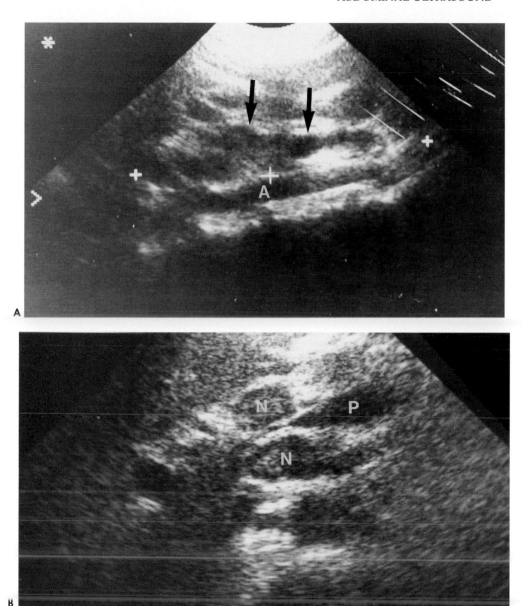

Figure 5–13. *A,* Sagittal image of aorta (*A*). Hypoechoic structures are lymph nodes (*arrows*). *B,* Porta hepatis nodes (N) compressing portal vein. Image is oblique parallel to long axis of portal vein (P).

multiple calcifications within it (Fig. 5–16). Dilatation of the pancreatic duct may also be seen in chronic pancreatitis secondary to obstruction of the pancreatic duct.

PANCREATIC CANCER

Adenocarcinoma of the pancreas is a relatively common tumor occurring in those over age 50. About two-thirds of adenocar-

cinomas of the pancreas occur in the head of the gland. About one-quarter occur in the body, with a small percentage occurring in the tail. The ultrasound evaluation of the pancreas is dependent upon adequate visualization. It is not always possible to get adequate visualization and, even in experienced hands, only about 70 percent of patients will have a study in which the pancreas is adequately seen. The classic

Table 5–2. INTRAPERITONEAL MASSES

COMMON
Hematoma
Abscess
Fluid in bowel
Pseudocyst of pancreas
Abnormal bowel
  Infarcted
  Infected
  Infiltrated (lymphoma)
  Obstructed
  Hematoma in wall
  Barium within
  Intussusception
Lymphoma
Fecaloma
Malignancy
  Ovary
  Colon
  Pancreas
  Gastric
Metastases

UNCOMMON
Duplication cyst
Mesenteric cyst
Lymphocele
Disseminated hydatid disease
Complex ascites
Abdominal tuberculosis
Omental tuberculosis
Crohn's disease
Echinococcosis
Omental cysts
Mesothelioma of omentum
Left ventricular aneurysm
Surgical transposition of ovary
Peritoneal inclusion cyst
Fat necrosis
Leiomyomatosis peritoneales disseminata
Ovarian vein thrombophlebitis
Mucocele of appendix
Tuberculous peritonitis
Cystic lymphangioma
Cystic mesothelioma
Sarcoma

Table 5–3. ABDOMINAL WALL MASSES

COMMON
Abscesses
Hematoma
Ventral hernia containing bowel

UNCOMMON
Seroma
Cellulitis
Tumors
  Desmoid
  Malignant fibrous histiocytoma
Urachal cyst
Endometrioma in cesarean section scar

pancreatic adenocarcinoma is a hypoechoic round lesion in either the head or the body of the gland (Fig. 5–17). There may be other causes for this appearance (Table 5–6). There may be associated pancreatic ductal obstruction and dilatation in about half of these patients. The pancreas does not have a serosal capsule, so spread from the pancreas to adjacent organs occurs early. This may be one reason why the cure rate for pancreatic carcinoma is low. Therefore, if pancreatic carcinoma is suspected, one must look for metastatic disease to the liver and obstruction of the common bile duct. Also, a search for metastatic disease to the lymph nodes in the adjacent celiac node plexus and porta hepatis regions must be made. In the past, obliteration of the fat around the superior mesenteric artery was taken as evidence of pancreatic cancer with local invasion. This is not a reliable way to differentiate between pancreatitis and pancreatic carcinoma. However, if the fat around the superior mesenteric artery is obliterated in the setting of known pancreatic carcinoma, it is a bad prognostic sign.

There is an important differential diagnosis to consider when dilatation of the pancreatic duct is identified along with dilatation of the common bile duct. This differential diagnosis includes pancreatic carcinoma in the head obstructing both ducts, ampullary carcinoma, or a stone lodged in the ampulla blocking both the common duct and the pancreatic duct. Occasionally, pancreatitis can lead to the obstruction of both ductal systems.

OTHER PANCREATIC NEOPLASMS

Cystic neoplasms of the pancreas have a better prognosis than the usual adenocarcinoma. They are divided into microcystic and macrocystic types. Microcystic cystadenomas were previously referred to as serous cystadenomas. These usually are well-defined, multilocular, multicystic masses. They may occasionally be calcified. About two-thirds occur in females over the age of 60. Microcystic cystadenomas are benign lesions and do not convert to cystadenocarcinomas. There is an association between this entity and von Hippel-Lindau syndrome. At ultrasound, the cysts may be too small to see and the pancreas may be echogenic due to multiple interfaces created by

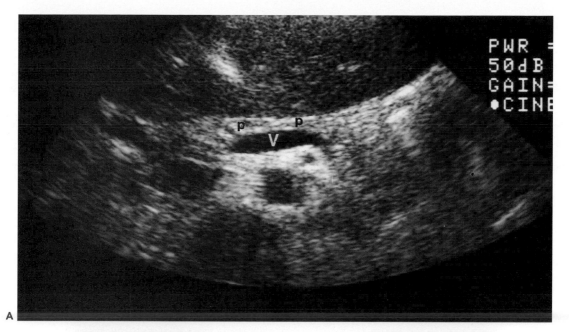

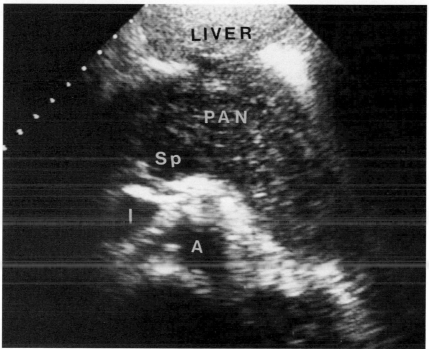

Figure 5–14. *A,* A normal pancreas (p) with the splenic vein (V) behind it. Pancreas should be more echogenic than liver and sits anterior to the splenic vein. *B,* Enlarged, hypoechoic pancreas (PAN). Sp = splenic vein. A = aorta. I = inferior vena cava.

the cysts. This echogenic appearance may occur for the same reason that echogenic kidneys occur in infantile polycystic kidney disease.

Macrocystic cystadenomas were previ-ously known as mucinous cystadenomas. They consist of between one and six cysts as compared to the microcystic type that is made up of many small cysts. Macrocys-tic cystadenomas occur in middle-aged to

Table 5-4. ECHOGENIC PANCREAS

COMMON
Chronic pancreatitis
Hemorrhagic pancreatitis

UNCOMMON
Cystic fibrosis
Obese patients
Diabetes
Steroid ingestion
Pancreatic insufficiency
Malabsorption
Hereditary pancreatitis

elderly patients. They are more common in the body and the tail of the gland. They should be excised because they are premalignant even when in the cystadenoma form. It can be difficult to differentiate a macrocystic cystadenoma or cystadenocarcinoma from a pancreatic pseudocyst.

Islet cell tumors may occur as part of the multiple endocrine neoplasia syndrome. These tumors can also occur as an isolated neoplasm. The most common type is an insulinoma or a B cell tumor. These are usually benign and are common in middle-aged patients who have hypoglycemia. The appearance of B cell tumors ranges from minute or even microscopic to huge masses. These tumors may be nonfunctioning. In that case, they grow to a larger size before they cause symptoms or are detected. About 30 percent of insulinomas are detectable by ultrasound.

Gastrinomas produce the Zollinger-Ellison syndrome. Insulinomas account for about 60 percent of all islet cell tumors while gastrinomas account for about 20 percent. These lesions are potentially malignant. Other types of islet cell tumors include glucagonomas, VIPomas and somatostatinomas.

The typical appearance of the islet cell tumor is of a hypoechoic lesion. They are not usually calcified. As the tumor becomes larger, it may have a complex appearance with calcifications or areas of liquefaction. The metastases from these tumors are usually echogenic. Intraoperative ultrasound with a high-frequency transducer has been used in an effort to detect these lesions. Approximately 80 percent of the lesions can be detected by this method.

FOCAL SPARING AND FATTY INFILTRATION

The pancreas frequently becomes infiltrated with fat, especially in the elderly, the obese, diabetics, and those with chronic pancreatitis, liver disease, malnutrition, or those on steroids. This causes the pancreas to become echogenic (Table 5-4). At times, all of the pancreas may undergo fatty change except for a small part of the head and uncinate process. This spared area may appear hypoechoic and may simulate a hypoechoic mass. Distinguishing between tumor and focal sparing may be difficult. Lack of dilation of the common bile duct and pancreatic duct, lack of symptoms, and lack of an increase in size of the pancreatic head all suggest that focal sparing may be occurring.

THE PEDIATRIC PANCREAS

Visualization of the pancreas is more often successful in the pediatric age group than in adults. Children should also be fasting, just as adults should. Table 5-7 gives normal pancreatic sizes for children of all ages. As in adults, pancreatic enlargement, decreased echogenicity, and dilatation of the pancreatic duct are indicators of pancreatitis. Trauma is a frequent cause of pancreatitis in the pediatric age group. The existence of a pancreatic pseudocyst should strongly suggest trauma. Before age 5, child abuse should be considered. Children also may develop pancreatitis as a result of cystic fibrosis, obstruction of the pancreatic duct as in gallstone pancreatitis, or pancreas divisum. Pancreas divisum is suggested if the pancreatic head is relatively enlarged, but this is usually a difficult diagnosis. Hyperparathyroidism can also lead to pancreatitis. In cystic fibrosis, the pancreas is relatively fat replaced and, therefore, is very echogenic. The pancreas may also become atrophied and develop calcifications. Frank pancreatitis does not occur often in cystic fibrosis, however.

Pediatric patients may get adenocarcinoma of the pancreas. When it occurs in this age group, it is usually very aggressive. Similarly, they may develop islet cell tumors, just as adults do.

PANCREAS DIVISUM

These patients present with recurrent bouts of pancreatitis. The embryologic dor-

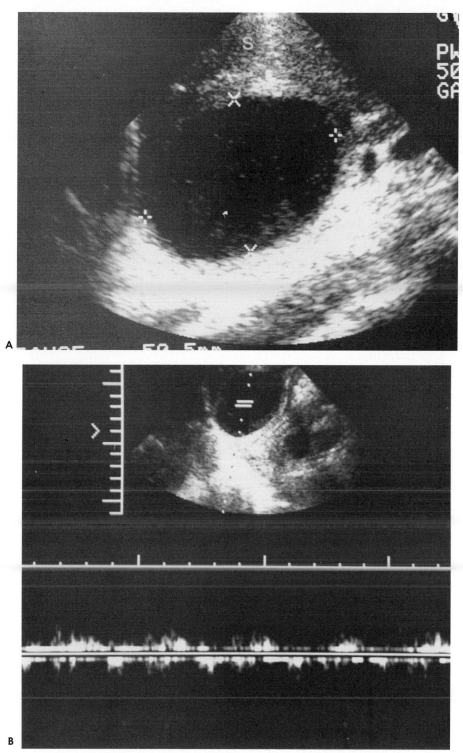

Figure 5–15. Sagittal images. *A*, Pancreatic pseudocyst. S = spleen. *B*, Similarly appearing lesion but Doppler showed a small amount of flow. This was a splenic artery aneurysm secondary to pancreatitis.

Table 5–5. CYSTIC LESIONS OF THE PANCREAS

COMMON
Pseudocyst

UNCOMMON
Posttraumatic cysts
Cystadenoma
Cyst adenocarcinoma
Islet cell tumors
Abscess
Duodenal cysts
Dilated distal common bile duct
Congenital cysts
Hematoma
Lymphoma
Left renal vein varix
Splenic artery aneurysm

sal-ventral pancreatic buds have failed to fuse, leading to a situation in which the accessory pancreatic duct (Santorini) that would normally drain only a small portion of the pancreas is forced to carry a large volume of pancreatic juices. If this duct is narrow, then pancreatitis may result. The main pancreatic duct (Wirsung) carries only a minority of pancreatic secretions in this situation (Fig. 5–18). Up to 10 percent of the population may have a variant of this condition. Treatment is sphincteroplasty of the accessory papilla. Diagnosis can be suggested by visualization of both a dorsal and ventral pancreatic duct. A secretin challenge test may be performed in which 1 unit/kg of secretin is injected intravenously and the pancreatic duct is monitored for 30 minutes. Enlargement of the pancreatic duct indicates resistance to the flow of pancreatic secretions and suggests the diagnosis of pancreas divisum.

Liver and Biliary System

BILIARY DISEASE

First, the common duct in the porta hepatis should be measured. This is near where the cystic duct inserts. Usually the common hepatic duct is measured but sometimes the common bile duct is measured. It is often difficult to tell which portion of the ductal system is being measured since the cystic duct cannot be identified. A common duct of 5 mm or less is within normal limits, while 6 mm and 7 mm are considered bor-

derline, and 8 mm is definitely abnormal. As patients age, the common bile duct may enlarge slightly, with a 6-mm common duct being acceptable in a 60-year-old but probably abnormal in a 20-year-old. A rule of thumb allows a 5-mm duct in a 50-year-old, 6 mm in a 60-year-old, etc. The common bile duct should not be larger than 2 mm in infants under the age of 1, or 4 mm in older children.

Some controversy exists about the status of the common bile duct after the gallbladder has been removed. Some think that the biliary system takes over the reservoir function normally performed by the gallbladder. Therefore, after the gallbladder has been removed, the common duct may enlarge slightly.

If there is doubt about whether a common duct is obstructed or not, then the flow of bile can be stimulated either by a meal or by injection into the blood of a cholecystokinin-type substance. When the bile flow is stimulated, an obstructed duct will become larger if measured 30 minutes to 1 hour after stimulation. An unobstructed duct should become smaller or remain the same when the sphincter of Oddi opens and bile is allowed to drain into the duodenum.

The intrahepatic biliary ducts should be examined carefully. In general, they will measure less than 2 mm in size. When scanning through the liver, they will not be seen unless a careful search is made. A bile duct should be seen with each portal venous structure. A portal venous structure is usually larger and has echogenic walls. When two parallel tubes are seen coursing through the liver, it is likely that one of the tubes is the portal venous system and the second tube is a dilated biliary system (Fig. 5–19 and Table 5–8). Experimentally, when the common bile duct is tied off, the bile duct will dilate over about 24 hours. However, many patients never dilate their intrahepatic ducts and manifest only a very large common bile duct. When the obstruction is removed, it may take 1 to 2 months before the bile duct returns to normal and, in some patients, it may never return to a completely normal caliber. Dilatation of the common bile duct may occur for reasons other than stones (Table 5–9).

Detecting common bile duct stones by ultrasound is difficult. Only about 60 to 70

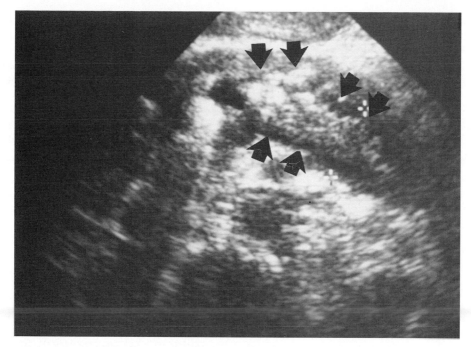

Figure 5–16. Transverse image. Arrows outline small pancreas with multiple calcifications of chronic pancreatitis.

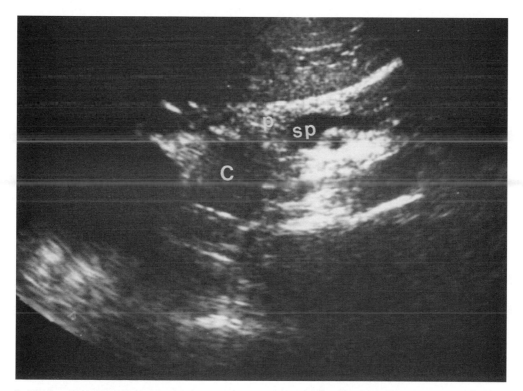

Figure 5–17. Transverse image. Hypoechoic lesion in pancreatic head is cancer. Often, a discrete hypoechoic lesion will not be seen but a portion of the pancreas will have a heterogeneous disorganized echo pattern associated with a mass. C = cancer; sp = splenic vein; p = pancreas.

Table 5-6. FOCAL MASS IN PANCREAS

COMMON
Carcinoma
Lymphomatous nodes
Pseudocyst
Pancreatitis, especially acute

UNCOMMON
Metastatic nodes
Cystadenoma
Cystadenocarcinoma
Islet cell tumor
Pancreatic phlegmon
Congenital cysts
Retention cysts
Abscess
Peripancreatic adenopathy
Sarcoidosis
Lipomatosis of pancreas

percent of common duct stones will be detected (Fig. 5-20). The specificity is about 90 percent: Air in the biliary tree, surgical clips, a mucus plug, the right hepatic artery crossing the common bile duct (Fig. 5-5), and sludge all can mimic intrahepatic stones or masses (Table 5-10).

Cholangiocarcinoma is an almost uniformly fatal disease that presents in older patients. These tumors may be either adenocarcinomas or squamous cell carcinomas. The most common site is in the common bile duct, with the more proximal biliary system being less commonly involved. Cholangiocarcinoma seen on ultrasound may present in one of three ways: (1) as an ill-defined infiltrating-type lesion that extends along the bile ducts (80 percent), (2) a bulky exophytic mass (15 percent), or (3) a polypoid intraluminal mass (5 percent). Predisposing factors include ulcerative colitis, clonorchiasis, Caroli's disease, and choledochal cysts.

One type of cholangiocarcinoma is a Klatskin tumor that occurs at the junction between the right hepatic duct and the left hepatic duct. Cholangiocarcinomas present with dilated intrahepatic ducts. Depending on the site of the tumor, the extrahepatic duct may be dilated down to the level of the tumor. In a Klatskin tumor, the dilated hepatic ducts do not merge at the hilum but run into a soft tissue mass. This nonunion is said to be relatively specific for a Klatskin tumor.

Mirizzi's syndrome causes bile duct obstruction. In this syndrome, the cystic duct inserts unusually low in the common duct system. Therefore, the cystic duct and the common hepatic duct run parallel for a brief distance. A stone lodges in the distal cystic duct, and the inflammation causes obstruction of the common hepatic duct. At ultrasound, two dilated tubes (common duct and cystic duct) may sometimes be seen (Fig. 5-21).

Caroli's disease is dilatation of the intrahepatic biliary system. It usually presents in childhood or in early adult years. It is associated with infantile polycystic kidney disease and congenital hepatic fibrosis. These patients get saccular bile duct dilatation intrahepatically and are predisposed to form stones and develop cholangitis. Obstruction is not the etiology of this disease. The dilated bile ducts may be quite large and actually resemble hepatic cysts.

Choledochal cysts occur more commonly in children and young adult females. The pathology is dilation of the extrahepatic biliary system. This large cyst in the porta hepatis may cause obstruction of the common bile duct. Intrahepatic bile duct dilatation is also frequently present. One hypothesis is that this is a result of insertion of the common bile duct into the pancreatic duct anomalously, with resultant reflux and saccular dilatation of the common bile duct. The other hypothesis is that there is a weakness in the bile duct wall. These patients have an increased risk of cholangiocarcinoma. At ultrasound, a cyst in the porta hepatis will be seen separate from the gallbladder (Fig. 5-22). In neonates, a choledochal cyst may be a congenital finding.

There are several types of cholangitis. Sclerosing cholangitis occurs in patients with ulcerative colitis, Riedel's struma, Crohn's disease, and retroperitoneal fibrosis. Ultrasound of the biliary system reveals biliary obstruction with thickening of the wall of both the intra- and extrahepatic bile ducts. In many cases, there may be no ultrasound findings and the disease may be undetectable by ultrasound.

Oriental cholangitis, or recurrent pyogenic cholangitis, is a disease found mainly in patients from Southeast Asia. They present with abdominal pain, fever, and recurrent episodes of jaundice and they are usually between the ages of 20 and 40. They have fibrosis around the bile ducts. These

**Table 5–7. NORMAL DIMENSIONS OF THE
PANCREAS AS A FUNCTION OF AGE**

Patient Age	MAXIMUM ANTEROPOSTERIOR DIMENSIONS OF PANCREAS (CM ± 1 STANDARD DEVIATION)		
	Head	Body	Tail
<1 month	1.0 ± 0.4	0.6 ± 0.2	1.0 ± 0.4
1 month–1 year	1.5 ± 0.5	0.8 ± 0.3	1.2 ± 0.4
1–5 years	1.7 ± 0.3	1.0 ± 0.2	1.8 ± 0.4
5–10 years	1.6 ± 0.4	1.0 ± 0.3	1.8 ± 0.4
10–19 years	2.0 ± 0.5	1.1 ± 0.3	2.0 ± 0.4

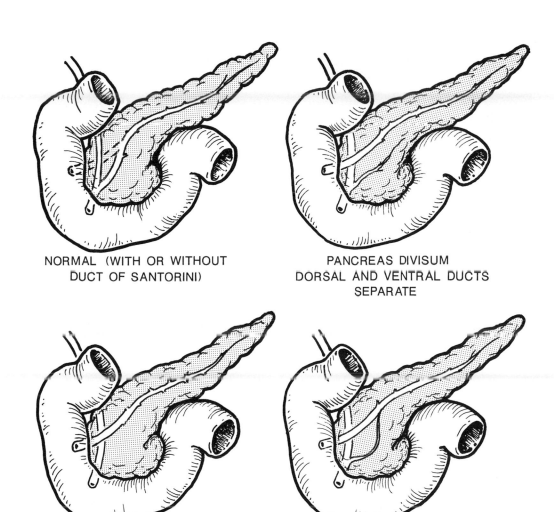

NORMAL (WITH OR WITHOUT
DUCT OF SANTORINI)

PANCREAS DIVISUM
DORSAL AND VENTRAL DUCTS
SEPARATE

PANCREAS DIVISUM
DORSAL DUCT ONLY
WIRSUNG ABSENT

FUNCTIONAL PANCREAS DIVISUM
FILAMENTOUS COMMUNICATION BETWEEN
DORSAL AND VENTRAL DUCTS

Figure 5–18. Various anatomic configurations of main pancreatic duct (Wirsung) and accessory duct (Santorini). (Modified from Warshaw A, et al. Evaluation and treatment of the dominant dorsal duct syndrome (pancreas divisum redefined). Am J Surg *159*:59, 1990, with permission.)

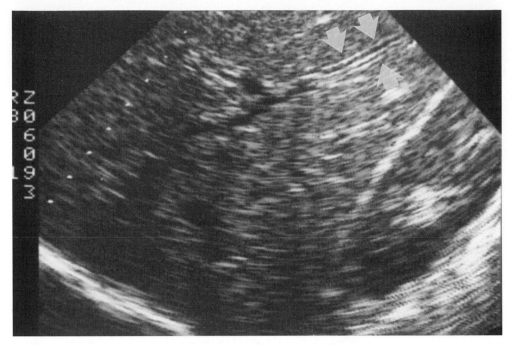

Figure 5–19. Between the arrows are two tubes. This is the "two tubes" sign of biliary obstruction. Sometimes normal patients will have parallel tubes similar to this if a 5-MHz or higher transducer is used.

Table 5–8. "TOO MANY TUBES" IN THE LIVER

Dilated intrahepatic bile ducts
   Biliary obstruction
   Caroli's disease
Dilated intrahepatic arteries
Angiodysplasia of hepatic artery

Table 5–9. ENLARGED COMMON DUCT

COMMON
Bile duct obstruction
   Biliary stone
   Pancreatic carcinoma
   Cholangiocarcinoma
   Ampullary carcinoma
   Lymphoma of pancreas
   Papilloma of common duct
   Choledochal cyst
   Biliary clonorchiasis
   AIDS
Recurrent pyogenic cholangitis
Sclerosing cholangitis
Oriental cholangitis

bile ducts may have stones or debris within them. This disease is felt to increase the risk of carcinoma of the bile ducts. It may occur secondary to dead parasites in the bile ducts with bile stasis. Ultrasound shows stones within the dilated intra- and extrahepatic ducts. The extrahepatic ducts are usually more dilated than the intrahepatic ducts. Portions of the liver may be atrophied and there may be gallstones. The dilated intrahepatic ducts may be difficult to recognize because they are filled with debris.

Suppurative cholangitis is a result of biliary obstruction usually secondary to stones or strictures. Carcinoma can also cause this condition. The obstructed bile becomes infected and the patients present with jaundice and fever. An early finding in suppurative cholangitis is sludge in the common duct. This may indicate that the patient's biliary ducts are becoming obstructed.

LIVER DISEASES

Benign liver diseases include cirrhosis, hepatitis, cysts, and parasites. The ultrasound diagnosis of cirrhosis can be difficult. The echo pattern becomes coarse and het-

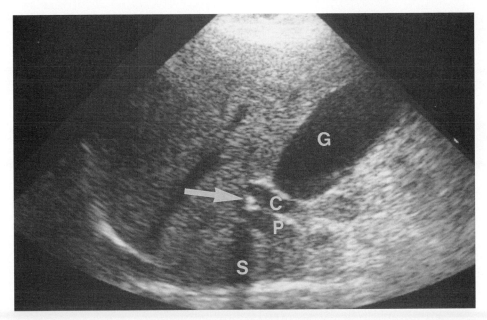

Figure 5–20. Sagittal image of common duct (C) with stone (*arrow*) within it. Note shadow (S). G = gallbladder, P = portal vein.

erogeneous instead of homogeneous. Early in the course of the disease the liver may be enlarged, but later it shrinks and becomes fibrotic. Fatty infiltration is part of this disease process. The surface of the liver will be irregular. Therefore, an irregular liver that is quite echogenic should suggest cirrhosis. As indicated, the liver may be either large or small. A search should be made for recanalization of the umbilical vein in the region of the falciform ligament.

Fatty infiltration of the liver may occur secondary to diabetes mellitus, alcohol use, obesity, steroids, parenteral nutrition, or

Table 5–10. ECHOES WITHIN THE COMMON DUCT

COMMON
Stone
Sludge

UNCOMMON
Pus
Clonorchiasis
Hemobilia
Pneumobilia
Recurrent pyogenic cholangitis
Calcification in head of pancreas
Cholangiocarcinoma
Feces
Hepatoma
Right hepatic artery crossing duct
Clips

chemotherapy (Fig. 5–23). It may be focal or diffuse. There are many causes of an echogenic liver (Table 5–11). Diffuse fatty infiltration manifests as a diffusely echogenic liver. Care must be taken that the gain settings are appropriate so that increased echogenicity of the liver is not produced artificially. Focal fatty infiltration may simulate a mass and be seen as a focal area of increased echogenicity (Fig. 5–24). This condition can sometimes be differentiated from neoplasm by its failure to displace intrahepatic blood vessels. However, neoplasms do not always displace vessels. Focal fatty sparing of the liver occurs when there is a normal area of liver parenchyma surrounded by a liver that is almost totally fat infiltrated in all other areas (Fig. 5–25). This typically occurs just anterior to the porta hepatis in the medial segment of the left lobe.

Hepatitis may produce a liver with either increased echogenicity or decreased echogenicity. If the echogenicity of the liver is decreased, the portal venus structures may stand out on the background of an echopoor liver. This is sometimes called a "starry sky" liver (Table 5–12) and is a common presentation for acute hepatitis. Increased echogenicity is more common with chronic hepatitis.

Benign cysts are common in the liver.

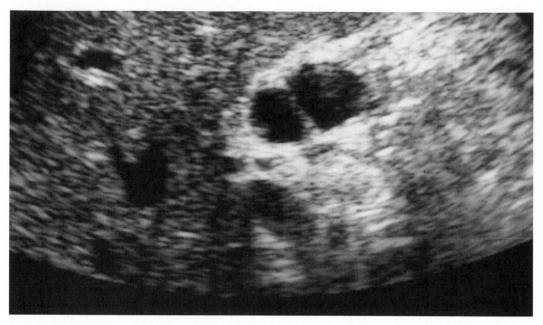

Figure 5–21. Transverse image through two dilated tubes: one is the dilated cystic duct and the other is the dilated common duct, which is being obstructed by a stone lodged in the distal cystic duct (Mirizzi's syndrome).

They should not be cause for concern as long as they meet all requirements for a simple cyst. They are thought to be bile duct developmental abnormalities. They are especially common after age 40. Table 5–13 gives a differential diagnosis for cystic liver lesions.

Echinococcal cysts occur in people after

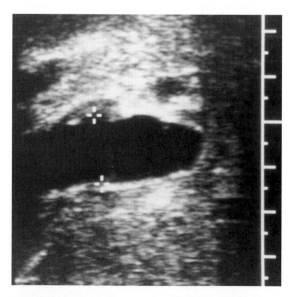

Figure 5–22. Choledochal cyst in the porta hepatis.

exposure to parasites, usually from dogs that have been used for herding sheep or cattle. Echinococcal cysts may take years to grow to a significant size. On ultrasound, these may be calcified or noncalcified simple cysts, cyst within cyst, honeycomb cysts, or solid masses; walls are commonly smooth. A double-line sign secondary to an interlaminated membrane within a larger cyst has been said to be specific for an echinococcal cyst. Small amounts of sand or gravel may be seen within the cyst. After adequate therapy, the cyst may become more solid or complex in appearance.

Bacterial abscesses are round and echolucent. They have irregular walls and may have debris within them.

Amebic abscesses occur when the parasite reaches the liver via the portal vein. On ultrasound, amebic abscesses typically appear as areas of decreased echogenicity and may have characteristics simulating a cyst (Fig. 5–26). Low-level echoes are seen within them. No discernible wall is seen. Many do not have these characteristics, however. These cysts are usually located peripherally and near the liver capsule.

Candida abscesses cause hypoechoic lesions. Classically, they are said to produce a target lesion: an area of decreased echo-

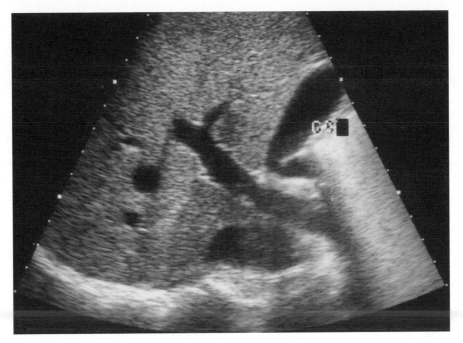

Figure 5–23. Fatty liver. Transverse image shows diffusely echogenic liver. The vessels and gallbladder stand out sharply against the echogenic liver.

Table 5–11. OVERALL INCREASED ECHOGENICITY OF LIVER

COMMON
Fatty infiltration
Fibrosis (cirrhosis)
Chronic hepatitis
Acute hepatitis

UNCOMMON
Diffuse tuberculosis

Liver congestion in Budd-Chiari syndrome

Diphenylhydantoin toxicity

AIDS

Inappropriate time gain compensation (TGC) curve

Glycogen storage disease

Infiltrating malignancy

Liver congestion from congestive heart failure

Wilson's disease

Reye's syndrome

Gaucher's disease

Schistosomiasis

Tyrosinemia

genicity with a small punctate echogenic focus in the center. However, this appearance is variable, and we have not often seen these target lesions.

The most common benign lesion in adults is a cavernous hemangioma (Fig. 5–27). These are endothelial vascular spaces in the liver that contain slowly flowing blood. They do not have large feeding vessels or large draining veins. They occur more often in the right lobe. Classically, they appear as an echogenic focus. Some of the larger lesions may have good through transmission. Doppler is not useful in characterizing these lesions because of the slow blood flow.

Focal nodular hyperplasia is more common in women than in men. This condition has been weakly linked to the use of birth control pills. It is usually echo poor but occasionally may be echogenic. The lesion appears as a focal lesion, usually solitary but occasionally multiple.

Benign liver adenomas have been linked to the use of birth control pills. They have a variable appearance ranging from hypoechoic to echogenic. They also present as a focal lesion.

Hepatomas may be unicentric, multicentric, or infiltrative. They are usually hypo-

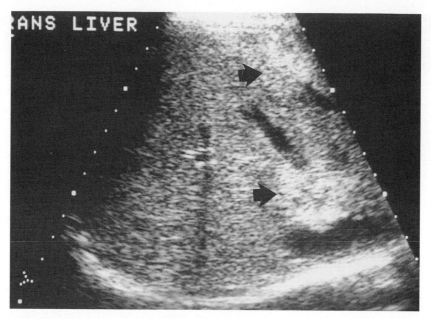

Figure 5–24. Poorly defined areas of increased echogenicity due to fatty infiltration.

echoic but may be mixed or even hyperechoic (Fig. 5–28). These tissues commonly have fatty elements in them and may also have fibrotic or necrotic elements in them, leading to the hyperechoic appearance. One particular type of hepatoma, called a fibro-lamellar hepatoma, has a central scar and calcification and tends to have a better prognosis. Hepatomas have a propensity to invade either the hepatic or portal venous system (Fig. 5–29).

Metastatic disease to the liver is more commonly hypoechoic but may also be hyperechoic or produce target lesions or even infiltrative patterns (Fig. 5–30). The infiltrative pattern may be very difficult to appre-

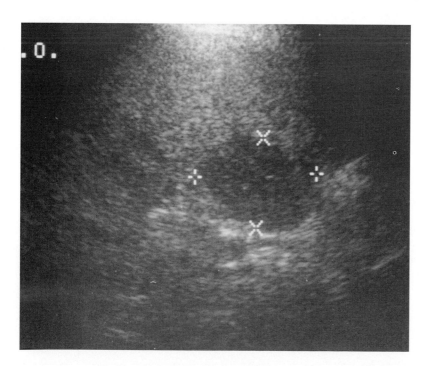

Figure 5–25. Focal fatty sparing simulates a mass.

Table 5–12. BRIGHT PERIPORTAL ECHOES (STARRY-SKY LIVER)

COMMON
Hepatitis

UNCOMMON
Hepatic Kaposi's sarcoma
Leukemia
Toxic shock syndrome
Burkitt's lymphoma
Oil embolism after lymphangiogram
Cholangitis
Mononucleosis
Cystic fibrosis
Biliary air
Periportal fibrosis
Right heart failure
Schistosomiasis

Table 5–13. INTRAHEPATIC CYSTIC LESIONS

COMMON
Simple cysts
Congenital cysts
Previous trauma
Segmental biliary obstruction
With adult polycystic kidney disease
Hemangioma

UNCOMMON
Caroli's disease
Abscesses
Bacterial
Amebic
Echinococcal
Biliary cystadenoma
Biliary cystadenocarcinoma
Cavernous hemangiomas
Necrotic tumor
Biloma
Hepatic foregut cysts
Choledochal cysts
Hepatic cystadenoma
Normal gallbladder
Pancreatic pseudocyst
Endometrioma
Posttraumatic biloma
Tuberculosis
Hematoma
Interposed bowel
AIDS
Hypoechoic lesions with septae
Mucocele of cystic duct remnant
Hepatic artery aneurysm
Pseudoaneurysm of anastomosis

ciate at ultrasound as the appearance will be vague areas of increased and decreased echogenicity scattered throughout the liver. There may be some distortion of hepatic structures such as the portal venous radicals. Breast cancer is a common primary that produces an infiltrative pattern. Gastrointestinal primaries, especially colon cancer, are prone to produce hepatic metastases. Calcifications occur in metastatic lesions from colon and other mucinous adenocarcinomas. Lymphoma usually has a hypoechoic appearance when it is focal but it often is infiltrative. The differential diagnosis for solid intrahepatic lesions is in Table 5–14.

In children, the most common primary liver tumor is hepatoblastoma. It usually occurs under age 3. The lesions may be calcified and are usually echogenic or have a mixed echodensity. Hepatoblastoma originates from primitive cells that resemble a fetal liver. It differs from hepatocellular carcinoma in that hepatocellular carcinoma originates from cells more closely resembling adult liver. Alpha-fetoprotein levels may be elevated in either hepatoblastomas or hepatomas. Primary liver tumors in older children tend to be hepatomas. A differential diagnosis for liver lesions in children is given in Table 5–15.

Infantile hemangioendothelioma usually occurs before age 6 months. These infants have a normal alpha-fetoprotein level that distinguishes them from hepatoma and hepatoblastoma patients. Hemangioendotheliomas are vascular tumors that occasionally produce congestive heart failure and may lead to platelet sequestration and a bleeding diathesis. These tumors are large and have a very mixed echo appearance on ultrasound, with areas of decreased and increased echogenicity.

One must remember that infants and children can have cavernous hemangiomas just as adults can.

Metastatic disease to the liver in the pediatric age group may come from neuroblastoma, Wilms' tumor, or leukemia. Neuroblastoma commonly metastasizes to liver whereas Wilms' more commonly metastasizes to lung and infrequently metastasizes to liver. These metastatic lesions in children may be echo poor to echogenic just as in adults but are more commonly echo poor.

LIVER TRANSPLANTS

Liver transplantation is a procedure that is becoming more available for primary bil-

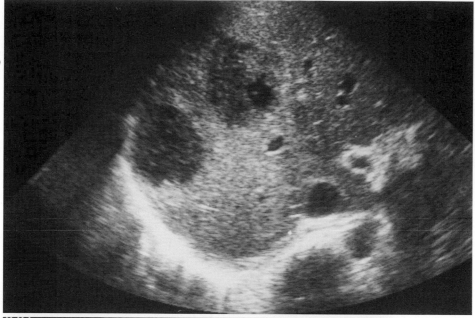

A

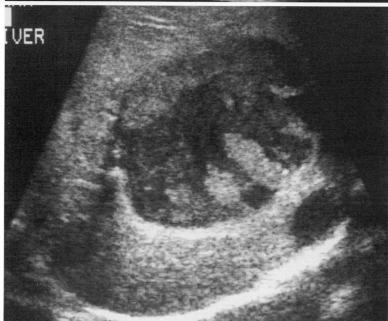

B

Figure 5–26. *A,* Two amebic abscesses. They are hypoechoic with no wall. Transverse image. *B,* More complex appearing amebic abscess on this transverse image.

iary cirrhosis, chronic hepatitis, sclerosing cholangitis, hepatic failure, and biliary atresia. Contraindications include cancer outside of the liver, uncontrollable infection outside of the liver, and intractable cardiac and/or pulmonary failure.

Ultrasound is mainly used after the transplant to evaluate for technical complications and suspected rejection. Color Doppler and pulsed Doppler are used to evaluate for portal venous thrombosis, which occurs in about 4 percent of transplants. Vena caval stenosis or thrombosis can occur either above the liver or below the liver. The suprahepatic type of vena caval lesion is difficult to treat and can cause hepatic dysfunction. These vena caval lesions are unusual, but color and pulsed Doppler should be used to evaluate the inferior vena cava. Hepatic artery thrombosis leads to he-

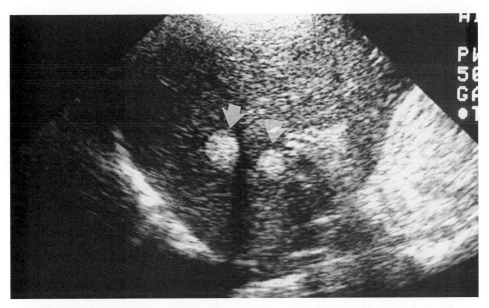

Figure 5–27. Two cavernous hemangiomas (*arrows*). Hemangiomas are usually echogenic. This appearance is not specific and has a differential diagnosis of metastasis, adenomas, focal nodular hyperplasia, or hepatoma.

patic necrosis, liver abscesses, and biliary strictures when it occurs in the early post-operative period and biliary strictures when it occurs late. This complication may occur in as many as 20 percent of children and about 5 percent of adults. Color Doppler and pulsed Doppler are used to prove patency of the hepatic artery. Hepatic artery stenosis is a common complication that leads to hepatic dysfunction. Color Doppler and pulsed Doppler are used to evaluate for areas of high velocity (>2 m/sec) and turbulence. Distal to a stenosis, a tardus-parvus wave form or slowed acceleration time may be found. The time from end-diastole to peak systole will be prolonged beyond 0.10 seconds. Doppler should be used to confirm patency of the hepatic veins.

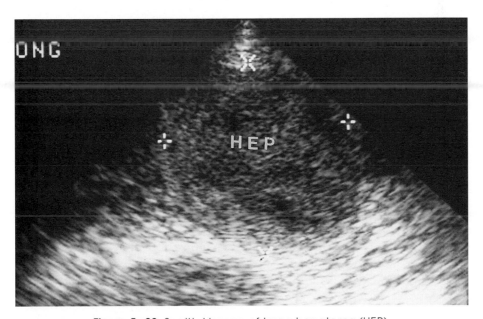

Figure 5–28. Sagittal image of large hepatoma (HEP).

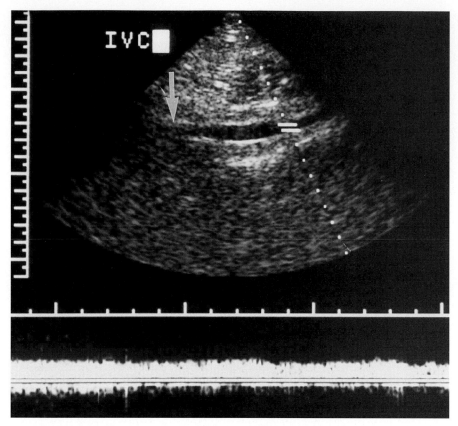

Figure 5–29. Sagittal image of inferior vena cava (IVC). Doppler shows flow in IVC but there is partial occlusion of the vessel by tumor clot (*arrow*) from a hepatoma.

Any intrahepatic or periportal fluid collections that are seen must be evaluated by Doppler to make certain they are not pseudoaneurysms originating from one of the many vascular anastomoses.

Gallbladder

NORMAL ANATOMY

The gallbladder can be reliably located on ultrasound. While it may usually be found simply by placing the transducer in the right upper quadrant and looking around, a more dependable way to find the gallbladder for those cases in which the gallbladder is small and shrunken and is not easily identified is needed. To locate the gallbladder, one should scan in the sagittal plane starting far laterally. The right lobe of the liver will be visible, as well as a portal venous branch in the anterior segment of the right lobe and a branch in the posterior segment of the right lobe. When the transducer is moved more medially, these two portal venous branches move closer and closer together and then merge to become the undivided segment of the right portal vein (Fig. 5–8). This is a short portion of right portal vein that is only about 3 cm in length. The gallbladder sits inferior to the undivided segment of the right portal vein. The gallbladder and the undivided right portal vein often will be connected by an echogenic line called the main interlobar fissure. This can be seen in about two-thirds of patients. If the gallbladder is not found in this location, then presume either that the gallbladder has been removed, the gallbladder never developed, or it is ectopic. Reasons for nonvisualization of the gallbladder are given in Table 5–16.

A small percentage of patients will have folds or kinks in their gallbladder. This is a normal developmental variant. The gallbladder sits anterior to the duodenal bulb.

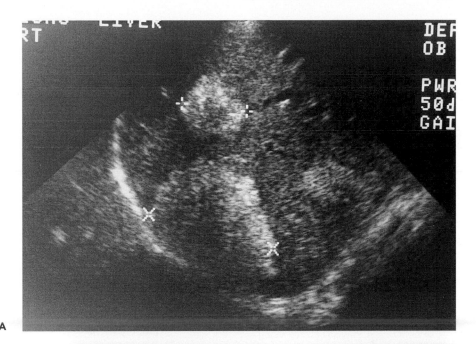

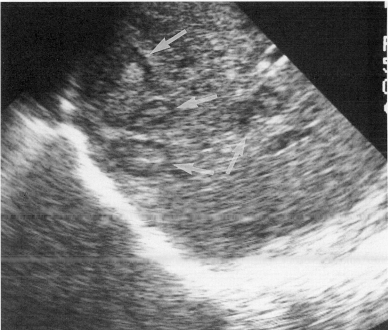

Figure 5–30. A, Hyperechoic metastases. These are usually from a mucinous adenocarcinoma, frequently colon. Carcinoid and choriocarcinoma are two other primaries that often produce hyperechoic metastases. B, Target lesions (arrows) secondary to metastases.

Gas from the duodenal bulb should not be mistaken for gallstones.

The gallbladder wall should be 3 mm or less in thickness and should be smooth and regular. Overall, the gallbladder should be less than 8 cm in length and 3.5 cm in width.

We emphasize that as high-frequency a transducer as possible should be used for

examining the gallbladder. This optimizes visualization of gallstones and their resultant shadow. The patient should have been fasting for a minimum of 4 hours and preferably 6 hours. We have scanned patients who have had only a cup of coffee and we saw no gallstones, and then re-scanned them after a true fast and found gallstones. Therefore, one must insist upon an absolute

Table 5–14. INTRAHEPATIC SOLID LESIONS

COMMON
Cavernous hemangioma
Metastases
Focal nodular hyperplasia
Adenomatous hyperplastic nodules
Focal spared areas
Hepatic adenomas
Focal fatty infiltration
Hepatoma

UNCOMMON
Capillary hemangioma
Abscess
Amebic abscess
Bile duct hamartomas
Fungal abscess
Extramedullary hematopoiesis
Candidiasis
Decreased portal flow
Echinococcal (hydatid) cysts
Granuloma from visceral larva migrans
Cholangiocarcinoma
Lymphoma
Tuberculosis
Leprosy
Wound abscess mimicking liver lesion
Hepatic artery aneurysm
Diphenylhydantoin toxicity
Regenerating cirrhotic nodules
Angiomyolipomas
Erythromycin-induced hepatitis
Hepatic Kaposi's sarcoma
AIDS
Fat in hepatocellular carcinoma
Multifocal cytomegalovirus or AIDS
Hematoma
Lipoma

Table 5–15. LIVER LESIONS IN CHILDREN

COMMON
Metastases
Neuroblastoma
Hodgkin's disease
Lymphoma
Cysts
Focal nodular hyperplasia
Adenoma
Regenerating nodules
Sarcoma, undifferentiated
Rhabdomyosarcoma
Angiosarcoma
Fibrosarcoma
Leiomyosarcoma
Teratocarcinoma
Hemangioma
  Capillary
  Cavernous
Infection
Abscess
Hepatoblastoma

UNCOMMON
Hepatoma
Biliary rhabdomyosarcoma
Mesenchymal hamartoma
Teratoma
Hamartoma
Cavernous transformation portal vein
Calcified ductus venosus
Fatty infiltration
Hemangioendothelioma

fast, although plain water should not interfere with the exam.

GALLSTONES

About 12 percent of adults have gallstones. Gallstones in and of themselves are not a reason to remove the gallbladder in an asymptomatic patient. Gallstones are composed of a mixture of cholesterol, calcium bilirubinate, and calcium carbonate. Visibility and formation of a shadow on ultrasound are less dependent upon the composition of the gallstone than on the size of the gallstone. A shadow will form if the stone is sufficiently wide to block the ultrasound beam. A stone that is dense on x-ray has a higher probability of attenuating a sound as it is a better reflector/absorber of sound. If it is not possible to demonstrate a

Table 5–16. NONVISUALIZATION OF GALLBLADDER

COMMON
Prior cholecystectomy

Calcification of near wall causing nonrecognition

Shrunken gallbladder from recent meal

UNCOMMON
Agenesis of gallbladder

Ectopic gallbladder

Anomalous shape of gallbladder

Gallbladder contracted or empty
  Severe hepatic dysfunction
  Biliary obstruction proximal to cystic duct

Microgallbladder

Shadowing from emphysematous cholecystitis

Sludge in gallbladder causing gallbladder to resemble liver

Situs inversus

Compression by adjacent mass

shadow, one should try a higher frequency transducer because it has a smaller beam width. Care must be taken to position the stone in the central portion of the beam with the focal zone of the transducer at the level of the stone.

Echodensities in the gallbladder that shadow and move with changes in a patient's position have nearly a 100 percent chance of representing gallstones. Structures that move but do not shadow still have a high probability of representing gallstones. Other causes of echoes in the gallbladder are listed in Table 5–17. Sludge balls may form in the gallbladder when the bile is very concentrated. These can occur in a patient who has been fasting, especially in one who has been fasting for a long period of time (Fig. 5–31). It can be very difficult to tell tumefactive sludge from nonshadowing gallstones. Given enough time, sludge will change shape. Therefore,

Table 5–17. ECHOES WITHIN GALLBLADDER

COMMON
Stones
Sludge

UNCOMMON
Gangrenous cholecystitis
Fold in gallbladder
Acute cholecystitis
Hemobilia
Empyema
Stone fragments after extracorporeal shock wave lithotripsy
Polyps, adenomatous or inflammatory
AIDS
Carcinoma
Hemorrhagic cholecystitis
Sarcoma of gallbladder
Metastases
Emphysematous cholecystitis
Mild of calcium
Clonorchiasis
Pus
Papilloma
Epithelial cysts
Ectopic pancreas
Ectopic gastric mucosa
Feces after fistula formation
Food particles after cholecystojejunostomy

one way to distinguish sludge from nonshadowing stones is to simply let the patient remain in one postural position for a period of time (sometimes as long as 15 minutes) and see if the sludge displays an appropriate layering effect. A stone will not change shape, while sludge will.

Children and infants do not often develop cholelithiasis but it does happen occasionally. It can happen when a child has been given a transfusion with resultant hemolysis or has hemolytic anemia or thalassemia. Furosemide and total parenteral nutrition also have been associated with cholelithiasis in children. Other diseases that may lead to gallstones include cystic fibrosis, liver disease, Crohn's disease, and sometimes even sepsis.

It can be difficult to distinguish between the shadow from a gallstone and shadow from bowel gas behind the gallbladder. In the past, it was thought that gallstones could be distinguished from gas because a stone had a clean shadow and bowel gas a dirty shadow. A clean shadow means that the gallstone should have absolutely no echoes behind it. However, it has been well shown that these criteria are not absolute and that there are gas bubbles that can produce a clean shadow. Likewise, gallstones can sometimes produce a dirty shadow, especially if they are small and do not completely block the beam or if there is gas within the gallstone. Changing the patient's position can help make this distinction.

ACUTE CHOLECYSTITIS

Acute cholecystitis is a result of an acutely inflamed gallbladder wall with infiltration of polymorphonuclear leukocytes. These patients usually present with fever, an elevated white count, and right upper quadrant pain.

In about 95 percent of patients with acute cholecystitis a gallstone is obstructing the cystic duct and causes the inflammation. A small percentage of patients will have no stone in the cystic duct and no stones in the gallbladder. These patients are said to have acute acalculous cholecystitis. Acute acalculous cholecystitis usually occurs in patients who have been burned or severely injured or who are severely ill for other reasons.

Ultrasound is about 95 percent accurate

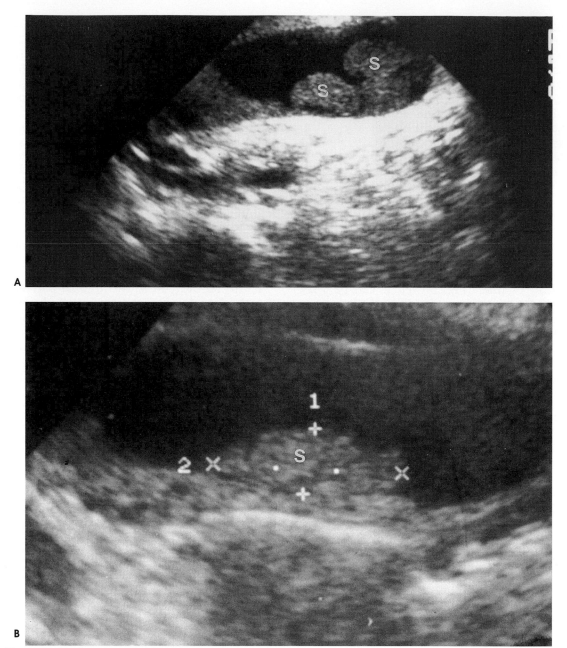

Figure 5–31. *A, B,* Tumefactive sludge (S) simulating a mass. (Courtesy of Dr. Arnold Miller, Shiprock, NM.)

in diagnosing acute cholecystitis. Major criteria for this diagnosis are gallstones and pinpoint tenderness directly over the gallbladder, known as a sonographic Murphy's sign. A sonographic Murphy's sign is elicited by identifying the gallbladder on ultrasound and then pushing with light pressure on the gallbladder. If the patient complains of pain, the transducer is moved 2 to 3 cm away so that the gallbladder is no longer underneath the transducer. Pressure is then once again applied. If the patient no longer has pain, then one may say that a sonographic Murphy's sign is present. Other signs of acute cholecystitis include a hydropic gallbladder or gallbladder dilatation and gallbladder wall thickening. Unfortunately, these findings are less specific.

Ultrasound is about 70 percent sensitive for acute acalculous cholecystitis. Acalculous cholecystitis has signs including an enlarged gallbladder, wall thickening, and focal hypoechoic regions in the wall of the gallbladder. There also may be fluid around the gallbladder. Finally, a sonographic Murphy's sign may be present.

Emphysematous cholecystitis occurs when there are gas-forming organisms in the gallbladder and can be diagnosed when gas is seen in the gallbladder. Stones may be absent but a sonographic Murphy's sign should be present. The presence of gas can be confirmed by either plain films or a CT. This is a surgical emergency. The shadowing structure (i.e., the gas) should move to the most anterior position in the gallbladder with changes in patient position. Emphysematous cholecystitis is more common in diabetic patients and is seen more often in males. Gangrene is a frequent complication of this condition. This ultimately may lead to a gallbladder abscess (Fig. 5–32).

Gangrenous cholecystitis is another entity associated with acute cholecystitis. Asymmetric irregular thickening of the gallbladder wall should be one sign that suggests gangrenous cholecystitis. Intraluminal membranes and fluid around the gallbladder also suggest a gangrenous gallbladder. These patients may not have a sonographic Murphy's sign but are more

likely to have diffuse abdominal pain. A striated gallbladder wall is another sign of gangrene and may presage gallbladder perforation (Fig. 5–33). A striated gallbladder wall may occur for other reasons (Table 5–18), as may fluid around the gallbladder (Table 5–19).

CHRONIC CHOLECYSTITIS

Chronic cholecystitis presents in a less fulminant manner than acute cholecystitis. The symptoms occur over a long period of time, usually as recurrent episodes of right upper quadrant pain that may be associated with meals. In chronic cholecystitis, there is no obstruction of the cystic duct, but instead there is abnormal functioning of the wall of the gallbladder. The gallbladder becomes ineffective at concentrating bile and the mucosal lining becomes damaged. Chronic cholecystitis usually occurs with gallstones.

The ultrasound criteria for chronic cholecystitis include gallstones and wall thickening. The gallbladder may be either contracted or very distended as a result of this disease. One particular form of chronic cholecystitis may be difficult to evaluate sonographically. This is when the gallbladder is not clearly seen in the gallbladder fossa but there are shadows from the gallbladder fossa. This occurs in chronic cholecystitis

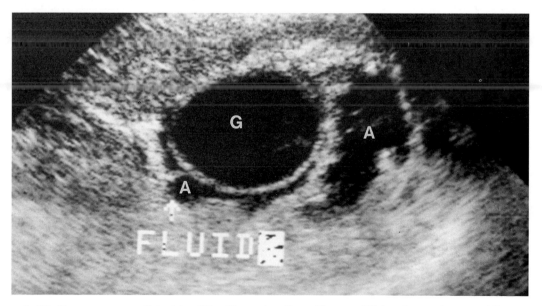

Figure 5–32. Gangrenous gallbladder (G) with perforation. Abscess (A) has formed around the gallbladder.

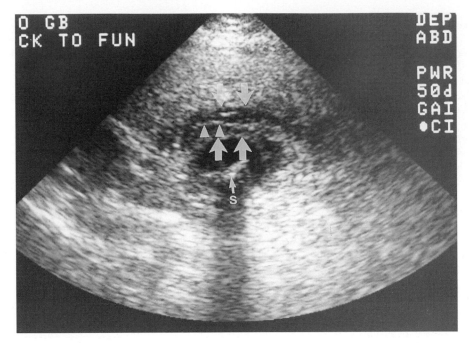

Figure 5–33. Striations in the wall of the gallbladder (*small arrowheads*) in gangrenous cholecystitis. *Large arrows* demarcate gallbladder wall. S = stone.

Table 5–18. STRIATED WALL THICKENING

Gangrenous cholecystitis
Liver disease
Congestive heart failure
Renal failure
Ascites
Low albumin
Pancreatitis
Adenomyomatosis
Blockage of gallbladder lymph or venous drainage

Table 5–19. PERICHOLECYSTIC FLUID

COMMON
Acute cholecystitis with or without perforation
Ascites

UNCOMMON
Associated with pancreatitis
Associated with peptic ulcer disease
Gallbladder torsion
After perforated appendix
Pericholecystic abscess
Hematoma
AIDS

when the gallbladder becomes contracted due to a poorly functioning mucosa. There will be a triad of signs consisting of wall, echo, and shadow (WES) in the absence of a well-defined gallbladder (Fig. 5–34).

ADENOMYOMATOSIS

Adenomyomatosis is a result of hyperplasia and proliferation of the mucosa of the gallbladder with extension of this mucosa into the muscular layer of the gallbladder and formation of Rokitansky-Aschoff sinuses. Adenomyomatosis may be diffuse and involve the entire gallbladder, or it may be focal and involve only small portions of the gallbladder wall. The Rokitansky-Aschoff sinuses may be identified as echolucencies in the wall. Small stones may develop within these echolucencies or diverticula.

Cholesterolosis is a result of a localized abnormality in the metabolism of cholesterol within the wall. It is not associated with hypercholesterolemia. Cholesterol polyps form and, on ultrasound, have an appearance of echogenic foci projecting into the lumen of the gallbladder from the wall (Fig. 5–35). This focus does not move with

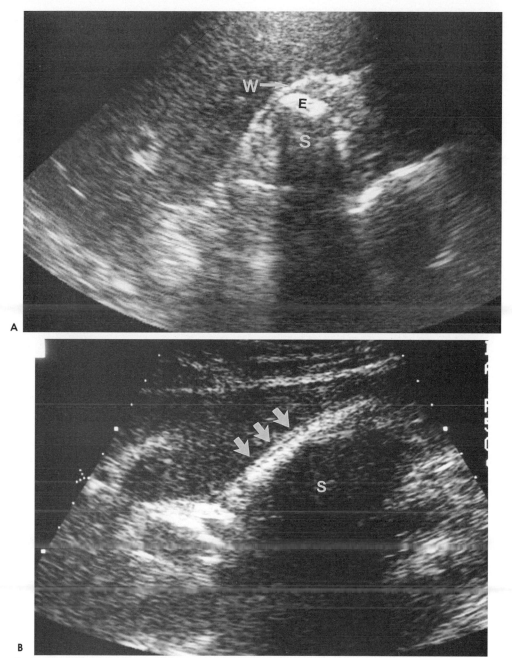

Figure 5–34. *A*, WES sign. W = wall, E = echo, S = shadow. *B*, Chronic cholecystitis with gallbladder filled with stones causing a dense shadow (S).

changes in patient position and does not cause a shadow.

GALLBLADDER CARCINOMA

Gallbladder carcinoma occurs in patients in their 50s and 60s. It is much more common in women. The majority of patients have gallstones. Usually this is an adeno-carcinoma. The gallbladder wall may be calcified on plain films in about one-quarter of the cases. Gallbladder carcinoma may grow into the lumen and form an intralu-minal mass in the gallbladder. The tumor usually extends outward from the gallblad-der to invade the liver and surrounding

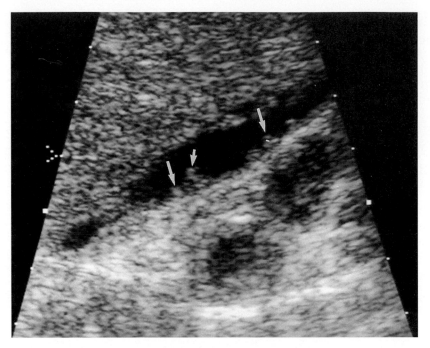

Figure 5–35. Cholesterol polyps (*arrows*).

structures. Occasionally, gallbladder carcinoma may be identified as a localized area of wall thickening. Gallbladder carcinomas usually are not diagnosed early and survival is poor.

Ultrasound may demonstrate an area of localized thickening of the gallbladder wall or a mass projecting either into the lumen (Fig. 5–36) of the gallbladder or outside of the gallbladder fossa. Almost half of these patients will have a large mass entirely replacing the gallbladder.

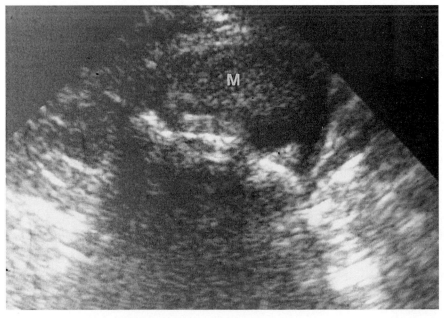

Figure 5–36. Mass in gallbladder (M) from gallbladder carcinoma.

METASTATIC DISEASE

Metastatic disease to the gallbladder may occur from tumors of the lungs, kidneys, or esophagus, and from malignant melanoma. On ultrasound, a gallbladder wall mass or an intraluminal mass may be seen.

DIFFUSE GALLBLADDER WALL THICKENING

This is a nonspecific finding seen in acute and chronic cholecystitis but also commonly seen in many other disease states (Table 5–20). A low serum albumin due to hepatic dysfunction may lead to gallbladder wall thickening. Many seriously ill patients and patients with acquired immunodeficiency syndrome (AIDS) will have this finding (Fig. 5–37).

PEDIATRIC DISEASE

In the neonate, making a distinction between biliary atresia and neonatal hepatitis is important. In biliary atresia, the biliary tract is hypoplastic to the point that there may be no significant extrahepatic ducts or even intrahepatic ducts. The gallbladder may not have developed, although about 20 percent of biliary atresia patients have at least a rudimentary gallbladder. Therefore, the identification of a gallbladder is not sufficient to rule out biliary atresia. Ultrasound is mainly used in these cases to look for other entities that would cause jaundice, such as obstructing masses or choledochal cysts. Nuclear medicine is the study of choice for biliary atresia. If a gallbladder is not seen at ultrasound, that absence is suggestive of biliary atresia but is still not diagnostic since the gallbladder may be small and contracted or bile flow may be so low as to prevent the gallbladder from filling.

Caroli's disease is dilatation of the bile duct system. Either the intrahepatic, the extrahepatic, or both bile duct systems may be dilated, although the intrahepatic system is more commonly involved.

Choledochal cysts may occur in neonates as a result of abnormal development. In children, choledochal cysts may result from reflux into the bile system with resultant damage to the wall of the common duct. With choledochal cysts, the patients often present with jaundice before age 20. At ultrasound, a large cyst will be seen in the porta hepatis. Communication with the common bile duct may be seen.

Acute cholecystitis does not occur often in childhood. The ultrasound signs are similar to those in an adult.

Gallstones in infants and children may be associated with furosemide, total parenteral nutrition, bowel resection, hemolysis, cystic fibrosis, liver disease, Crohn's disease, and sepsis.

Table 5–20. GALLBLADDER WALL THICKENING

COMMON
Gallbladder wall fold
Acute cholecystitis
Chronic cholecystitis
Hepatic dysfunction
Congestive heart failure
Hepatitis
Partial contraction after eating
Tumefacient sludge
Gangrenous cholecystitis
Alcoholic hepatitis
Hypoalbuminemia
Cirrhosis

UNCOMMON
Polyps
Carcinoma of gallbladder
Metastasis
Adenomyomatosis of gallbladder
Renal disease
Sepsis
Ascites
Papillary adenomas
Biliary pus
Biliary clot
Gallbladder torsion
Varices
Chronic renal failure
Acute pyelonephritis
Mononucleosis
Primary sclerosing cholangitis
Hemobilia
AIDS
Hemorrhagic cholecystitis
Xanthogranulomatous cholecystitis

Liver Doppler

Doppler can be used to evaluate the hepatic veins and portal veins. The portal veins are frequently large in patients with portal hypertension, but this is a variable finding and the size of the vein cannot be used as an indicator of direction of flow or portal venous pressure. Doppler can be used to indicate the direction of flow, however (Fig. 5–38A). Collateral vessels, includ-

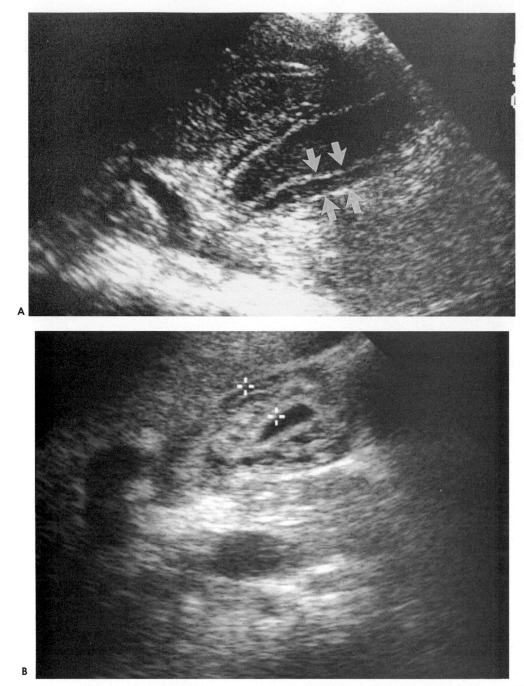

Figure 5–37. *A,* Gallbladder wall thickening (*arrows*) in patient with AIDS. *B,* Gallbladder wall thickening from acute hepatitis. This wall went from normal to this thickness over 1 week.

ing the coronary-gastroesophageal vessels and paraumbilical veins may be identified (Fig. 5–38*B*). In an effort to identify a recanalized umbilical vein or a paraumbilical vein, the left portal vein should be identified and then a search should be made for a

vessel extending from the left portal vein to the abdominal wall via the ligamentum teres. This will run inferiorly along the abdominal wall and terminate at the umbilicus.

Portal venous thrombosis may occur as a result of hepatoma, pancreatic carcinoma,

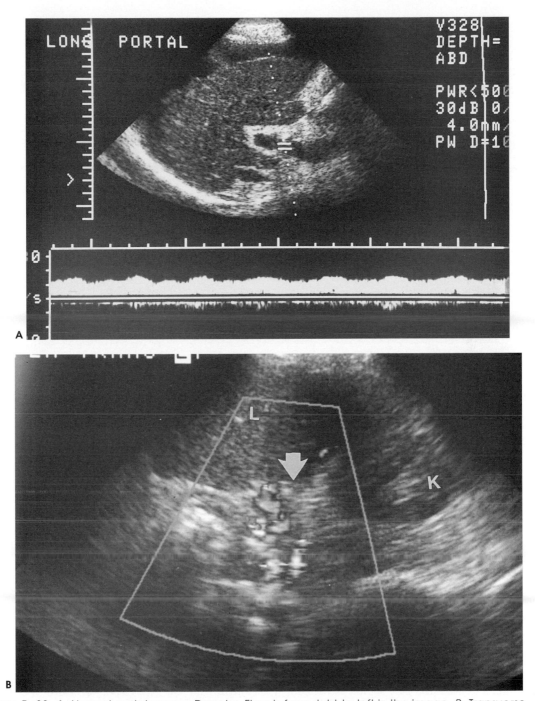

Figure 5–38. *A*, Normal portal venous Doppler. Flow is from right to left in the image. *B*, Transverse image left upper quadrant. L = left lobe of liver, K = left kidney. *Arrow* shows flow (by color Doppler) in collateral vessels around stomach. Patient had portal hypertension.

pancreatitis, cirrhosis, and polycythemia, and this can be diagnosed with color Doppler and pulsed Doppler. In children, portal venous thrombosis may be associated with dehydration, umbilical vein catheterization and sepsis. Thrombus may sometimes be identified within the lumen and it may be hypoechoic to hyperechoic (Fig. 5–39). This also occurs in liver transplants.

Budd-Chiari syndrome, or hepatic veno-

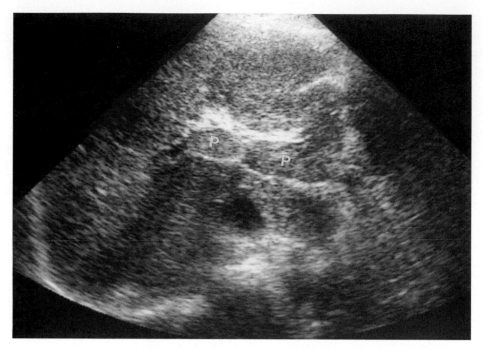

Figure 5–39. Clot in portal vein (P).

occlusive disease, may involve the major hepatic veins or the inferior vena cava. This may be a result of congenital webs but can also be acquired secondary to tumor masses or clotting abnormalities. Patients who have had chemotherapy prior to bone marrow transplants are especially at risk. Patients with liver transplants are also at risk.

On color Doppler, the veins will normally be identifiable. With Budd-Chiari, they may be seen to be lacking in flow and filled with echogenic thrombus. Extrahepatic collaterals may be seen and the intrahepatic vena cava may be narrowed. The hepatic veins may have a smaller caliber than usual but this can be secondary to enlargement and edema of the liver from diseases other than Budd-Chiari syndrome, such as hepatitis. After an acute thrombosis of the hepatic veins, intrahepatic venous collaterals may open. These serpiginous vessels may be seen but their direction will not be toward the inferior vena cava when their course is followed. Flow in the portal vein may be reversed.

Liver and Biliary Tree in AIDS

In AIDS, the liver is enlarged in about 40 percent and is echogenic in about 45 per-cent of patients. A smaller percentage have a hypoechoic liver. This increased echogenicity may be the result of fatty infiltration due to a poor nutritional status or treatment with drugs. Hepatitis may lead to a fatty liver and may coexist with AIDS. Hyperechoic periportal bands have also been reported and may be the result of tumor infiltration. Kaposi's sarcoma may appear as small echogenic masses, although these may sometimes be echo poor. Similarly, AIDS-related lymphoma may cause either hyper- or hypoechoic masses. AIDS masses from lymphoma are often focal as opposed to lymphoma masses non-AIDS patients, which they more often infiltrate. Punctate highly reflective foci without shadows may be due to *pneumocystis carinii*, cytomegalovirus, fungi, or *Mycobacterium avium-intracellulare*. Hypoechoic masses may be due to lymphoma or Kaposi's sarcoma as mentioned above as well as pyogenic or mycobacteria abscesses.

Biliary tract diseases include acalculous cholecystitis, papillary stenosis, and a type of cholangitis resembling sclerosing cholangitis. Thickening of the gallbladder wall and dilatation of the gallbladder are common. Both intra- and extrahepatic ductal dilatation are also common.

Lymphadenopathy in the upper abdomen is a frequent finding. Kaposi's sarcoma may cause lymphadenopathy. Lymphoma may cause hypoechoic masses in the spleen and kidney.

Spleen

EXAMINING THE SPLEEN

The spleen is usually scanned in both the longitudinal and transverse planes and is usually visualized via a posterolateral intercostal approach with the patient in the supine position. Normally, the spleen should be homogeneous and either equal to or slightly less echogenic than the liver.

Splenic size has been evaluated using various methods. All of these depend on some combination of height, width, and thickness to estimate splenic volume. We determine the length and, if it is more than about 13 cm, try to estimate splenic volume qualitatively. We have found it difficult to use any of the several indices suggested for determining if the spleen is enlarged. The spleen is an irregular organ and it is difficult to consistently decide on an axis in which to make a measurement or several measurements. There is a long differential diagnosis for splenomegaly, which is given in Table 5–21.

NEOPLASTIC DISEASE OF THE SPLEEN

The most common spleen neoplasm is a hemangioma. Many of these are isoechoic with the spleen and are not identifiable, and they may have calcifications. These lesions may range from echogenic, and an appearance similar to that seen in liver hemangiomas, to echo poor or complex. Large fluid-filled cystic spaces will lead to a relatively hypoechoic to complex pattern. Color flow Doppler may help to determine that the cystic spaces contain blood.

Lymphangiomas may have an ultrasound appearance of multiple cystic spaces replacing much of the spleen. Splenic hamartomas can also occur in the spleen and may range from hypoechoic to hyperechoic to complex cystic.

The spleen may be involved in either non-Hodgkin's or Hodgkin's disease. The involvement may take the form of either focal lesions or diffuse splenic involvement without evidence of a focal tumor. Focal le-

Table 5–21. ENLARGED SPLEEN

COMMON
Lymphoma
Portal hypertension
Mononucleosis
Leukemia
Hodgkin's disease

UNCOMMON
Herpes simplex viremia
Epstein-Barr virus
Cytomegalic virus
AIDS
Metastases
Gaucher's disease
Acute splenic sequestration crisis
Splenic abscess
Multiple myeloma
Wilson's disease
Myelofibrosis
Malaria
Reticulum cell sarcoma
Kala-azar
Still's disease
Glycogen storage disease
Hereditary spherocytosis
Hepatitis
Hemangioma/hemangiosarcoma
Septicemia
Sickle cell disease
Brucellosis
Hemolysis
Typhoid
Tuberculosis
Typhus
Sarcoid
Amyloid
Rheumatoid arthritis
Lupus
Wolman's disease
Syphilis
Lymphangioma
Subacute bacterial endocarditis
Rupture or fracture in trauma
Echinococcosis
Extramedullary hematopoiesis
Hepatic venous occlusion
Passive congestion of congestive heart failure
Q fever
Rocky Mountain spotted fever
Tularemia
Cat-scratch fever
Candidiasis
Histoplasmosis
Coccidioidomycosis
Cysticercosis
Schistosomiasis
Leishmaniasis
Toxoplasmosis

sions are usually hypoechoic in comparison to the surrounding spleen. A diffusely involved spleen may be more hypoechoic than expected when compared to the adjacent liver. In comparison to the pathologic examination of the spleen in patients with lymphoma and Hodgkin's disease, ultrasound is not especially sensitive.

Splenic metastases most often come from breast, lung, ovary, stomach and melanoma. These are usually hypoechoic focal lesions.

SPLENIC INFECTION

Calcifications in the spleen occur commonly secondary to prior infection by granulomatous diseases such as tuberculosis or histoplasmosis (Table 5–22).

Splenic abscesses usually occur due to hematogenous spread. Whenever a splenic abscess is encountered, then a bacterial endocarditis must be one of the first considerations. Abscesses may also come from trauma. Direct extension from adjacent organs such as the kidney or stomach may also occur. The ultrasound pattern is that of a complex, irregular hypoechoic lesion in the spleen. Gas may be seen within the abscess and there may be hyperechoic foci.

Fungal abscesses usually have a similar pattern, although a wheel-within-a-wheel appearance has been described for *Candida*. This wheel-within-a-wheel pattern consists of a fibrotic rim with pus and necrotic debris in the center. Echinococcosis may form hypoechoic to anechoic lesions in the spleen. These are predominantly cystic.

In AIDS, hyperechoic foci may be identified. It is not clear as to the etiology of

these foci, but *Pneumocystis carinii* is a prime consideration, although *Mycobacterium avium-intracellulare* is a possibility. Ultrasound seems to be more sensitive than CT for these lesions. Finally, cytomegalovirus is reported as causing a similar pattern. Therefore, if hyperechoic foci are seen in the spleen, infection secondary to AIDS should be considered. Splenomegaly is a very common manifestation of AIDS. AIDS-related lymphoma may lead to hypoechoic splenic masses.

Other causes of focal splenic abnormalities are listed in Table 5–23.

Table 5–22. CALCIFICATIONS IN SPLEEN

COMMON
Tuberculosis
Histoplasmosis
Splenic artery atherosclerosis
Posttraumatic cyst

UNCOMMON
Hydatid cyst
Phleboliths in hemangioma
Brucellosis
Sickle cell disease
Thorotrast
Infarct, healed
Healed abscess

Table 5–23. FOCAL ABNORMALITIES OF THE SPLEEN

COMMON
Abscess
Prior granulomatous disease
Cysts
Metastases
Infarct
Hematoma
Infarction

UNCOMMON
Candida or other fungus
Lymphoma
Hemangioma
Tuberculosis
Cat-scratch fever
Left lobe of liver mimicking fluid collection
Hydatid disease
Extramedullary hematopoiesis
Gaucher's disease
Splenic sequestration crisis

Table 5–24. CYSTS IN SPLEEN

COMMON
Congenital
Posttraumatic cyst

UNCOMMON
Parasitic
Neoplastic
Lymphangiomas
Cavernous hemangiomas
Abscess
Hematoma
Capillary hemangioma
Epidermoid cyst
Hamartoma
Rupture with fissure
Hydatid disease
Splenic sequestration crisis

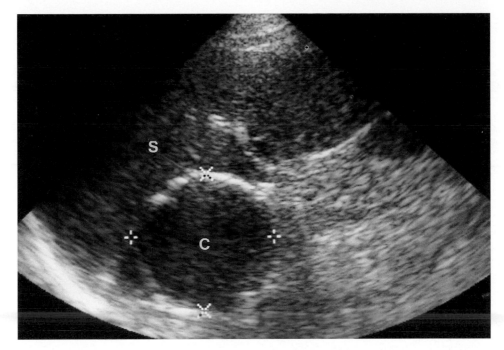

Figure 5–40. Long image of spleen (S) showing cyst (C) with calcified wall. This is posttraumatic.

Table 5–25. BOWEL WALL THICKENING

COMMON
Carcinoma
Intussusception
Lymphoma
Hematoma
Inflammatory disease
Crohn's disease
Ulcerative colitis
Low albumin state

UNCOMMON
Leiomyosarcoma
Typhoid
Schönlein-Henoch purpura
Diverticulitis
Whipple's disease
Pseudomembranous colitis
Duodenal ulcer
Amebic colitis
Campylobacter jejuni enteritis
Adenoma
Postradiation
Ischemia
Pancreatitis
Strongyloidiasis
Lymphangioma
Adjacent abscess
Amyloidosis
Giardia
Behçet's syndrome
Ameba
Tuberculosis
Metastases
Carcinoid tumors
Polyposis syndrome

CYSTS

Echinococcal cysts have already been mentioned. They are indistinguishable from the other types of cysts that occur in the spleen (Table 5–24). Other cysts of the spleen include epithelial-lined cysts, which are thought to be congenital, and nonepithelial-lined cysts, which are thought to be posttraumatic in nature. Posttraumatic cysts may calcify (Fig. 5–40). Occasionally, a pancreatic pseudocyst may interpose itself into the spleen and simulate a splenic cyst.

SPLENIC TRAUMA

Ultrasound is not usually the test of choice for evaluating suspected traumatic injury to the spleen. However, hypoechoic areas within the spleen or peripheral lucencies consistent with fluid may be seen after splenic rupture. Fractures of the spleen may also be seen as hypoechoic linear areas. Blood from splenic trauma can vary in appearance, ranging from hyperechoic to hypoechoic, with the echogenicity decreasing as time goes by.

SPLENIC INFARCTION

Splenic infarction may occur secondary either to emboli or to thrombosis. It is more

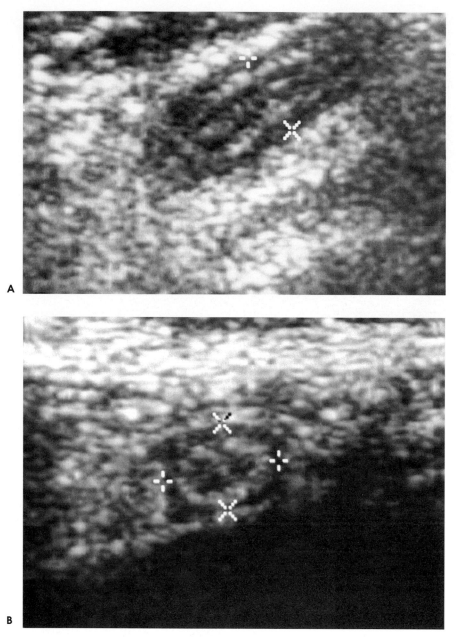

Figure 5–41. *A,* Longitudinal image of appendix. Crosshairs measure the appendix at 10 mm. The appendix could not be compressed. Appendicitis. *B,* Transverse image of same enlarged, noncompressible appendix.

likely to occur in patients who have inflammatory processes such as pancreatitis in adjacent organs. Sickle cell patients also are prone to develop splenic infarction. If a smooth-bordered, wedge-shaped, hypoechoic to anechoic area is seen, then an infarction should be suspected. However, some infarctions may be spherical and focal and can simulate previously mentioned types of lesions. Abscess is in the differential diagnosis when this appearance is seen.

In a splenic sequestration crisis in sickle cell patients, the spleen becomes enlarged suddenly.

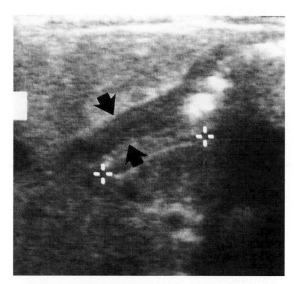

Figure 5–42. Hypertrophic pyloric stenosis. *Arrows* show preferred measurement of one wall. In this case it was greater than 4 mm, indicating pyloric stenosis. The crosshairs are measuring the pyloric length, but this is a less reliable measurement.

ACCESSORY SPLEENS AND SPLENOSIS

Accessory spleens consist of congenital splenic tissue located outside of the spleen itself. Splenosis is a result of seeding of splenic tissue on the surfaces of other organs secondary to trauma. In our experience, evaluation of accessory spleens and splenosis is best accomplished with other imaging modalities. Technetium-99m sulfur colloid or technetium-labeled, heat-denatured red cells are useful, as well as CT.

Stomach, Bowel, and Appendix

Abnormally dilated loops of bowel are a common incidental finding. If mechanical obstruction is present, the waves of peristalsis may be visible, although this is not the only cause of a hyperactive bowel. Normal bowel wall is less than 4 mm thick. If the wall is thickened, then any number of diagnoses may be considered (Table 5–25).

Ultrasound of the appendix is an accurate way to diagnose appendicitis. A noncompressible, sausage-shaped, blind-ending pouch is the diagnostic finding. On a transverse view of the appendix, the entire organ should be no more than 6 mm thick and the wall should be no more than 3 mm thick (Fig. 5–41). When this organ is identified, pressure is applied via the transducer (we use a linear 5 MHz). If the lumen can be obliterated by pressure, then the appendix is normal. In appendicitis, the walls are inflamed and rigid and cannot be compressed. Identification of an appendicolith is also suggestive of appendicitis. We scan in three planes: sagittal, transverse, and oblique (oriented perpendicular to the iliac vessels). We identify the cecum, iliac vessels, iliacus and psoas muscles, and iliac bone as normal structures. Overall accuracy is about 90 percent. We frequently cannot identify a normal appendix. We consider this inability to see the appendix as diagnostic of a normal organ. A retrocecal appendix may be difficult to see even if it is enlarged and inflamed by appendicitis.

Hypertrophic pyloric stenosis (HPS) occurs in the first few months of life, usually in male infants. Using ultrasound, the pylorus may be found anterior to the pancreas. The stomach is often filled with fluid because of the obstructing pylorus. The thickness of the entire pylorus will be greater than or equal to 13 mm, the thickness of one wall will be 4 mm or greater, and the entire pyloric channel will be 17 mm or longer in HPS (Fig. 5–42). We consider the single wall measurement of 4 mm or greater to be the most accurate reliable indication of this condition (mnemonic – 4 mm + 13 mm = 17 mm).

Suggested Readings

Goldberg BB. Textbook of Abdominal Ultrasound. Baltimore, Williams & Wilkins, 1993.
Mittelstaedt CA. General Ultrasound. New York, Churchill Livingstone, 1992.
Seminars in Ultrasound, CT, and MR. Vol 5, no. 4, 1984.

CHAPTER 6

Renal Ultrasound

Technique

The kidneys are usually scanned using a 3.5-MHz transducer. In some thin patients, it may be possible to use a 5.0-MHz transducer. It is preferable to have the patient in a fasting state, but it is not absolutely necessary.

The right kidney can often be imaged from an anterior subcostal approach. If this is unsuccessful, then an approach from the right flank with a coronal imaging plane is almost always successful. In a few patients, these two techniques may not work, and then it may be useful to have the patient stand, causing the kidney to move to a more inferior location. Other methods include having the patient go into a left decubitus position with the right side up and attempt to image the kidney coronally. Finally, the pillow can be removed from under the patient's head and placed under the patient's left flank with the patient still in a decubitus position. This has the effect of forcing the right flank into a convex shape and opening up the rib interspaces. The left kidney may be imaged in a similar fashion. The left kidney is usually harder to see, and at times may be impossible to see in spite of trying the above techniques. We usually have the most success with the patient in a right decubitus position with the left side up while scanning in a coronal plane. Both kidneys are usually situated so that the upper pole is more posterior and medial than the lower pole. At least three to six longitudinal images should be obtained in an attempt to cover all portions of the kidney. After the longitudinal images have been obtained (either coronally or sagittally), then three to six transverse images should be obtained.

Anatomy

The kidneys are usually situated so that the lower pole is more anterior and lateral than the upper pole. Therefore, care should be taken to obtain the longest possible axis. We consider kidneys between 9 cm and 13 cm on ultrasound to be within normal limits. We expect to see smaller kidneys in smaller patients. Older patients also tend to have smaller kidneys. The peripheral portion of the kidney or cortex is usually less echogenic than adjacent normal liver in adults (Fig. 6–1). Neonatal and infant kidneys have a renal cortex that is more echogenic and approximately equal to liver and spleen. The medullary pyramids are seen inside the cortex. They are hypoechoic and can be very prominent in neonates and infants (Fig. 6–2).

Some diseases increase cortical echogenicity but spare the medullary pyramids, and this also makes the medullary pyramids appear very hypoechoic in comparison to the cortex (Tables 6–1 and 6–2). Other diseases increase the echogenicity of the medulla or decrease the echogenicity of the cortex (Tables 6–3 and 6–4). The central portion of the kidney is very echogenic and consists of renal sinus fat. In infants there is less renal sinus fat and this area is less echogenic. It is difficult to judge the thickness of renal parenchyma because the amount of renal sinus fat varies. Patients with a large amount of renal sinus fat appear to have a decrease in cortical thickness that may not be real. In judging whether or not atrophy is present, the thickness of parenchyma external to the medullary pyramids should be estimated. Usually, the contour of the normal kidney is smooth, although fetal lobulation can be a normal finding. Fetal lobulation appears as undulations along the outer margin of

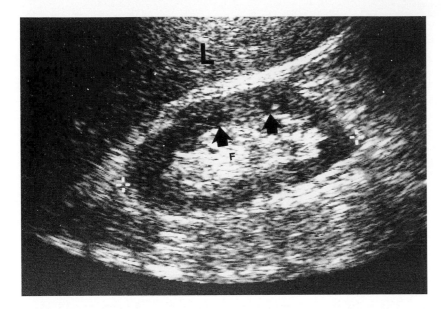

Figure 6–1. Normal kidney. Cortex is hypoechoic compared to liver (L). Medullary pyramids are faintly visible (arrows). Renal sinus fat (F) is echogenic.

the kidney and can sometimes be differentiated from scarring or focal cortical thinning by the fact that lobulation should extend around the entire periphery of the kidney. The renal pelvis and calices are usually not identified in the normal examination. Normal patients may have mild separation of the walls of the renal pelvis. A measurement of up to 5 mm of renal pelvis wall separation is normal. Obviously, if any calices are dilated, hydronephrosis is probably present. Some believe that the walls of the renal pelvis should be apposed and that any separation of the walls is indicative of hydronephrosis. However, the use of these criteria will frequently result in a false diagnosis of hydronephrosis.

If color Doppler is used to identify renal vessels, then the renal veins will lie anterior to the renal arteries. The left renal vein can usually be identified by finding the take-off of the superior mesenteric artery in a transverse imaging plane and then looking just caudal and posterior to that structure. The right renal vein will usually come into the inferior vena cava at a similar level as the left renal vein. The arteries are more difficult to identify, and over 20 percent of pa-

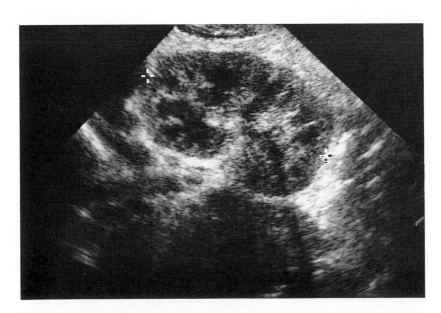

Figure 6–2. Normal neonatal kidney. Cortex is echogenic, medullary pyramids are prominent.

Table 6-1. INCREASED CORTICAL ECHOGENICITY COMPARED TO MEDULLA

COMMON	COMMENT
Acute glomerulonephritis	
Chronic glomerulonephritis	
Nephrosclerosis	
Diabetic nephropathy	
Acute tubular necrosis	
Transplant rejection	
UNCOMMON	
Lupus erythematosus	
Alport's syndrome	
Papillary necrosis	
Preeclampsia	
Amyloidosis	
Nephrocalcinosis	
Renal vein thrombosis	
AIDS	
Acute cortical necrosis	Calcified, echogenic cortex
Leukemic infiltration	Bilateral
Beckwith-Wiedemann syndrome	
Hypercalcemia	
Oxalosis	

tients will have multiple renal arteries. Technical difficulties in identifying the renal arteries and the presence of multiple renal arteries have inhibited the use of ultrasound and Doppler for evaluating renal artery stenosis and other diseases of these vessels.

Normal variations in the kidney anatomy include a dromedary hump. This is a bulge from the lateral contour of the left kidney, hypothesized to be a result of pressure from the adjacent spleen. A junctional defect is a small indentation in the cortex of the right kidney at the junction between the upper third and the lower two-thirds (Fig. 6-3). This can sometimes occur on the left kidney. This is an embryologic remnant.

A column of Bertin may create the appearance of a mass. This is cortical tissue extending between the medullary pyramids (Fig. 6-4) and is sometimes called a renal pseudotumor. These usually occur in the middle portion of the kidney and usually indent the renal sinus. A pseudotumor should have echogenicity identical to that of the adjacent renal cortex. If the echogenicity is different, then a renal cell carcinoma or other type of renal tumor must be considered. If there is doubt, then computed tomography (CT) with intravenous contrast may be useful to determine if it is a renal neoplasm or a column of Bertin. A column of Bertin will enhance similar to the remainder of the cortex. A duplicated collecting system may be manifested by a longer

Table 6-2. INCREASED ECHOGENICITY—NO DISTINCTION BETWEEN CORTEX AND MEDULLA

COMMON	COMMENTS
Chronic pyelonephritis	
Chronic glomerulonephritis	
UNCOMMON	
Focal acute bacterial nephritis	
Acquired immunodeficiency syndrome (AIDS)	Usually in drug users
Healing infarct	
Infantile polycystic kidney disease	
Renal tubular ectasis	
Adult polycystic kidney disease	
Medullary cystic disease	
Acquired cystic disease of dialysis	

Table 6–3. ECHOGENIC MEDULLA

Tamm-Horsefall proteinuria
Sepsis
Dehydration
Candida
Renal tubular necrosis
Williams syndrome
Gout
Sjögren's syndrome
Medullary sponge kidney
Primary aldosteronism
Lesch-Nyhan syndrome
Glycogen storage disease type I
Wilson's disease
Pseudo-Bartter's syndrome
Hypokalemia
Medullary nephrocalcinosis
   Hyperparathyroidism
   Chronic pyelonephritis
   Chronic glomerulonephritis
   Distal renal tubular acidosis
   Milk-alkali syndrome
   Malignancy with bone involvement
   Hypervitaminosis D
   Primary hypercalcemia
   Sarcoidosis
   Renal tubular acidosis
   Medullary sponge kidney
   Medullary cystic disease

Table 6–4. DECREASED CORTICAL ECHOGENICITY

Acute pyelonephritis
Renal vein thrombosis
Transplant rejection
Lupus nephritis
Multicentric renal cell carcinoma
Lymphoma of kidneys

than usual kidney, with the renal sinus fat being separated into two discrete clumps. This does not mean that there is a complete duplication of the renal collecting system, but may simply indicate a partial duplication.

RETROPERITONEAL ANATOMY

The kidneys lie in the retroperitoneum. The retroperitoneum is divided into three spaces. The anterior pararenal space includes the pancreas, the ascending and descending colon, and the retroperitoneal portion of the duodenum (Fig. 6–5). The perirenal space includes the kidneys and adrenal glands. The posterior pararenal space lies behind the kidneys and contains only fat. The psoas muscle and quadratus lumborum muscle are contained within their own fascia and do not lie within the posterior pararenal space. The fascial planes that surround the kidneys are sometimes called Gerota's fascia, although others use the name Zuckerkandl's fascia for the layer that surrounds the kidney posteriorly and separates the kidney from the posterior pararenal space. The anterior pararenal and posterior pararenal spaces have potential communication inferiorly because the leaves of Gerota's fascia and Zuckerkandl's fascia are only loosely apposed inferiorly in the region of the iliac crest. Therefore, there is always a potential for infectious processes to communicate between these two spaces.

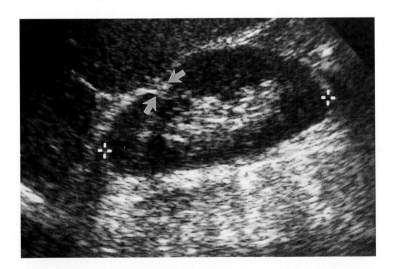

Figure 6–3. Junctional defect (*arrows*). This is not a scar but a site of fusion of upper and lower anlages during development. It is common in children.

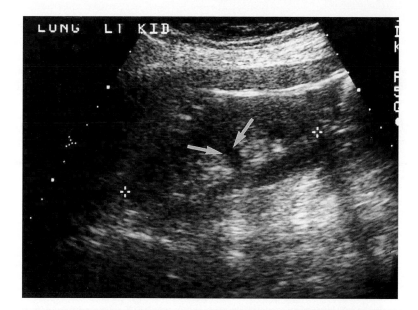

Figure 6–4. Column of Bertin. This is cortical tissue extending between medullary pyramids into the renal sinus fat (*arrows*).

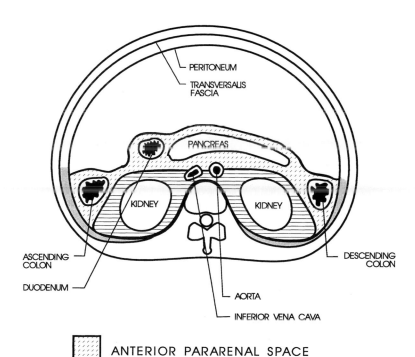

Figure 6–5. Three compartments of retroperitoneum. (Adapted from Meyers MA. Dynamic Radiology of the Abdomen, 4th ed. New York, Springer-Verlag, 1994, with permission.)

PERITONEUM
TRANSVERSALIS FASCIA
PANCREAS
KIDNEY
KIDNEY
ASCENDING COLON
DESCENDING COLON
DUODENUM
AORTA
INFERIOR VENA CAVA

ANTERIOR PARARENAL SPACE
PERIRENAL SPACE
POSTERIOR PARARENAL SPACE

Cystic Disease of the Kidney

RENAL CYSTIC DISEASE

Simple renal cysts occur in approximately 50 percent of people over age 50. Younger patients may also have simple renal cysts. A simple renal cyst has little significance. The ultrasound criteria for simple renal cysts include the following:

1. increased through transmission,
2. no internal echoes,
3. imperceptible walls,
4. round or spherical shape, and
5. a well-defined far wall.

A cyst that meets these criteria needs no further evaluation. If a cyst does not meet these criteria, then it is possibly a complex cyst or a solid mass, and further work-up is indicated. Aspiration may be necessary to

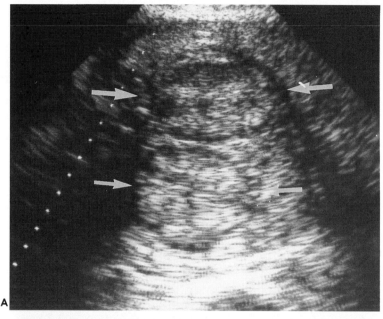

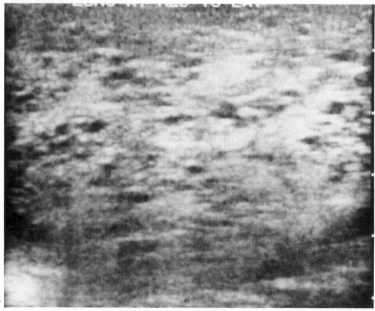

Figure 6–6. *A,* Echogenic kidneys of infantile polycystic kidney disease (IPKD). Coronal images of kidneys are outlined by arrows. *B,* Magnified image of kidney in IPKD. Note the cysts that are actually ectatic tubules. *Illustration continued on opposite page*

make certain that no carcinoma is present. Sometimes, complex cysts are followed with ultrasound examinations every 3 to 6 months. Alternatively, CT scanning with and without intravenous contrast can be useful in an effort to determine whether or not a neoplasm is present.

A hyperdense cyst may be visible on a CT scan. The differential diagnosis is a hyperdense renal cell carcinoma versus a hemorrhagic cyst. Ultrasound can help solve this dilemma. A hemorrhagic renal cyst should still be predominately cystic on ultrasound, in spite of the presence of blood in the cyst fluid although some internal echoes may be seen. If ultrasound indicates that the mass is probably solid, then it should be presumed to be a hyperdense renal cell carcinoma. In general, renal cysts arise from cortical tissue.

Other cystic structures seen in the kidney may include caliceal diverticula or a parapelvic cyst. Cysts can also be confused with hydronephrosis when multiple dilated calices are present. Differentiation between multiple cysts and hydronephrosis is made by determining whether or not the cystic structures communicate with the renal pelvis. Communication with the renal pelvis indicates that the cystic structures are actually dilated calices and the diagnosis is hydronephrosis. Parapelvic cysts are seen in the vicinity of the renal hilum. They do not communicate with the collecting system and they do not arise from cortical tissue. It is thought that they are of lymphatic origin.

ADULT POLYCYSTIC KIDNEY DISEASE

Adult polycystic kidney disease (APKD) is an autosomal dominant disease, most often seen in adults. It may occasionally be seen in children or even neonates. Usually, both kidneys are enlarged and contain multiple cysts. About one-third of patients will have cysts in the liver. Cerebral aneurysms are present in about one-fifth of patients. Most patients, but not all, will have a history of cyst disease in the family. It is not always possible to differentiate multiple simple cysts associated with old age from adult polycystic kidney disease. The cysts will sometimes contain echogenic debris from previous hemorrhage. These patients classically present with bilaterally enlarged kidneys, abdominal pain, and hematuria. However, that classic presentation is seen in a minority of patients.

AUTOSOMAL RECESSIVE POLYCYSTIC KIDNEY DISEASE

This condition almost always involves both kidneys. There are four subcategories based on the age at presentation: perinatal, neonatal, infantile, and juvenile. The younger the age at presentation, the less the life expectancy. Those in whom the disease presents between the ages of 1 and 5 years (juvenile) may survive up to age 50 or beyond. The less severe the renal involvement, the more severe the hepatic fibrosis and hepatosplenomegaly.

The sonographic appearance includes bilateral symmetrically enlarged echogenic kidneys and loss of cortical medullary distinction (Fig. 6–6). The renal border is irregular and indistinct. In a minority of patients, the cortex demonstrates normal echogenicity and an abnormally echogenic medulla. The cysts, which represent ectatic tubules, cannot be visualized in most patients, but occasionally a patient will have identifiable cysts surrounded by a thin rim

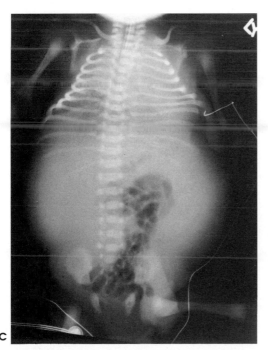

Figure 6–6. *Continued. C,* Radiograph showing hypoplastic thorax due to IPKD.

of cortex. The increased echogenicity is caused by the numerous tiny cysts that create a multitude of reflective interfaces.

MULTICYSTIC DYSPLASTIC KIDNEY

In multicystic dysplastic kidney (MCDK) disease, renal cysts form from dilated collecting tubules. This is usually unilateral, but in 40 percent of cases, there is an abnormality of the other kidney. MCDK may be the result of atresia of the ureteral bud during embryogenesis. Sonographically, these patients present at an early age. There is an abdominal mass that resembles a cluster of grapes on ultrasound (Fig. 6–7). The minority of kidneys in patients with MCDK are small or normal in size. The abdominal mass may ultimately regress and even disappear. The diagnosis is most often made in childhood, but is sometimes made in adults.

MEDULLARY CYSTIC DISEASE

Patients with medullary cystic disease present as juveniles or young adults with anemia, salt wasting, and, ultimately, renal failure. Multiple small cysts will be present in the medullary portion of both kidneys; however, these cysts frequently cannot be detected by ultrasound. There will be increased medullary echogenicity causing the medullary pyramids to have the same echogenicity as the adjacent renal sinus fat. This may cause the kidney to look like it

has a very broad and extensive area of renal sinus fat. Small cysts can be visualized sometimes. The cysts can be as large as 1 cm. The kidneys are usually normal or slightly decreased in size. Ultimately, the entire kidney becomes echogenic when failure is advanced.

MEDULLARY SPONGE KIDNEY

A medullary sponge kidney is of limited clinical significance. On intravenous urography, ectatic collecting tubules may sometimes be seen. Stones can form in these collecting tubules and calcium may be deposited in the interstitium of the medulla. At ultrasound the medullary pyramids can become very echogenic but the tubules cannot be visualized.

ACQUIRED CYSTIC KIDNEY DISEASE OF DIALYSIS

Patients undergoing either hemodialysis or peritoneal dialysis may develop cysts of varying size in their native kidneys. The cortex of these kidneys is usually quite echogenic. Some nephrologists recommend periodic screening of native kidneys in patients on dialysis because of an increased incidence of adenomas or renal cell carcinomas. If a complex cyst is seen during such screening, CT should be done to determine if there is a solid component to the mass and to determine if any part of

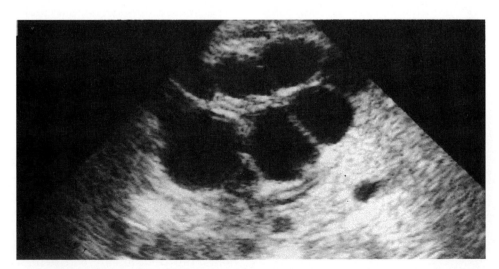

Figure 6–7. Multiple cysts of multicystic dysplastic kidney in a newborn.

the complex cyst resembles a renal cell carcinoma.

OTHER CYSTS

The differential diagnosis for cystic masses is listed in Table 6–5. Cysts may be associated with chromosomal trisomies and may also be seen with tuberous sclerosis. Zellweger's syndrome and Turner's syndrome also are associated with small cortical cysts. Congenital megacalices may simulate cysts. These are calices that are dilated but not obstructed, probably as a result of poorly developed renal pyramids.

Inflammatory Disease of the Kidney

PYELONEPHRITIS

Acute bacterial pyelonephritis occurs when bacteria ascend from the bladder. It may be secondary to reflux. *Escherichia coli* is the most common organism and females are more commonly affected than males. The kidneys of most patients with acute pyelonephritis are normal in appearance sonographically. In a minority of patients, the kidney may be enlarged. There may be diffuse or focal areas of decreased echogenicity. Segmental areas of decreased echogenicity secondary to pyelonephritis have been called lobar nephronia, or focal bacterial nephritis. Occasionally, increased echogenicity is seen in the infected area. A helpful sign in pyelonephritis is the failure of the inflamed kidney to slide on the psoas muscle when the patient breathes (Fig. 6–8).

Liquefaction of the infected area can lead to a renal abscess. Abscesses tend to have an appearance more suggestive of a fluid collection (i.e., they show through transmission). Patients with decreased immunity, such as diabetics, may develop emphysematous pyelonephritis. This is a fulminant process leading to destruction of the kidney. Nephrectomy is usually the treatment of choice. Mortality can be high without nephrectomy. Shadowing echogenic foci, caused by gas, are sometimes seen in the renal sinus or in the renal parenchymal. It is important to be aware that reverberation artifact may be associated with the gas and to not mistake the gas bubbles for stones.

Pyonephrosis indicates pus in the collecting system. This occurs in an obstructed kidney that becomes secondarily infected. This condition requires either percutaneous or surgical drainage. The ultrasound findings show echogenic debris or a fluid-debris level in a hydronephrotic kidney.

Fungal abscesses usually occur in immunocompromised patients, especially diabetics. A fungal abscess is usually secondary to *Candida*. The ultrasound appearance is identical to that of bacterial renal abscess. Occasionally, a spherical echogenic structure representing a fungus ball may be seen in a dilated collecting system. Differential diagnoses are given in Table 6–6.

Xanthogranulomatous pyelonephritis (XPG) almost always occurs in patients who have renal stones, either partially or totally obstructing the renal collecting system. The ultrasound appearance of XPG is that of a complex mass with renal stones. The diffuse type results in renal enlargement and multiple hypoechoic areas. The tumefactive type may simulate a tumor. The tumefactive type is a focal process involving only a portion of the kidney and on ultrasound presents as a complex mass with an associated stone. This condition is thought to result from chronic infection in the face of obstruction by a calculus. It may

Table 6–5. CYSTIC MASSES

COMMON
Simple cysts
Focal hydronephrosis
Abscesses
Hematomas
Peripelvic cysts

UNCOMMON
Adenocarcinoma
Urinoma
Vascular malformations
Focal pyelonephritis
Xanthogranulomata
Renal artery aneurysm
Calyceal diverticula
Cysts with mural tumor
Renal pyramids
Adult polycystic kidney disease
Multicystic dysplastic kidney
Postdialysis cysts
Angiomyolipoma
Urinoma
Renal artery psuedoaneurysm
Lymphangioma
Metastases
Multilocular cystic nephroma

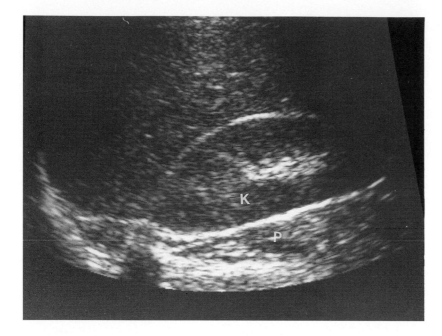

Figure 6–8. Coronal image of kidney (K). Psoas muscle = P. When patient breathes, the kidney should slide freely on the psoas. In pyelonephritis, the kidney and psoas may move together as though they are adherent.

also be a result of inadequate antibiotic treatment. This condition is more common in diabetics and females. In the diffuse type, the parenchyma is replaced by multiple hypoechoic masses in the cortical medullary area. These appear as fluid-filled at ultrasound and may have debris within them. The kidney is generally enlarged.

Chronic pyelonephritis, or reflux nephritis, is thought to be a result of chronic reflux with progressive destruction of the interstitium of the kidney. Infection is probably a part of this chronic reflux. These processes scar the kidney. There is usually an increase in echogenicity, irregularity and thinning of the cortex secondary to the scar, and a decrease in kidney size.

Renal tuberculosis is usually a blood-borne disease. However, most patients with renal tuberculosis do not have either active pulmonary tuberculosis or an abnormal chest radiograph. This process usually involves both kidneys. There is frequently diffuse disease with destruction of both kidneys and calcification. Multiple focal lesions are identified, which are usually hypoechoic but may be hyperechoic or complex. The kidney may also show hydronephrosis, and there may be debris within the dilated collecting system.

Trauma

Although ultrasound of trauma patients can be used to evaluate the kidneys, CT with intravenous contrast is a preferable method. The ultrasound findings following renal trauma can include perinephric fluid if the kidney has been contused or fractured. The differential diagnosis of perinephric fluid is given in Table 6–7. If the fracture extends through the collecting system, so that urine is leaking, then there should be a large amount of perinephric fluid. If the trauma is severe enough, then the perinephric space may be violated, and there may be fluid in the pararenal spaces, either anteriorly or posteriorly. Color Doppler of the kidney can indicate whether or not there is still flow to the kidney, and

Table 6–6. ECHOES WITHIN COLLECTING SYSTEM

COMMON
Fungus ball
Stones
Blood clots
Transitional cell carcinoma
Infected obstructed system (pyonephrosis)
Emphysematous pyelonephritis
Nephrostomy tube
Stent

UNCOMMON
Gas (emphysematous pyelonephritis)
Sloughed papillae

Table 6–7. PERIRENAL FLUID

COMMON
Blood, after trauma
Blood, after biopsy
Spontaneous decompression of obstructed system

UNCOMMON
Urinoma
Lymphocele
Perinephric abscess
Herniated bowel
Pancreatic pseudocysts
After percutaneous stone removal
Abscess
Blood associated with tumor or vascular abnormality

thereby rule out a complete artery avulsion. It may be difficult to identify hematomas in either the perirenal space or in the posterior pararenal space. This is because the echogenicity of hematomas can vary. A hematoma may range from echolucent to echogenic in appearance depending on hematoma age, how well confined the hematoma is, and how much it is diluted by serous fluid.

Tumors of the Kidney

RENAL CELL CARCINOMA

Renal cell carcinoma is typically a lesion seen in older patients, but it is not unusual to see patients in their 30s and occasionally even in their 20s with renal cell carcinoma. A small percentage occur in childhood. The term renal adenoma refers to a small renal cell carcinoma. The course of renal adenomas is uncertain, but they should be considered an early form of a renal cell carcinoma. A size of 3 cm is used to differentiate between a renal adenoma and renal cell carcinoma.

On ultrasound, renal cell carcinoma typically appears as a mass that is hypoechoic or isoechoic in comparison to the remainder of the kidney (Fig. 6–9). Approximately 1 percent of renal cell carcinomas have a cystic or complex appearance. Not all of these will have a mural nodule, and therefore, it may be very difficult to distinguish a complex cyst from a renal cell carcinoma with cystic components. A small percentage of renal cell carcinomas will be hyperechoic relative to the adjacent kidney. Calcifica-tions within a mass do not exclude renal cell carcinoma and should actually increase concern that a mass is malignant. The differential diagnoses for solid and complex cystic masses are listed in Tables 6–8 and 6–9.

Doppler can be used to increase the certainty of a diagnosis of a renal cell carcinoma. Renal cell carcinoma has neovascularity and abnormal vessels with atrioventricular shunting, probably due to lack of a capillary bed and the fact that the abnormal vessels do not have a muscular wall. Therefore, between 80 and 90 percent of renal cell carcinomas will show high velocity flow within them. In addition, these will be low impedance vessels, and they will have high diastolic flow also. A significant caveat is that some inflammatory masses may also have neovascularity and atrioventricular shunting and can have similar Doppler features. As many as 20 percent of renal cell carcinomas may be relatively hypovascular, and it may be difficult to detect the abnormal vessels using Doppler. Therefore, failure to find high-flow vascularity in a mass does not exclude renal cell carcinoma. So, the presence of high-flow vessels with low impedance supports a diagnosis of renal cell carcinoma, but does not confirm the diagnosis, and the failure to identify this type of vessel does not exclude the diagnosis.

Whenever a mass is identified and renal cell carcinoma is suspected, the ipsilateral renal vein should be examined for tumor clot and the suprarenal inferior vena cava should also be examined for tumor clot. The contralateral kidney should also be thoroughly examined. One final note. Most renal cell carcinomas will disturb the contour of the kidney and lead to a contour abnormality. If a lesion is hypoechoic, but does not disturb the contour, then care should be taken to make sure that it is not actually a medullary pyramid.

ANGIOMYOLIPOMAS

An angiomyolipoma is a renal hamartoma that usually consists of smooth muscle cells, abnormal blood vessels, and fat. They are common in patients with tuberous sclerosis. However, they may occur in patients of any sex or age.

Ultrasonographically, they are usually

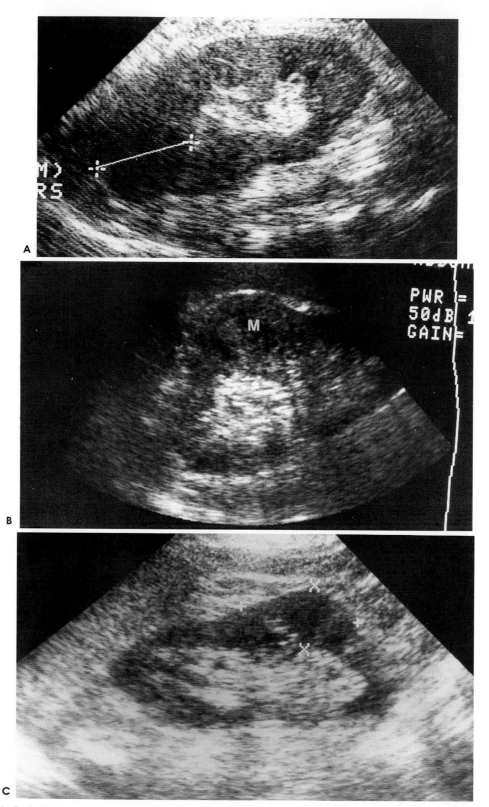

Figure 6–9. *A,* Hypoechoic renal cell carcinoma. *B,* Hypoechoic mass (M) distorts renal contour on this longitudinal image. This is another renal cell carcinoma. *C,* Third example of a hypoechoic renal cell carcinoma.

Table 6–8. SOLID MASSES IN KIDNEY

COMMON
Adenocarcinoma

UNCOMMON
Lymphoma
Hematoma
Calcified cyst
Abscess
Angiomyolipoma
Transitional cell carcinoma
Sinus lipomatosis
Leukemic infiltrate
Neurofibroma
Extramedullary hematopoiesis
Carcinoid of kidney
Oncocytoma
Malakoplakia

hyperechoic in comparison to the adjacent renal cortex (Fig. 6–10). It should be noted, however, that a hyperechoic renal mass is not pathognomonic for angiomyolipoma. The differential diagnosis includes renal cell carcinoma, metastatic disease, lymphoma, oncocytoma, lipoma, and cavernous hemangioma. CT performed with thin cuts may detect fat within a renal lesion and can definitively establish the diagnosis. Occasionally, the lower transmission speed of sound through the fat in these tumors can make structures behind the tumor appear to be posteriorly displaced. Doppler of the tumor may show high flow, but will usually not have the extremely high flow seen in renal cell carcinoma.

Table 6–9. COMPLEX MASSES IN KIDNEY

COMMON
Adenocarcinoma
Hematomas
Abscesses

UNCOMMON
Infarcts
Infected cysts
Hemorrhagic cysts
Pyonephrosis
Peripelvic cysts
Xanthogranulomatous pyelonephritis
Focal bacterial pyelonephritis
Angiomyolipoma
Lymphoma
Transitional cell carcinoma
Multicystic dysplastic kidney
Lymphangioma
Multilocular cystic nephroma

MULTILOCULAR CYSTIC NEPHROMA

This is an uncommon tumor seen in boys under 4 years of age and in women over the age of 50. It appears as a mass consisting of multiple fluid-filled spaces with thick septations. This is a relatively benign lesion, but it may occasionally metastasize and grow and is considered premalignant. On ultrasound, it generally appears to be a bundle of cysts separated by septa. Calcifications may be present in the septa. These neoplasms may mimic cystic renal cell carcinoma. Treatment is surgical removal of the mass.

ONCOCYTOMA

This is a benign tumor occurring in the older age groups, more commonly in males. These tumors do not metastasize or invade the renal veins. They may, however, grow. On ultrasound, they appear as a solid mass that is usually hypoechoic like a renal cell carcinoma. Occasionally, a central echogenic scar may be identified, and this suggests the diagnosis.

TRANSITIONAL CELL CARCINOMA

These tumors usually occur in the bladder. A small percentage (less than 10 percent) may occur in the renal pelvis. They usually have the sonographic appearance of a hypoechoic mass within the collecting system. These tumors can be very difficult to recognize unless there is dilatation of the renal pelvis or calices. If the tumor infiltrates into the kidney itself, it appears as a mass in the region of the renal sinus fat. These tumors may be confused with a hypertrophied column of Bertin. Ultrasound is not a sensitive method of detecting these tumors. The differential diagnosis of renal pelvic masses is listed in Table 6–10.

RENAL METASTASES

The most common sources of metastases to the kidneys are lung cancer, colon cancer, malignant melanoma, and breast cancer. There will frequently be multiple lesions. These are usually hypoechoic and have a poorly defined border.

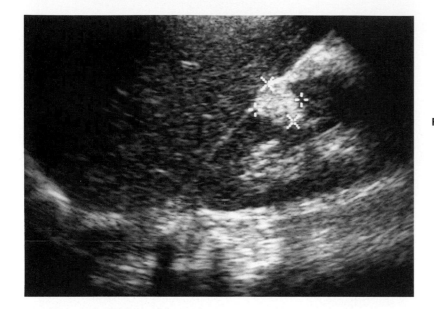

Figure 6–10. Sagittal image of kidney showing echogenic mass in midportion. This is echogenic fat of an angiomyolipoma. The fat is not usually this echogenic.

RENAL LYMPHOMA

Renal lymphoma may be due to primary renal lymphoma or it may be metastatic disease from lymphoma in other sites. Non-Hodgkin's lymphoma is more common than Hodgkin's lymphoma as a cause of renal lymphoma. The kidneys are usually enlarged on ultrasound and contain multiple bilateral hypoechoic renal masses. The differential diagnosis for enlarged kidneys with multiple masses is given in Table 6–11.

Other Renal Diseases

Acute tubular necrosis may be caused by numerous etiologic agents, including hypotension and drug toxicity. The ultrasonographic appearance may range from normal to that of an enlarged hyperechoic kidney, with the cortex being echogenic in comparison to the medullary pyramids.

Acute cortical necrosis is less common than acute tubular necrosis. Acute cortical necrosis usually occurs after shock or hypotension and is common in trauma patients and in postpartum patients with complicated deliveries. On ultrasound, the renal cortex may be hypoechoic early in the disease process, but later, with recovery, may be echogenic and may even have calcifications within the cortex.

GLOMERULONEPHRITIS

With glomerulonephritis, regardless of the type, the usual ultrasound appearance is that of an echogenic kidney. Early in the disease process, the kidneys may be en-

Table 6–10. RENAL PELVIC MASSES

COMMON
Transitional cell carcinoma
Stones
Peripelvic cyst

UNCOMMON
Neurofibroma
Squamous cell carcinoma of pelvis
Adenocarcinoma of pelvis
Lymphoma
Renal vein varices
Fungus balls
Hematoma
Matrix calculus

Table 6–11. KIDNEYS: ENLARGED BILATERALLY, MULTIFOCAL LESIONS

COMMON
Adult polycystic kidney disease
Multiple, simple cysts

UNCOMMON
Acquired cystic disease
Hodgkin's disease/lymphoma of kidney
Bilateral renal cell carcinoma
Multiple hamartomas
Metastases

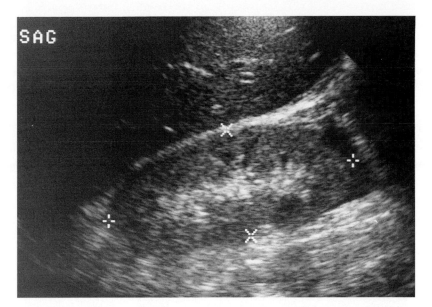

Figure 6–11. Longitudinal image of kidney. Kidney is more echogenic than liver. Almost any disease that damages the kidneys may lead to echogenic kidneys.

larged, but in the later stages of the disease, the kidneys are usually small.

Almost any disease process that damages the kidneys and causes renal failure may lead to echogenic kidneys that are small (Fig. 6–11). The differential diagnosis for echogenic kidneys is given in Table 6–2. It should be noted that the echogenicity of the kidney is not a reflection of the severity of the disease process and is not a sensitive indicator as to whether or not a disease is present. Many patients with renal failure and medical renal disease have normal-appearing kidneys. The differential diagnosis for small bilateral kidneys with a smooth contour is given in Table 6–12 while the differential diagnosis for unilateral small kidneys is given in Table 6–13.

AMYLOIDOSIS

Amyloidosis appears as bilateral renal enlargement in kidneys that are abnormally echogenic. In the later stages of the disease, the kidneys may be small.

STONES AND CALCIFICATIONS

Nephrocalcinosis indicates that there is calcification of renal parenchyma. Stone dis

Table 6–12. KIDNEYS: SMALL, BILATERAL, SMOOTH CONTOUR

COMMON
Hypertensive nephropathy
Generalized arteriosclerosis
Nephrosclerosis

UNCOMMON
Atheroembolic renal disease
Chronic glomerulonephritis
Renal papillary necrosis
Alport's syndrome
Medullary cystic disease
Late amyloidosis
Hypotension
Bilateral renal artery stenosis
Radiation nephritis
Postobstructive atrophy, bilateral
Postinflammatory atrophy
Reflux atrophy
Bilateral infarcts
Renal cortical necrosis
Lead poisoning

From Davidson AJ. Radiology of the Kidney. Philadelphia, WB Saunders, 1985, with permission.

Table 6–13. KIDNEYS: SMALL, UNILATERAL, SMOOTH CONTOUR

COMMON
Reflux atrophy

UNCOMMON
Renal artery stenosis or ischemia
Chronic renal infarction
Radiation
Congenital hypoplasia
Postobstructive atrophy
Postinflammatory atrophy
Heminephrectomy

From Davidson AJ. Radiology of the Kidney. Philadelphia, WB Saunders, 1985, with permission.

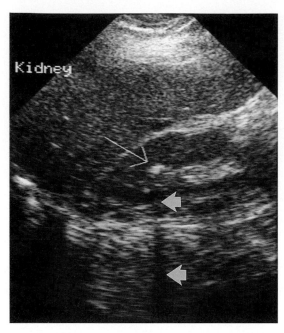

Figure 6–12. Renal stone (*thin arrow*) causing a shadow (*thick arrows*).

Table 6–14. INTERNAL ECHOGENIC AREAS

COMMON
Renal stones
Renal calcifications
Calcifications too small to shadow

UNCOMMON
Renal cell carcinoma
Renal gas
Fat-filled postoperative cortical defect
Tuberculosis with calcifications
Renal tubular acidosis
Medullary sponge kidney
Hyperoxaluria
Sarcoidosis
Milk-alkali syndrome
Hypervitaminosis D
Hyperparathyroidism
Calcification in cysts
Calcification in adenocarcinoma
Carcinoma with paraneoplastic syndrome
Metastatic carcinoma to bone
Calcification in xanthogranulomatous
   pyelonephritis
Papillary necrosis
Echinococcus with calcification
Calcified multicystic dysplastic kidney

ease means that there are stones in the collecting system. Stones or calcifications should be echogenic and should show posterior shadowing (Fig. 6–12). However, very small stones or calcifications may not show posterior shadowing. The highest frequency transducer possible should always be used in an effort to detect shadowing. Patients may have both stones and nephrocalcinosis. Nonradiopaque stones will still be echogenic and have a shadow. The most sensitive technique for the detection of renal stones is CT without contrast. Ultrasound has a somewhat lower sensitivity estimated at about 80 percent. The differential diagnosis for echogenic foci within the kidney is given in Table 6–14.

HYDRONEPHROSIS

Ultrasound is sensitive and accurate for the detection of hydronephrosis. When the hydronephrosis involves only the renal pelvis, it is usually considered to be mild. Moderate hydronephrosis involves the renal pelvis with some dilatation of the calices. Severe hydronephrosis involves marked dilatation of the calices and cortical thinning. Normal kidneys, however, may have minimal separation of the walls of the renal pelvis, especially after the intake of large volumes of fluid. We allow up to 5 mm of separation of the walls of the renal pelvis before considering it to be abnormal. Normal patients with full bladders may also have pelvic or pelvocalyceal dilatation. If it is suspected that overdistention of the bladder is the cause of the hydronephrosis, then the bladder should be emptied, and the kidneys rescanned. We have used pulsed Doppler of interlobar arteries to distinguish between dilated nonobstructed collecting systems and the dilated system due to obstruction. A resistive index greater than .75 implies obstruction.

It may, at times, be difficult to tell hydronephrosis from multiple renal cysts. Multiple renal cysts should not have a clear connection to the renal pelvis and should have septa separating them. Parapelvic cysts can also cause confusion and likewise should not connect to the renal pelvis. Hydronephrosis may be mimicked by congenital megacalices. Sonography cannot reliably make the distinction between these two entities, although Doppler may help as mentioned previously. Occasionally in acute obstruction, the pelvis and calices may not have yet dilated and therefore may appear normal. Likewise, obstruction in dehy-

Table 6–15. DILATED COLLECTING SYSTEM

COMMON
Urinary obstruction
Reflux
Distended bladder

UNCOMMON
Infection causing aperistalsis
Diuresis
Extrarenal pelvis
After relief of obstruction
After diuretics
After contrast injection
Overhydration
Megacalices
Papillary necrosis
Diabetes insipidus
Postinflammatory calyceal clubbing
After extracorporeal shock wave lithotripsy

Table 6–16. MIMICS OF DILATED COLLECTING SYSTEM

COMMON
Central renal cysts
Parapelvic cysts
Multiple simple cysts

UNCOMMON
Lucent renal pyramids
Lumbar meningomyelocele
Pancreatic pseudocyst
Renal artery aneurysm
Sinus lipomatosis
Hypoechoic renal lymphoma

drated patients or in a patient with renal failure may not manifest as a dilated pelvis or calices. The causes of a dilated collecting system are listed in Tables 6–15 and 6–16.

Pregnant patients frequently have hydronephrosis, especially on the right side. This may be secondary to an enlarged uterus obstructing the ureter where it crosses the pelvic brim. Another hypothesis is that the peristalsis in the ureters is reduced by hormonal changes, but this would not explain why hydronephrosis is predominant on the right side. We routinely look at the kidneys for hydronephrosis during obstetric ultrasound. If hydronephrosis is present, an attempt should be made to identify the ureters at the bladder base to determine if they are dilated at this level or to determine if the level of obstruction is proximal to the base of the bladder. An attempt may also be made to follow the ureters from the kidney into the pelvis, but this is only rarely successful.

Renal Transplant Evaluation

Evaluation of a renal transplant is performed visually by looking for changes in the appearance of the transplant and also

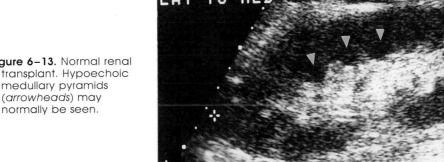

Figure 6–13. Normal renal transplant. Hypoechoic medullary pyramids (*arrowheads*) may normally be seen.

by Doppler evaluation of arcuate, interlobar, and hilar vessels (Fig. 6–13). Small collections of fluid around the transplant in the immediate postoperative period are usual. These are not significant unless they are causing obstruction or are compressing the kidney. They usually resolve.

However, there is one significant cause of a postoperative fluid collection that is quite significant, and that is a urinoma. A urinoma simply represents a leak of urine, usually at an anastomotic site. Urinomas typically occur within the first days after a transplant. Nuclear medicine examinations can be useful in evaluating a urinoma because radioactive material will be extravasated into the perirenal fluid.

Lymphoceles develop around transplants. These have a different time course, usually appearing between one and six months after the transplant. Sonographically, they are echolucent with septa, may become quite large, and can sometimes cause obstruction (Fig. 6–14). They may need to be surgically drained or excised, although sometimes percutaneous aspiration and drainage will be curative.

Abscesses may develop around a transplant, but these are usually the result of infection of a pre-existing fluid collection.

It is not unusual for a well-functioning normal transplant to have slight separation of the walls of the renal pelvis. This does not indicate obstruction. Due to the position in which the transplant lies, urine does not drain from the renal pelvis as well as from the renal pelvis of a native kidney. In addition, the peristalsis of the transplanted ureter may not be as good as in a native ureter. Therefore, some separation of renal pelvis walls does not necessarily indicate obstruction. In addition, an overly full urinary bladder may result in an appearance indicating hydronephrosis, and the transplant should be checked with the bladder both full and empty.

Acute tubular necrosis (ATN) presents in the immediate posttransplantation period. Sonographically, ATN cannot be differentiated from rejection. In both conditions, the kidney may be enlarged and may become more globular in shape as opposed to the normal elliptical shape. This is a manifestation of edema. The renal sinus fat may become less echogenic because it is dispersed by the swollen, edematous kidney

(Fig. 6–15A). Therefore, there is no longer a clump of renal sinus fat.

In addition, the renal cortex may become hypoechoic, although it occasionally may become hyperechoic. As a result, the medullary pyramids may become more prominent. The pyramids may increase in height, becoming thicker than the overlying cortex (Fig. 6–15B). This may give an increased distinction between cortex and medulla or there may be a decreased distinction with blurring of the cortex and medulla and an overall increase in the kidney's echogenicity. Thickening of the walls of the renal pelvis is also a sign of rejection. All of the above sonographic signs are nonspecific and can be seen with other transplant problems. In general, they simply reflect an edematous transplant.

Cyclosporine toxicity may also produce an enlarged kidney. Generally, the cortical echogenicity is increased, but it may be variable with cyclosporine.

Doppler has long been used to evaluate renal transplants. Usually, an interlobar or arcuate artery is identified in the upper pole, midpole, and lower pole of the transplant. A good wave form is obtained. A resistive index is usually used as an indicator as to whether or not disease is present. The resistive index equals peak systolic velocity minus end-diastolic velocity over peak systolic velocity. In general, a resistive index below .70 is normal. In cases of rejection, ATN, obstruction, cyclosporine toxicity, or compression of the transplant, the resistive index may increase. Initially, it was thought that the resistive index was a sensitive and specific way to diagnose rejection, but it is now accepted that this is a nonspecific indicator of a renal transplant problem. Changes in resistive indices, when compared to previous examinations in the same patient, may be a better indicator of disease than the absolute resistive index. A high resistive index reflects poor diastolic flow.

It is important to check the hilar vessels of the transplant to make sure that there is no evidence of renal artery occlusion. We also try to get a Doppler tracing of the renal vein to make sure it is open because renal vein thrombosis is a serious complication, usually occurring in the postoperative period. Reversal of diastolic flow in the main renal artery is an indicator of renal vein thrombosis. However, it is nonspecific, and

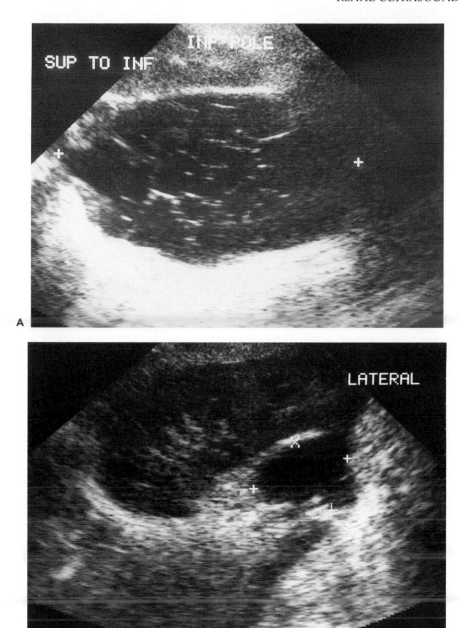

Figure 6-14. *A,* Lymphocele. This lymphocele is hypoechoic with multiple septae. *B,* This lymphocele sits near the hilum of transplant. This lymphocele could be confused with a dilated renal pelvis.

may also be seen with other problems such as rejection, ATN, or a renal artery embolus.

Doppler of the main renal artery is useful to evaluate for arterial stenosis and thrombosis. Hypertension suggests arterial stenosis. In addition, the transplanted kidney may not show the normal increase in size after it is transplanted. Stenosis is suggested when velocities exceed 200 cm/sec.

Many renal transplant patients undergo multiple renal biopsies. Therefore, they are at risk for developing arteriovenous fistulas and pseudoaneurysms. Color Doppler ultrasound can be used to search for these two complications. If an arteriovenous fistula develops, the venous wave may change to an "arterialized" pattern (Fig. 6-16).

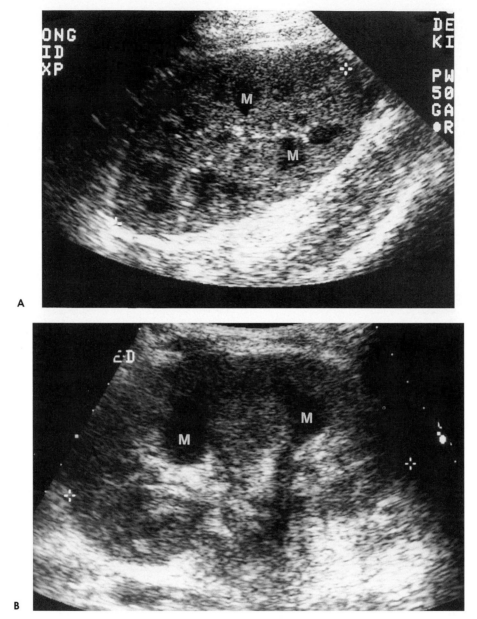

Figure 6–15. *A*, Transplant rejection. Kidney is swollen as manifested by an increase in width. The cortex is increased in echogenicity and the medullary pyramids (M) have become enlarged and prominently hypoechoic. The renal sinus fat is no longer seen in an echogenic clump. *B*, Tall pyramids in transplant rejection. (M = pyramids.)

Doppler of the Native Kidneys

Numerous investigators have attempted to use duplex Doppler to evaluate renal vascular disease. In recent years, attempts have been made to utilize color Doppler to evaluate the renal arteries. In general, this is difficult and requires great persistence. The examinations sometimes exceed one hour. Most ultrasonographers have not been successful in using this technique with sufficient accuracy to make it an adequate screening examination. Various techniques, including the peak systolic velocity, the ratio of peak systolic velocity in the renal

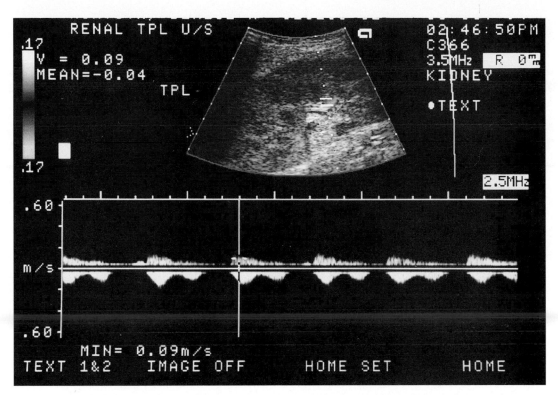

Figure 6–16. Doppler gate includes both main renal artery (above baseline) and main renal vein (below baseline). Trace of venous flow has become "arterialized" because of arteriovenous fistula.

artery to that in the aorta, and the resistive index in the renal artery, have been used to evaluate the kidneys. Recently, the rate of upstroke of the systolic peak has been tried as an indicator of renal artery stenosis. This is known as the tardus-parvis waveform. This waveform occurs distal to a stenosis and the time from end-diastole to peak systole is greater than .08 seconds. This waveform can be evaluated in the renal parenchyma, obviating the need for identification of the main renal artery. However, this method has not gained wide acceptance. A serious problem with the evaluation of renal arteries on color Doppler is the fact that over 20 percent of patients may have multiple renal arteries, and it is difficult to know which patients have multiple renal arteries and to know precisely where the additional renal arteries originate.

Evaluation of the renal veins for thrombosis has some problems similar to evaluating the renal arteries. An increase in intrarenal impedance may result when the venous outflow from the kidney is obstructed. This leads to an elevation in the resistive index, but, of course, this is a non-

specific finding. Renal vein thrombosis may cause complete reversal of diastolic flow when the renal artery wave form is evaluated, a finding that can be helpful in diagnosing renal vein thrombosis.

Arteriovenous fistulas frequently occur in the kidney, especially as a complication of renal biopsy or trauma. These can lead to hematuria or hypertension, and if enough blood is shunted, can lead to high output cardiac failure. On ultrasound, an echolucent mass that has a multiloculated cystic appearance may be seen. This appearance is the result of a cluster of arteries and veins. By using color flow, these can be demonstrated to be vascular in nature, and the correct diagnosis made.

Bladder

For successful transabdominal ultrasound examinations of the bladder, it is necessary that the bladder be well distended with urine. A Foley catheter can be inserted and the bladder filled in a retrograde fashion. As with other organs, the bladder must

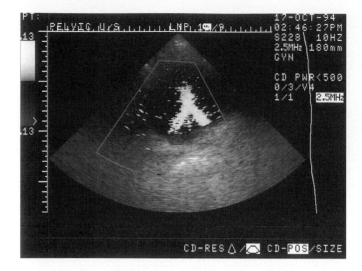

Figure 6–17. Transverse color Doppler image showing ureteric jets. See color plate 4.

be examined in at least two planes. The entire wall of the bladder must be visualized and when the bladder is adequately distended, the wall should be no more than 3 mm thick. A nondistended bladder wall may be considerably thicker. When measuring the bladder, care must be taken not to include the peritoneum of the anterior peritoneal reflection on the superior portion of the bladder, and adjacent organs such as the rectum should not be included. Note that urine may periodically enter the bladder from the ureters and may cause echoes to arise at the ureteric orifice. This phenomenon has been called ureteric jets (Figure 6–17).

The bladder may be abnormally thickened, either focally or diffusely (Table 6–17). Focal increases in bladder wall thickness may be secondary to tumors. Transitional cell carcinoma is the most common bladder neoplasm, and any mass or any area of focal thickening that is seen should include transitional cell carcinoma as a possible diagnosis. However, numerous other diseases can also produce focal thickening of the bladder, including blood clots, stones, debris, and scar from prior surgery. Endometriosis and neurofibromatosis can also produce areas of focal thickening. Thickening at the base of the bladder near the prostate gland in a male should raise the question of invasive prostate carcinoma. Most commonly, diffuse thickening can be caused by a bladder outlet obstruction and cystitis.

Other bladder tumors include bladder papillomas, which are benign but premalig-

nant for transitional cell carcinoma. Squamous cell carcinoma is responsible for a small percentage of primary bladder cancers. Masses in the bladder may be due to hematomas (Fig. 6–18), bladder stones, or debris from infection (Table 6–18). A word of caution: It is common to see pseudomasses in the bladder that are actually caused either by reverberations within the bladder or by beam width artifacts (see Fig. 1–27).

Table 6–17. BLADDER WALL THICKENING

COMMON
Transitional cell carcinoma
Blood clot
Neurogenic bladder

UNCOMMON
Secondary to diverticulitis of bowel
Cyclophosphamide-induced cystitis
Crohn's disease involvement of bladder
Colovesical fistula
Vesicovaginal fistula
Cystitis glandularis
Candida cystitis
Extension of prostate cancer
Bladder outlet obstruction
Malakoplakia
Leukoplakia
Neurofibroma
Hemangioma
Schistosomiasis
Pheochromocytoma
Endometriosis
Adjacent abscess
Hematoma in wall

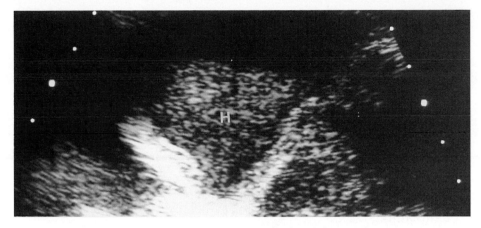

Figure 6–18. Transverse bladder image showing hematoma (H).

Prostate Ultrasound

TECHNIQUE

Ultrasonography of the prostate is performed using a transrectal ultrasound transducer. The transducer is covered by a condom to prevent contamination of the transducer itself. On many machines, either a water bath is located between the transducer and the condom or gel is placed in the condom to provide acoustic coupling. Prior to the ultrasound examination, a digital rectal examination is performed using lubricating jelly. In addition, the prostate is palpated to make certain there are no rectal

Table 6–18. BLADDER MASSES

COMMON
Transitional cell carcinoma
Blood clot
Cystitis
Stones

UNCOMMON
Ureterocele
Foley catheter balloon
Bladder diverticulum
Pheochromocytoma
Endometriosis
Chloroma
Metastases
Neurofibroma
Extension of prostate cancer
Foreign body
Wall hematoma
Polyp
Fungus ball
Leiomyoma
Leiomyosarcoma
Schistosomiasis

masses and to assess the overall size of the prostate and palpate for hard areas in the prostate, which may be an indicator of cancer. In addition, nodules can be palpated and their location noted. Many institutions prep the patient by having the patient take a cleansing enema prior to exam. This is not absolutely necessary; however, it is preferable not to have stool within the rectal vault. Many patients, especially older ones, do have stool in that area, and a cleansing enema may be helpful.

The digital rectal examination will lubricate the anus. A small amount of lubricant is placed on the transducer, and the transducer is inserted into the rectum. It is frequently useful to aim the tip of the transducer posteriorly toward the sacrum so that the transducer will slide past an enlarged prostate gland. Once the transducer has been inserted, then the operator must take care to make certain that contact is maintained between the transducer and the prostate gland. With some types of machines, it is possible to use the same transducer to scan in both the sagittal and axial planes. This is not possible with other machines and a different transducer must be used to obtain the second view. The transducer may be either end firing or side firing. Usually, a 5.0- or 7.5-MHz transducer is used.

ANATOMY

The prostate gland is divided into zones (Fig. 6–19). The transitional zone is adjacent to the urethra and is the site of benign pros-

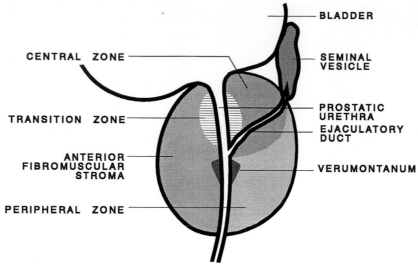

Figure 6–19. Prostate zonal anatomy. (Modified from Rifkin MD. Ultrasound of the Prostate. New York, Raven Press, 1988, with permission.)

tatic hypertrophy. The peripheral zone accounts for the largest portion of the prostate gland. This lies peripherally next to the rectum. Approximately 70 percent of prostate cancers originate in this area. Finally, the central zone is located at the top of the prostate or base. Ejaculatory ducts pass through this region.

The seminal vesicles may be identified at the top (base) of the prostate gland (Fig. 6–20). In the axial plane, they resemble a bow tie. In the sagittal plane, they resemble a small projection sticking off of the top of the prostate. The apex of the prostate gland is located inferiorly.

Multiple images should be obtained in both the sagittal and transverse planes. The overall size and shape of the gland are evaluated. Hypoechoic areas can be indicative of prostate cancer, but these can also simply be secondary to benign prostatic hypertrophy (Table 6–19). Significant numbers of prostate cancers may be hyperechoic or isoechoic. There is some controversy as to whether or not biopsy of hypoechoic areas is any more useful than random biopsies. The seminal vesicles should be symmetric in their relationship to the prostate gland. Calcifications can frequently be seen in the prostate, and these probably originate from prostatitis. Corpora amylacea may be identified as hyperechoic areas in the prostate in some patients. These are the results of

inspissated secretions and are formed from glycoproteins.

In patients who have prostatic hypertrophy, it is common to see cysts (Table 6–20). These are usually of no significance. Some congenital cysts may be identified, including utricle cysts that are near the midline, and müllerian duct cysts, which may extend lateral to the midline from the region of the verumontanum to near the seminal vesicle. Ejaculatory duct cysts are the result of dilatation of the ejaculatory duct. When an ejaculatory duct cyst is aspirated, it will contain spermatozoa, whereas müllerian duct cysts do not contain spermatozoa. Cysts may be identified in the seminal vesicle. These are of little significance. Cysts may be the result of infection.

When cancer is suspected, an evaluation should be performed to determine if the cancer has spread outside of the prostate. The borders of the prostate are often referred to as a prostate capsule. Although there is no true capsule surrounding the prostate, vessels and nerves run in the margins of the prostate and the fat around the prostate is compressed, leading to a pseudocapsule.

INDICATIONS FOR PROSTATE BIOPSY

There are those who advocate screening the entire elderly male population, much as

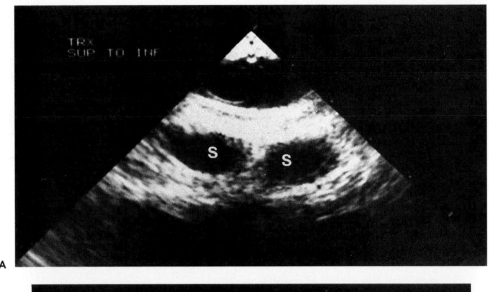

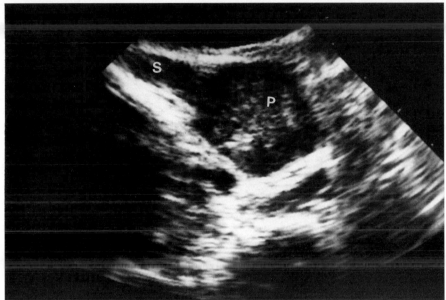

Figure 6–20. Seminal vesicles. *A,* Transverse image just superior to the prostate shows both right and left seminal vesicles. *B,* Longitudinal image. The two seminal vesicles should be symmetric. Lack of symmetry implies invasion by cancer. S = seminal vesicle, P = prostate.

women are screened with mammography. It is doubtful that this would be efficacious. The natural course of prostate cancer is not completely understood at this time, and it may be that many patients who have biopsy proof of prostate cancer will have a disease with a benign course. Definite indications for prostate ultrasound and biopsy include a palpable nodule and elevated prostate-specific antigen or elevated acid phosphatase levels. Ultrasonog-

raphy has also been used to stage a known prostate cancer.

TECHNIQUE OF BIOPSY

Ultrasound-guided prostate biopsy is most often performed using a needle-firing gun that attaches to the side of the transducer. Biopsy guidelines on the ultrasound screen show the path of the needle. We usually use an 18-gauge or 19-gauge needle.

Table 6–19. HYPOECHOIC LESIONS OF THE PROSTATE

COMMON
Cancer
Benign prostatic hypertrophy
Prostatitis
UNCOMMON
Malakoplakia
Cysts
Abscess

The gun projects this needle approximately 2 cm into the prostate. A core biopsy is then obtained. We usually perform six biopsies per gland, three on each side, in the superior, middle, and inferior portions of the gland. For this procedure, the patient is placed in the left lateral decubitus position.

The complications of prostate biopsy include infection and hemorrhage. Hemorrhage may result from a laceration of a periprostatic artery. If this occurs, the patient will usually have sufficient bleeding such that the rectal vault will fill with blood over the course of one hour. Therefore, we hold our patients in the waiting room for approximately one hour after the biopsy. Defecation of a large amount of blood is indicative of this complication. Approximately half of all patients will have some blood in the urine or stool. This may last for several days. Patients may also have blood in their ejaculate. We had one patient in whom blood in the ejaculate continued for a month.

The other possible complication is sepsis. Patients should be premedicated with an antibiotic. It is unclear as to which antibiotic should be used. Although some clinicians favor norfloxacin, prostate levels of antibiotic are better with ciprofloxacin, and that

Table 6–20. CYSTS IN PROSTATE

COMMON
Seminal vesicle cysts
After prostatitis
With benign prostatic hypertrophy
UNCOMMON
Müllerian duct cysts
Utricle cysts
Abscess
Hydroureter
Cystocele
Parasitic cysts
With carcinoma

is the drug that we currently use. We prescribe 500 mg orally the night before and the morning of an examination and follow that with another dose the evening after the exam. In addition, we give an 80-mg dose of gentamicin sulfate immediately before the biopsy, but this regimen is not in widespread use. However, we have had patients become septic when only norfloxacin or ciprofloxacin was used.

PATHOLOGY

Sonographically, prostate cancer is classically hypoechoic. However, as indicated, it may be hyperechoic or even isoechoic. Disturbance of the capsule and asymmetry of the seminal vesicles should be looked for in an effort to identify extension outside the prostate gland.

With benign prostatic hypertrophy, the gland will be generally enlarged and may be quite asymmetric. The echo pattern is a combination of increased and decreased echogenicity. Calcifications may be seen. Benign prostatic hypertrophy may lead to hypoechoic nodules resembling carcinoma. Even though benign prostatic hypertrophy originates in the transitional zone, the changes in the gland may appear to be in the peripheral zone, causing it to be confused with prostate cancer. Prostate cancer frequently does coexist with benign prostatic hypertrophy, however.

Chronic prostatitis may give a very heterogeneous-appearing gland with areas of increased and decreased echogenicity.

In patients with acute prostatitis, the gland is frequently exquisitely tender. The gland may be swollen and edematous, leading to a hypoechoic appearance. Ultrasound can be used to guide aspiration of any cystic or complex cystic cavities that resemble an abscess.

LOCATION OF PROSTATE CANCER

About 70 percent of prostate cancer is located in the peripheral zone. Twenty percent will be in the transitional zone, and another 10 percent in the central zone.

Adrenal Gland

Ultrasonography of the adrenal glands is sometimes useful. Often, an incidental ad-

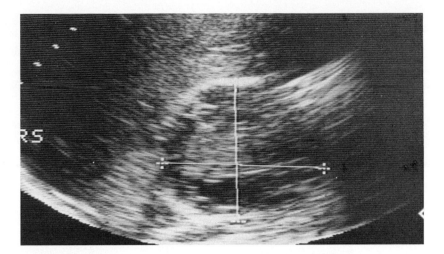

Figure 6–21. Adrenal metastasis. Transverse image. Large complex-appearing mass.

renal mass is found. CT and magnetic resonance imaging are the primary imaging techniques for looking at the adrenal glands. The right adrenal gland lies superior and slightly medial to the right kidney and directly behind the vena cava. The left adrenal is medial to the upper pole of the left kidney.

PATHOLOGY

The most common cause of an adrenal mass is a nonfunctioning adenoma. These are commonly found at autopsy and as incidental findings at the time of CT. When a mass is identified in the adrenal gland, ultrasound cannot distinguish between a nonfunctioning adenoma, a functioning ade-

Table 6–21. MASSES IN ADRENAL GLAND

COMMON
Hyperplasia
Adenomas
Metastases

UNCOMMON
Cysts
Abscesses
Ganglioneuromas
Pheochromocytomas
Adrenal cortical carcinoma
Invasion from renal tumor
Prominent diaphragmatic crus
Myelolipoma
Neuroblastoma
Lymphoma
Hemorrhage
Hydatid disease

noma, or even an adrenocortical carcinoma (Table 6–21).

Adrenocortical carcinomas are very malignant. They may occur in either sex at any age. About 50 percent of these secrete hormones. On ultrasound, they are usually homogeneous. If they become large, they may necrose and lead to a complex cystic appearance. Calcifications may also be seen after necrosis.

Myelolipomas are benign hamartomas of the adrenal gland containing fat and elements from the bone marrow. They occur in the older age groups. Ultrasound may show an echogenic mass. CT is a better test if myelolipoma is suspected because it may detect fatty components and this allows a pathognomonic diagnosis.

Adrenal cysts may result from previous hemorrhage with resorption of the clot and subsequent cyst formation. These frequently calcify.

Adrenal metastases are common, especially from lung cancer (Fig. 6–21). Metastases may be very small or up to 10 or 15 cm in size. The appearance is nonspecific. Sonographically, the mass will usually be heterogeneous, but it may be cystic or homogeneously solid.

Pheochromocytomas are located in the adrenal gland in about 90 percent of cases. These lesions are usually several centimeters in diameter and are well defined. Necrosis may lead to a complex cystic appearance on ultrasound, or there may be echogenic areas within the lesion.

Hemorrhage within the adrenal glands usually occurs in the neonate (Fig. 6–22),

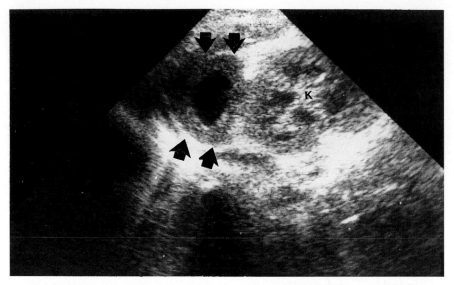

Figure 6–22. Longitudinal image. Adrenal hemorrhage in neonate (*arrows*). Liquefaction has begun. K = kidney.

but occasionally trauma or infection (especially meningococcemia) may lead to adrenal hemorrhage in an adult. This is more often right-sided and unilateral in an adult. The adrenal gland will appear echogenic on ultrasound. Over time, the size of the adrenal mass will shrink as the hemorrhage is reabsorbed.

Adrenal hyperplasia usually will not be detected by ultrasound. This condition leads to bilateral enlargement of the adrenal glands. Occasionally, multiple bilateral nodules may be seen with hyperplasia. These nodules tend to be very small in size and not appreciated at ultrasound.

Infection of the adrenal glands, such as tuberculosis or histoplasmosis, can cause enlargement of the adrenal. The adrenal masses are usually hypoechoic to complex cystic.

Scrotal Ultrasound

ANATOMY

The testicles descend from the abdomen through the inguinal ring to lie in the scrotum during the last trimester of gestation. They bring with them a sac of peritoneum from the abdominal cavity. This sac of peritoneum lines the walls of the scrotum and covers the testes and the epididymis. This is the tunica vaginalis with a parietal layer on the outside lining the scrotal wall and a visceral layer on the inside reflected over the testes and epididymis. This two-layer tunica vaginalis does not completely surround the testes because in the posterior portion of the testicle, there is a bare area where vessels and ducts enter. The testis is attached to the scrotal wall along its posterior surface. The testicle is surrounded by a protective layer of dense fibrous connective tissue, known as the tunica albuginea. The tunica albuginea invaginates into the testicle as a structure known as the mediastinum testes (Fig. 6–23). At the mediastinum testes, arteries enter and veins leave the testicle. Seminiferous tubules exit the mediastinum and they provide a pathway for sperm into the efferent ductules that, in turn, connect to the head of the epididymis. The head of the epididymis is located at the upper pole of the testicle (Fig. 6–24). The body of the epididymis runs inferiorly from the head of the epididymis down the back side of the testicle. The tail of the epididymis is located at the lower pole of the testicle posteriorly. This, in turn, connects to the ductus deferens, which runs back up the scrotum to enter the spermatic cord. The head of the epididymis is sometimes called the globus major, while the tail may be called the globus minor.

The testicle itself should be homogeneous in appearance. Sometime during the ultra-

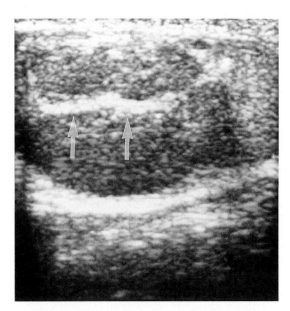

Figure 6–23. Longitudinal image of testicle shows echogenic line that is mediastinum testes (*arrows*).

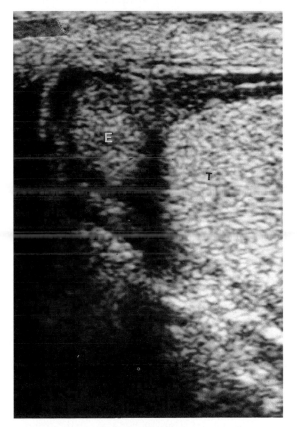

Figure 6–24. Longitudinal testicle (T). Head of epididymis (E) sits on top of upper pole and has echogenicity similar to the testicle. It is about 1 cm or less in size.

sound examination, a transverse image with both testicles on one frame should be obtained so that the echogenicity of the two testicles can be compared. The tunica albuginea is an echogenic line surrounding the testicle. The body and tail of the epididymis may not be identified. The mediastinum testes frequently can be seen as a dense echogenic line (Fig. 6–23).

Four testicular appendages exist:

1. The appendix testes, sometimes known as the hydatid of Morgagni, is a remnant of the müllerian ducts. This structure can sometimes be identified between the head of the epididymis and the upper pole of the testicle. It lies between the parietal and visceral layers of the tunica vaginalis. If torsed, a small hypo- or hyperechoic mass may be seen.

2. The appendix epididymis. This is a remnant of the mesonephros. It can become torsed but often cannot be visualized by ultrasound. If seen, it is a small mass adjacent to the epididymis.

3. The paradidymis (organ of Giraldes) also is a mesonephric remnant in the region of the lower spermatic cord, but is not seen by ultrasound.

4. The vas aberrans (organ of Haller), the third mesonephric remnant located at the junction of the body and tail of the epididymis, also is not seen on ultrasound.

TECHNIQUE

Scrotal ultrasound is performed by placing the patient supine. A towel is usually placed over the penis, which is moved upward so it lies on the lower abdominal wall. A towel can also be placed across the thighs and behind the scrotum so that the scrotum is supported by the towel. A high-frequency (7.5-MHz) transducer is used to obtain multiple sagittal and transverse images.

NORMAL TESTES

Ultrasound of the normal testes reveals two homogeneous, egg-shaped structures. Most patients will have a few milliliters of fluid around at least one of the testes. This is a normal finding and should not be considered to be a pathologic hydrocele. The head of the epididymis can be identified in a posterior location at the upper pole of the testicle. It will measure approximately 1 cm in diameter. It should be isoechoic to the testis. The remainder of the epididymis is harder to identify. The body of the epididymis is a smaller, hypoechoic structure extending from the head to the slightly more bulbous tail. Color Doppler of the testicle should reveal low-resistance flow in the spermatic cord. The resistive index should be between .5 and .7. Flow should be seen in the central portion of the testicle (i.e., the mediastinum testes). This is low-velocity flow and may be difficult to detect.

TESTICULAR TUMORS

Testicular tumors are usually found in 20- to 35-year-olds. They are dramatically more common in undescended testicles. Most intratesticular tumors are malignant, whereas most extratesticular tumors are benign. An intratesticular tumor may originate from a germ cell or it may originate from one of the stromal supporting cells. The tumors are classified as in Table 6–22.

The mixed type, which account for about 40 percent of the total, were previously called teratocarcinomas. The ultrasound appearance of most of these tumors is usually that of a hypoechoic mass or masses (Fig. 6–25). Embryonal cell carcinomas tend to be more heterogeneous and disorganized in appearance. Teratomas tend to have a mixed cystic and solid appearance with some calcifications (Table 6–23).

Most metastatic lesions appear as hypoechoic, well-defined masses, although a heterogeneous, disorganized appearance to the testicle may also result from an infiltrating type of metastatic lesion. The most common metastases to the testicle come from leukemia and lymphoma (Fig. 6–26). After treatment for these two diseases, the testicle may provide a reservoir of disease because the gonadal blood–testicle barrier may leave tumor in the testicles that has not been effectively treated by chemotherapy.

Extratesticular tumors include the adenomatoid tumor (Table 6–24). It is usually located in the region of the tail of the epididymis. It may also be found in the spermatic cord. Adenomatoid tumors are usually solid, well-defined masses with echogenicity similar to that of the testicle. Adrenal rests may be found in the cord or around the testicle. These are benign tumors. They may be either hypo- or hyperechoic and are of minimal significance. Sperm granulomas occur in patients who have had a vasectomy. They present as a solid hypoechoic mass around the epididymis, usually near the tail. Spermatoceles occur because of obstruction of epididymal ducts. They are hypoechoic, avascular, spherical, and have good through transmission.

A hydrocele may be idiopathic, posttraumatic, or postinfectious. Occasionally a hydrocele will be associated with a tumor. Hematoceles follow trauma. Varicoceles are dilated venous channels in the spermatic cord (Fig. 6–27). These may lead to warming of the testicle with resultant sterility. Color flow Doppler should indicate that there is flow in this dilated, cylindrical-shaped structure and result in the diagnosis of a varicocele. The Valsalva maneuver will cause the flow to decrease and the varicocele to increase in size.

Testicular cysts are usually thought to be of no significance. Rarely, a carcinoma may have cystic components, but its appearance should be different from that of a simple, well-defined cyst. Calcifications in the testicle are manifest as multiple small echogenic foci usually scattered throughout both testicles (Table 6–25). These have been reported to have an association with germ-cell tumors. Regressed germ-cell tumors may also calcify. However, testicular microlithiasis (tiny, almost indiscernible calcifications) has been reported to be a benign condition. It is not clear that the ultrasonographer can make a reliable distinction between these two conditions.

INFECTIOUS LESIONS

Infections of the testicle usually result from epididymitis, although diseases such as tuberculosis can occasionally infect the testicle. Epididymitis presents as an en-

Table 6–22. CLASSIFICATION OF TESTICULAR TUMORS

GERM CELLS	STROMAL CELLS
Seminomas–40%	Sertoli cell
Mixed–30%	Leydig cell
Embryonal cell–20%	Mesenchymal cell
Teratomas–5%	
Choriocarcinoma–rare	

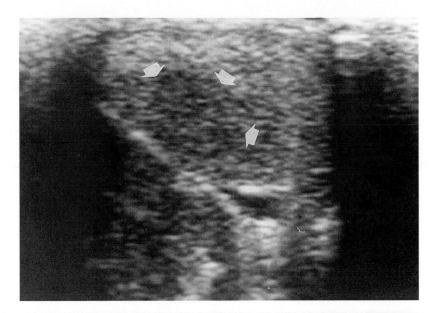

Figure 6-25. Hypoechoic seminoma demarcated by arrows.

Table 6-23. ABNORMAL ECHOGENICITY OF TESTES

COMMON
Seminoma
Embryonal cell carcinoma
Choriocarcinoma
Mixed germ cell lesions
Lymphoma
Leukemia

UNCOMMON
Teratocarcinoma
Teratoma
Epidermoid cyst
Torsion
Metastases
Epididymal tumors
Hematoma
Abscess
Infarcts
Leydig's cell tumors
Lipomas
Sertoli's cell tumors
Sarcoidosis
Adrenal rests
Postsurgical defects
Tunica albuginea cysts
Brucellosis
Myeloma of testicle
Plasmacytoma
Focal orchitis
Malakoplakia
Lipoma
Fibrosis
Adenomatoid tumor

larged epididymis, usually with an associated hydrocele (Fig. 6–28A). The hydrocele may have debris and septa in it. An abscess may result from the epididymitis. Color flow Doppler is useful in examining the patient with epididymitis because the epididymis should have increased flow (Fig. 6–28B). This may allow distinguishing it from other processes. If the epididymitis progresses into an abscess, then a complex lesion will be identified in the testis itself. This may be complex cystic or may simply be hypoechoic. Other complications include testicular infarct, atrophy, and infertility.

TESTICULAR TORSION

Torsion most commonly occurs in 12- to 18-year-olds. Cold weather, sexual activity, and trauma may precede torsion presumably due to cremasteric contraction. Polyorchidism and undescended testicles also predispose. Color Doppler may be used in the diagnosis of testicular torsion. Gray scale images usually will reveal an enlarged, edematous testis acutely. As the torsion becomes chronic, the testicle may shrink and become atrophic. Color Doppler of torsion will reveal that there is no flow in the parenchyma or mediastinum of the testis itself, although there may be peripheral collateral flow along the outside margins of the testicle. Care must be taken to set the instrument to detect slow flow. Epididymal enlargement may also occur early in the

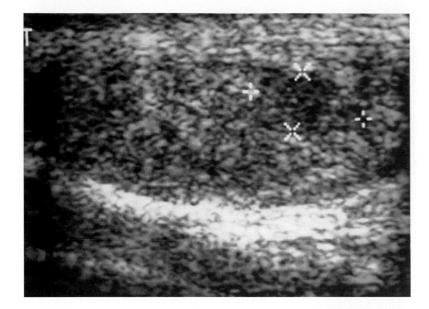

Figure 6-26. Ill-defined hypoechoic lymphoma of the testicle.

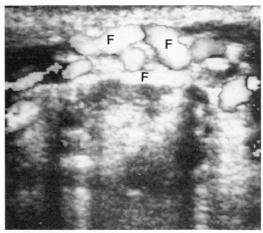

Figure 6-27. Longitudinal image above testicle. Color Doppler image (but photographed in black and white) shows flow (F) in varicocele.

Table 6-24. FLUID AND MASSES, EXTRATESTICULAR

COMMON
Primary hydrocele
Reactive hydrocele
Varicoceles
Ascites
Hematoceles
Spermatocele
Epididymitis

UNCOMMON
Cysts
Herniated bowel
Epididymal cysts
Pyoceles
Adenomatoid tumor
Extratesticular seminoma
Leiomyomas
Fibromas
Adrenal rests
Lipomas
Chronic epididymitis
Metastases
Rhabdomyosarcoma of funiculus
Sarcoidosis
Sperm granuloma
Mesothelioma of tunica vaginalis
Bowel herniation into scrotum
Polyorchidism
Fibrolipoma of cord
Lymphangioma
Mesothelioma of tunica albuginea

Table 6-25. CALCIFICATION IN TESTES

IN NORMALS
With cryptorchidism
Klinefelter's syndrome
With testicular tumors
With pulmonary alveolar microlithiasis
Epidermoid cyst
Tuberculosis
Granulomatous orchitis
Old hematoma
Phlebolith in varicocele

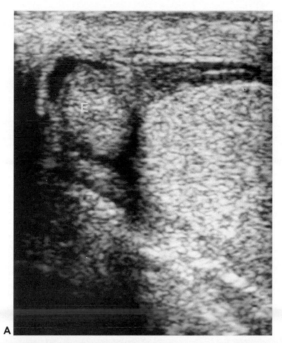

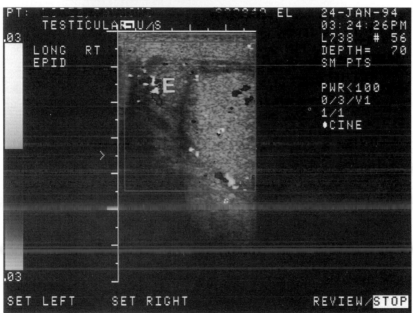

Figure 6–28. *A,* Enlarged hypoechoic epididymis consistent with epididymitis (E). *B,* Color Doppler image shows enlarged epididymis (E) with increased flow consistent with epididymitis. See color plate 5.

course. Between 24 hours and 10 days, the testicle will have a disordered heterogeneous echo appearance. Ultimately, in chronic torsion, the testicle will shrink in size. Partial and intermittent torsion can still have normal blood flow at color Doppler. Color Doppler has a sensitivity of about 85 per-

cent and specificity of about 95 percent. In other words, some torsed testicles may have apparently normal flow.

Torsion of the appendix testes has been reported sometimes to cause a hypoechoic extratesticular mass near the upper pole. Several of these cases have had an echogenic rim.

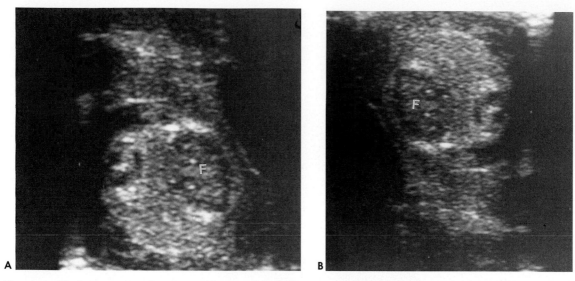

Figure 6–29. *A,* Transverse image of fractured testicle (F). *B,* Different patient. Another example of a fracture (F).

TRAUMA

After trauma, ultrasound may be used to look for a testicular fracture or intratesticular hematoma (Figs. 6–29). Ultrasound is quite sensitive for these conditions.

Pediatric Renal Ultrasound

When infants are being examined, it is wise to start the examination with a look at the bladder. The bladder will fill and empty intermittently; it must be examined when it is full. After examining the bladder, then the kidneys can be examined.

ANATOMY

In the neonatal period, the renal cortical echogenicity is frequently equal to that of the liver, unlike in the adult where the kidney is relatively hypoechoic. The medullary pyramids are hypoechoic and more prominent than in an adult, and the renal sinus fat is less prominent, probably because a neonate has less overall body fat and thus has less renal sinus fat. By 6 months of age, most infants have a renal cortex that is less echogenic than liver.

The renal size should be checked against a table of normal renal size by age, so it can be determined if the kidneys are appropriate for the patient's age (Table 6–26).

Embryologically, the kidney develops from the fusion of two metanephric elements. The site of fusion may lead to a small indentation in the renal cortex called the junctional defect (Fig. 6–3). This is an echogenic focus on the margin of the kidney. This junctional defect may be con-

Table 6–26. SONOGRAPHIC RENAL LENGTH VERSUS AGE

AGE (yr)	SIZE (cm)	AGE (yr)	SIZE (cm)
0	5	6	8.1
0.2	5.4	8	8.6
0.4	5.7	10	9
0.6	6.1	12	9.4
0.8	6.5	14	9.9
1	7	16	10.3
2	7.2	18	10.8
4	7.7		

Standard deviation = .69 cm under age 1
= .79 over age 1
From Rosenbaum DM, Korngold E, Teele RL. AJR 142:467–469, 1984, with permission.

nected to the renal hilum by an echogenic line called the interrenicular septum, which is also a result of this fusion. These are normal findings and should not be confused with pathology.

CONGENITAL ABNORMALITIES

Renal agenesis may occur bilaterally with an incidence of about 1 in 4,000 live births. These infants die quickly of pulmonary hypoplasia. Ultrasound shows no kidneys. Care must be taken not to mistake an enlarged hyperplastic adrenal gland sitting in the renal fossa for a kidney. In cases of unilateral renal agenesis, care is also necessary to avoid mistaking an adrenal gland for a kidney. These patients are at increased risk for anomalies of the reproductive system and also of the cardiovascular or gastrointestinal systems.

Pancake and horseshoe kidneys are other abnormalities that may occur. These may be difficult to visualize and may simulate the appearance of bowel. The lower poles of a horseshoe kidney are often connected by only a fibrous band that may be impossible to see at ultrasound. If the lower poles of both kidneys deviate medially and the renal pelvis faces anteriorly, then a horseshoe kidney may be present. Cross-fused renal ectopia is when both kidneys are on the same side of the retroperitoneum and the ureter from the ectopic one crosses the midline and enters the bladder normally. This kidney will frequently be fused to the lower pole of the nonectopic kidney. This condition can be very difficult to recognize at ultrasound.

Duplications of the renal collecting system are common. They may be either incomplete or complete. In complete duplication, there are two complete collecting systems with two ureters entering the bladder. The lower pole ureter usually enters in a normal location, but frequently has a shorter course within the wall of the bladder, and therefore, may be prone to reflux. The upper pole ureter inserts in a distal location toward the base of the bladder and is prone to obstruction. The upper pole ureter, which is ectopic, may insert into areas other than the bladder, including the vagina, uterus, or urethra in girls and into the urethra, seminal vesicle, or vas deferens in boys. If the ectopic ureter inserts below the external sphincter, then urinary incontinence results. This distal ectopic ureter may be complicated by ureterocele. Also, the distal ureter can be stenotic, and the result of either a ureterocele or a stenosis may be obstruction. Therefore, it is typical for the upper pole moiety to be obstructed. However, the lower pole of the ureter may also be dilated due to reflux.

In an incomplete duplication, there are two renal pelvises, but somewhere along the course of the ureter, there is fusion with the result of only a single ureter entering the bladder. These are common and are usually of no significance clinically. They are recognized sonographically by two clumps of echogenic fat in the renal pelvis (Fig. 6–30).

URETEROPELVIC JUNCTION OBSTRUCTION

Obstruction at the ureteropelvic junction is the most common etiology of upper urinary tract obstruction in children. At ultrasound, multiple cystic structures will be identified. There will be communication between the cysts since they represent calices. The renal pelvis should be identifiable. When an attempt is made to identify the proximal ureter as it leaves the renal pelvis, it will either be nonidentifiable or will be of normal caliber. The parenchyma of the kidney may have abnormal echogenicity or even contain cysts. This may be a result of renal dysplasia secondary to the obstruction. If the ureter is enlarged, then the possibility of reflux as a cause of the hydronephrosis should be considered. This will require examination of the ureters by a retrograde study.

MEGAURETER

Megaureter may be either primary or secondary. Secondary megaureter is due to obstruction, a neurogenic bladder, or very high urinary flow. Primary megaureter occurs either because of fibrous tissue obstructing a portion of the ureter or a portion of the ureter that is lacking smooth muscle and, therefore, has no peristalsis. The entire ureter may be dilated down to a distal segment that is not functioning properly or only a segmental portion of the ureter may be involved, and therefore, a small portion may be dilated. It is not unusual to have

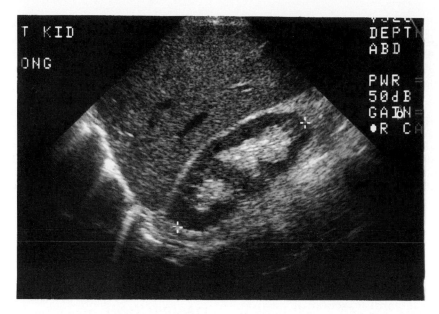

Figure 6–30. Renal sinus fat is divided into two clumps of echogenic fat indicating duplication of the collecting system.

dilatation of the pelvis and calices of the ipsilateral kidney. When the dilated ureter is identified, then it is important to attempt to determine if there is an obstructing lesion present. This is not always possible with ultrasound. The ureter should be followed from the renal pelvis to the base of the bladder, if possible, but only in a small percentage of patients can this be done.

EAGLE-BARRETT SYNDROME

The Eagle-Barrett syndrome, or prune belly, consists of a deficiency of the muscles of the anterior abdominal wall, hypotonic dilated ureters, a large bladder, and a urachus extending from the bladder domes. In addition, there is associated bilateral cryptorchidism and dilatation of the prostatic urethra. These findings are secondary to decreased or deficient muscle fibers throughout the genitourinary tract. These patients have dilated ureters and a large bladder. They may have dilated calices and pelvis. The kidneys may be dysplastic in appearance.

POSTERIOR URETHRAL VALVES

Posterior urethral valves are mostly a male disorder. These membranous valves are in the proximal portion of the urethra and cause obstruction of the urethra and ul-

timately the bladder. Dilatation of the proximal urethra, bladder, ureters, and kidneys may result. The posterior urethral valves cannot be seen with ultrasound, but a dilated proximal urethra may be seen if ultrasound is performed as the patient empties his bladder. A cystogram is the optimal study for evaluation of this problem.

NEUROGENIC BLADDER

A neurogenic bladder may result from a patient with a meningomyelocele or some other cause of spinal cord dysfunction. Usually, the bladder is dilated, and this may result in dilatation of the ureters and proximal collecting systems. The bladder will usually have a thick, irregular wall.

RENAL CYSTIC DISEASE

Multicystic dysplastic kidney is usually a unilateral disease, although the patient may have associated ureteropelvic junction obstruction on the opposite side. On ultrasound, the kidney will have multiple cysts of varying size, and the renal parenchyma may look quite dysplastic. The ureter is small or atretic, and the renal artery is either small or absent. The kidney functions minimally or not at all. The cysts will be separated by septa. The kidney is usually enlarged. Over the long term, these kidneys tend to atrophy, and the current thinking is that surgical removal may not be necessary.

Infantile polycystic kidney disease presents with enlarged, poorly functioning kidneys. The kidneys are enlarged on ultrasound, and are usually echogenic (Fig. 6–31). The cysts in this disease are 1 to 2 mm and up to 1 cm in diameter. On ultrasound, it may not be possible to discretely identify cysts. Infantile polycystic kidney disease is associated with biliary ductal ectasia with periportal fibrosis. In general, the worse the renal disease, the less severe the hepatic fibrosis. Patients who present early in renal failure tend to have minimal hepatic fibrosis, but the children who present in late childhood with renal disease frequently have severe hepatic fibrosis. It should be noted that some patients do have macroscopic cysts that can be seen on ultrasound in the region of the medullary pyramids. The liver may become quite echogenic in this disease secondary to the hepatic fibrosis.

Autosomal dominant polycystic kidney disease includes large cysts that can be seen on ultrasound. This disease may present in childhood. Cysts may also be found in the liver, pancreas, and spleen.

Acquired cystic disease occurs in patients on either hemodialysis or peritoneal dialysis. They may develop macroscopic cysts in their kidneys. These can usually be identified with ultrasound. The incidence of adenomas and carcinomas in these kidneys is increased.

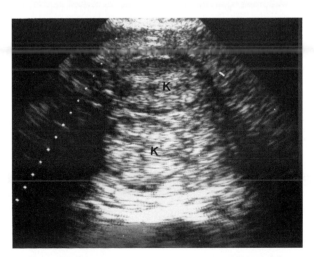

Figure 6–31. Echogenic enlarged kidneys (K) in infantile polycystic kidney disease. Coronal image.

INFLAMMATORY DISEASE OF THE KIDNEY

Infection

Acute pyelonephritis is an ascending infection from the bladder via reflux. Usually, the ultrasound will show normal kidneys. However, sometimes the kidney will be swollen and may have decreased echogenicity secondary to edema. Occasionally, thickening of the wall of the renal pelvis may be seen. Acute lobar nephronia is a focal pyelonephritis leading to a localized area of decreased echogenicity. This localized area may be mass-like in appearance. The mass may liquify and develop a renal abscess. With adequate antibiotic treatment, the mass in the area of decreased echogenicity will disappear.

Sonography of an abscess shows as a focal area of decreased echogenicity with an appearance resembling that of fluid. Pyonephrosis occurs when the debris is identified in the collecting system secondary to infection (Fig. 6–32). This occurs in an obstructed system.

Chronic pyelonephritis is probably the end result of reflux plus infection with scarring of both the collecting system and renal parenchyma. Patients may develop fungus balls in the collecting system. These are usually due to *Candida* and are common in diabetics. A mass will be seen, but there will be no shadowing.

Noninfectious Renal Disease

Glomerulonephritis is a form of inflammatory disease that is usually not infectious. It may occur after streptococcal infection. Acute glomerulonephritis will usually lead to large edematous kidneys. The echogenicity may be either increased or decreased. Medullary pyramids may be spared so that they are much more hypoechogenic than the echogenic cortex. Renal diseases have been divided into two categories based on whether or not cortical medullary differentiation is lost or is retained (see Tables 6–1 and 2).

With chronic glomerulonephritis and most of the chronic nonobstructive, noninfectious renal diseases, the kidneys ultimately become small and echogenic.

Children with a urinary tract infection are

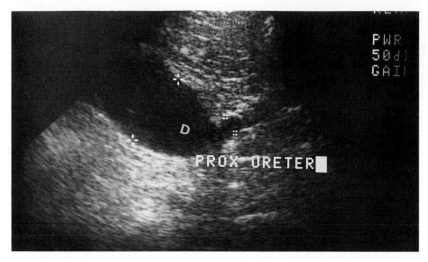

Figure 6–32. Dilated renal pelvis and proximal ureter. Faint echoes due to debris (D) indicate pyonephrosis.

evaluated for vesicoureteral reflex and anatomic abnormalities. A voiding cystourethrogram (VCUG) is usually the test of choice as about 20 percent of these children will have reflux. While ultrasound can detect reflux if it distends the renal pelvis and calices, it is not sensitive at detecting reflux into ureters. However, ultrasound is still useful when a first urinary tract infection has occurred because it may detect anatomic abnormalities such as renal ectopia and duplicated collecting systems. Some of these children may have had previous silent infections and scarring of the kidneys may be seen.

When renal hydronephrosis is detected by fetal ultrasound, a renal ultrasound and VCUG should be performed after delivery. These tests are done to detect reflux and anatomic anomalies. The ultrasound should not be done on day one because a relative physiologic dehydration may mask hydronephrosis and the kidneys may look normal. Even though there is pressure to perform the ultrasound immediately after birth so the infant may go home, the study should be done between day three and day seven.

PEDIATRIC CALCULUS DISEASE

Several pediatric diseases develop diffuse bilateral punctate calcifications. These include renal tubular acidosis, hyperparathyroidism, and hypervitaminosis D. In these diseases, the calcifications are usually confined to the medulla. Chronic glomerulonephritis may cause cortical calcifications diffusely and bilaterally. Furosemide therapy can also cause calcifications in the kidneys, which may be seen in both the cortex and medulla and may be bilateral.

Renal stones from other causes are seen less frequently than in adults. The appearance is similar to that in adults, with an echogenic focus with shadowing behind it. Ultrasound is less sensitive than plain films or CT for the detection of calculi.

RENAL VEIN THROMBOSIS

Renal vein thrombosis is usually seen in the neonatal period and is associated with dehydration, but may also be associated with hypercoagulable states, such as polycythemia. It occurs more often in infants of diabetic mothers. The kidney will be enlarged with a distorted appearance with areas of increased and decreased echogenicity and loss of the cortical medullary differentiation. Only rarely will thrombus be seen in the renal vein or inferior vena cava. However, Doppler may be unable to detect flow in the renal veins, and there may be reversed diastolic flow when pulsed Doppler of the ipsilateral renal artery is performed. Over time this kidney may become an end-stage kidney with decrease in size and an increase in echogenicity, or the process may resolve, and the kidney may resume a normal appearance.

RENAL TUMORS

Wilms' tumor usually occurs between ages 2 and 5 years. This is a large tumor that frequently distorts the kidney and the collecting system. It is usually homogeneous ultrasonographically but may have some inhomogeneous hypoechoic areas. Bilateral Wilms' tumors may be present in less than 10 percent of cases. Wilms' tumors are associated with Beckwith-Wiedemann syndrome, congenital hemihypertrophy, aniridia, or neurofibromatosis. Like a renal cell carcinoma, this tumor may spread into the renal vein and then into the inferior vena cava. The echogenicity of this tumor is usually slightly less than that of the adjacent normal kidney. Nephroblastomatosis is a congenital renal lesion that is a precursor of Wilms' tumor. It may be found in up to one-third of kidneys with Wilms' tumor and is also found in the diseases that have a high predisposition to Wilms' tumor. The kidneys involved with nephroblastomatosis are usually normal in size, although they may have lobules secondary to the nephroblastomas. Frequently, these areas of nephroblastomatosis are not recognizable on ultrasound because the echogenicity is nearly identical to that of the adjacent renal parenchyma.

Neuroblastoma is the second-most common childhood abdominal tumor after Wilms'. It occurs at a slightly earlier age, usually before age two. Neuroblastoma will have a heterogeneous echo appearance with multiple areas of increased echogenicity and calcification. It is much less well defined than Wilms'. It also may be associated with Beckwith-Wiedemann syndrome. Other diseases with which it is seen include Klippel-Feil, fetal alcohol syndrome, fetal Dilantin syndrome, and Hirschsprung's disease.

A mesoblastic nephroma is a fetal renal hamartoma that resembles Wilms' tumor. It is usually found in the first few months of life when a mass is detected. Ultrasound shows a hypoechoic mass. The mass may resemble a Wilms' tumor. It is distinguished from Wilms' by the young age of the patient. It has a favorable outcome.

Renal cell carcinoma is rare in the pediatric age range. It usually presents as a hypoechoic mass.

Angiomyolipoma is a hamartoma. These tumors can hemorrhage. They are associated with tuberous sclerosis. On ultrasound, the mass will have areas of varying echogenicity. Hyperechoic regions are probably secondary to fat. There may also be cysts in these kidneys, and the kidneys may be enlarged. CT is an accurate way to confirm the presence of fat and make the diagnosis.

Multilocular cystic nephroma is an uncommon lesion that has predominantly benign behavior. It usually occurs in males less than 4 years of age. There is a second peak incidence in adult females. On ultrasound this lesion usually is a large mass with multiple anechoic areas separated by a septa. The appearance is similar to that of multicystic dysplastic kidney.

Renal lymphoma occurs more often in non-Hodgkin's lymphoma than Hodgkin's disease. It usually presents as multiple hypoechoic nodules. These should be seen in both kidneys. They may show through transmission. Occasionally, a renal lymphoma will infiltrate a kidney, and no nodule will be seen. This usually happens when there is disease in adjacent lymph nodes.

Leukemic infiltrates may occur in the kidneys. The kidneys will become enlarged and have a distorted architectural appearance. Occasionally, hypoechoic nodules are identified.

Whenever a renal ultrasound is performed, the bladder should also be examined. The bladder wall, if the bladder is well distended, should be 2 mm or less in thickness in children. The bladder wall may become thickened any time the bladder is obstructed. Cystitis may also result in thickening of the bladder wall. Patients with neurogenic bladders may have thickening of the bladder wall. Rarely, congenital polyps may be seen projecting into the bladder. Usually if a mass is in the bladder in the pediatric age group, then either hematoma or a fungus ball should be suspected.

Suggested Readings

Davidson AJ, Hartman DS. Radiology of the Kidney and Urinary Tract. 2nd ed. Philadelphia, WB Saunders Company, 1994.

Fernbach SK, Feinstein KA. Selected topics in pediatric ultrasonography. Radiol Clin North Am 30: 1011–1031, 1992.

Jafri SZ, Madrazo BL, Miller JH. Color Doppler ultrasound of the genitourinary tract. Curr Opin Radiol 4:16–23, 1992.

Mittelstaedt CA. General Ultrasound. New York, Churchill Livingstone, 1992.

CHAPTER 7

Ultrasound of the Female Pelvis

Ultrasound of the female pelvis consists of the evaluation of the uterus, ovaries, and adjacent adnexae. Patients are scanned when the bladder is full, unless endovaginal scanning is used.

Anatomy

The uterus is predominantly smooth muscle. It has a homogeneous appearance and is normally long and thin. It may be in a neutral position or may be anteverted, anteflexed, retroverted, or retroflexed. Anteverted or retroverted means that the uterus is straight but is tilted either anteriorly or posteriorly. Anteflexed or retroflexed means that the uterus has a bend in it between the uterine body and the cervix and the bend either allows the fundus to bend anteriorly or posteriorly depending on whether or not it is anteflexed or retroflexed (Fig. 7–1).

In most patients, an endometrial stripe can be identified. The appearance of the endometrial stripe varies depending on the time in the menstrual cycle (Fig. 7–2). Immediately after menses, the line will be a single echogenic line (Fig. 7–2A). Early in the proliferative stage of the menstrual cycle the echogenic line becomes surrounded by a hypoechoic functional layer (Fig. 7–2B). Later on in the proliferative stage, as ovulation nears, this functional layer becomes very thick, with a thin echogenic line going down the middle of it (Fig. 7–2C). The thin line represents the endometrial canal. Finally, the secretory endometrium just before menses is a thick, bright echogenic layer (Fig. 7–2D). In a woman of reproductive age, the endometrial stripe should be no thicker than 14 mm, including the echogenic stripe and the surrounding hypoechoic layers. In a postmenopausal female, we use 6 mm as an upper limit, although estrogens may increase this to 10 mm. The differential diagnosis for a thick endometrial stripe is given in Table 7–1.

The uterus has three portions. The part above the entrance of the tubes is called the fundus. The cervix consists mostly of fibrous tissue and is at the lower end of the uterus. Between the cervix and the fundus is the body.

The uterus should be measured from the cervix to the tip of the fundus for length. Width and anteroposterior diameter may also be measured. We use an upper limit of normal for length of about 11 cm for premenopausal women and about 10 cm for postmenopausal women. Normal uterine sizes are given in Table 7–2. The differential diagnosis for an enlarged uterus is given in Table 7–3.

The ovaries are located posterolaterally to the uterus. The internal iliac artery can frequently be used as a marker as the ovaries often lie anterior to this artery. However, in a woman who has been pregnant, the uterus may have pushed the ovaries to the upper pelvis, and they may not have returned to their previous location. Therefore it is best to consider that the ovary may be found in any location throughout the pelvis. Ovarian volume is calculated by multiplying height × width × length and multiplying by .52. This is the formula for a prolate ellipsoid. Under age 5, the ovary should have a volume less than 1 ml. The ovary gradually increases in size during puberty. In a female of reproductive age, the ovary may be 9.8 ± 5.8 cu cm. The 95 percent confidence range is 2.5 to 21.9 cu cm.

143

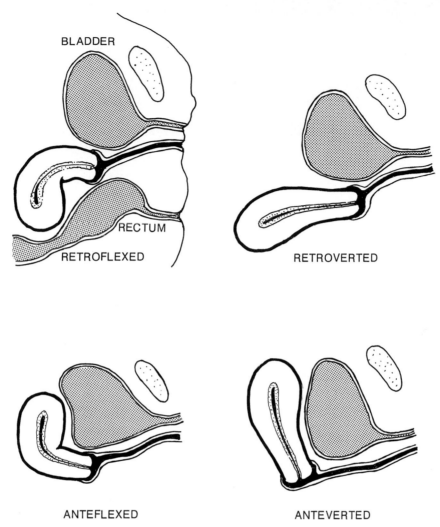

Figure 7–1. Sagittal schematics. An anteflexed or retroflexed uterus has a bend or flexion point in the uterus itself. With an anteverted or retroverted uterus, there is no bend in the uterus but the entire uterus angles either anteriorly or posteriorly. Pubic bone is dotted structure. Pubic bone is depicted to right of bladder.

Table 7–1. THICK ENDOMETRIAL STRIPE

Secretory endometrium
Endometrial hyperplasia
Endometrial carcinoma
Endometritis
IUD
Retained products of conception
Gestational trophoblastic disease
Hematometra
Pyometra
Adenomyosis
Tamoxifen
Early intrauterine pregnancy
Ectopic pregnancy
Endometrial polyps

The 95 percent confidence interval for premenarchal is .2 to 9.1 and for postmenopausal is 1.2 to 14.1 cu cm.

Congenital Anomalies of the Uterus

Congenital anomalies of the uterus may be secondary to failure of the müllerian duct to develop, failure of the two müllerian ducts to fuse, or failure of the median septum of the uterus to resorb (Fig. 7–3).

When the müllerian duct does not develop, the uterus becomes hypoplastic or

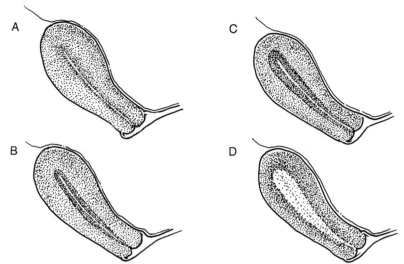

Figure 7–2. *A,* Immediately after menses, a single echogenic line is seen. *B,* Proliferative stage: hypoechoic functional layer develops around echogenic line. *C,* Near ovulation, functional layer thickens. *D,* Secretory endometrium just before menses. A thick bright stripe is present. (From Forrest TS, Elyaderani MK, Muilenburg MI, et al. Cyclic endometrial changes: US assessment with histologic correlation. Radiology *167*:233–237, 1988, with permission.)

Table 7–2. UTERINE LENGTHS BY AGE

GROUP	LENGTH	WIDTH	A-P
Neonatal	3.4 ± .6 cm	1.2 ± .5 cm	
Infants to age 7	3.2 ± .4 cm	.7 ± .15 cm	
Premenopausal, nulliparous	7.1 ± .8 cm	4.6 ± .6 cm	3.3 ± .8 cm
Premenopausal, parous	8.9 ± 1.0 cm	5.8 ± .8 cm	4.3 ± .6 cm
Postmenopausal	7.9 ± 1.2 cm	4.9 ± .8 cm	3.2 ± .7 cm

Data from Orsini LF, Saladri S, Pilu G, et al. Pelvic organs in premenarcheal girls: real-time ultrasonography. Radiology *153*:113–116, 1984; Nussbaum AR, Sanders RC, Jones MD. Neonatal uterine morphology as seen on real-time US. Radiology *160*:641–643, 1986; Platt JF, Bree RL, Davidson D. Ultrasound of the normal nongravid uterus: correlation with gross and histopathology. J Clin Ultrasound *18*:15–19, 1990; Miller EI, Thomas RH, Lines P. The atrophic postmenopausal uterus. J Clin Ultrasound *5*:261–263, 1977.

aplastic. If both müllerian ducts do not develop, then uterine aplasia occurs. If one müllerian duct does not develop, then uterus unicornis unicollis (only a single uterine horn and cervix) develops.

Table 7–3. ENLARGED UTERUS

COMMON
Pregnancy
Postpartum state
Leiomyomas
Endometritis

UNCOMMON
Carcinoma
Hydrometrocolpos
Arteriovenous malformation of uterus
Adenomyosis

If the müllerian ducts are not fused, then a uterus didelphis results. In this case there are two vaginas, two cervices, and two uteruses. This may sometimes be diagnosed by an indentation in the superior portion of the uterus. Lesser degrees may lead to uterus bicornis bicollis in which there is a single vagina but two cervices and two uterine horns or uterus bicornis unicollis in which there is a single vagina, a single cervix, and two uterine horns.

If the median septum does not resorb, there may be two compartments to the uterus. However, the difference between this and the müllerian duct anomaly is that there is little or no indentation in the superior portion of the uterus.

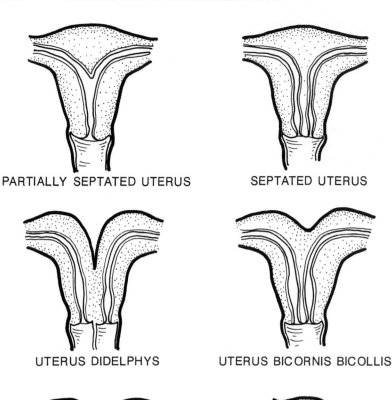

PARTIALLY SEPTATED UTERUS   SEPTATED UTERUS

UTERUS DIDELPHYS   UTERUS BICORNIS BICOLLIS

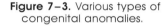

Figure 7–3. Various types of congenital anomalies.

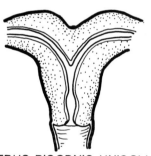

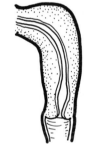

UTERUS BICORNIS UNICOLLIS   UTERUS UNICORNIS

If two endometrial stripes are seen, then it is important to determine which type of anomaly is present, if possible. Two stripes usually means there is a müllerian duct abnormality and it is necessary to determine if there are two cervices and two vaginas. The differentiation between a septate and a bicornuate uterus is important because a septated uterus can now be treated for infertility in an outpatient setting, resulting in a short recovery time. The bicornuate uterus still requires an abdominal surgical approach, if surgical therapy is performed. Ultrasound has been useful in distinguishing between these two conditions, but visualization of the notch at the superior portion of the uterine fundus is better performed by magnetic resonance imaging

(MRI). Sometimes one horn will have a pregnancy in it and the second horn will have an endometrial stripe and the diagnosis can be made (Fig. 7–4).

A T-shaped uterus may be the result of diethylstilbestrol exposure. At ultrasound, the uterus will be thin without a usual bulbous fundus.

In infants, hydrocolpos (watery fluid) or hematocolpos (bloody fluid) refers to a fluid-filled vagina due to obstruction from vaginal atresia, a septum, or imperforate hymen. If both vagina and uterus are fluid filled, then the term is hydrometrocolpos or hematometracolpos. If only the uterus is fluid filled, then the term is hematometras. If vaginal obstruction is present, then there frequently are other congenital anomalies.

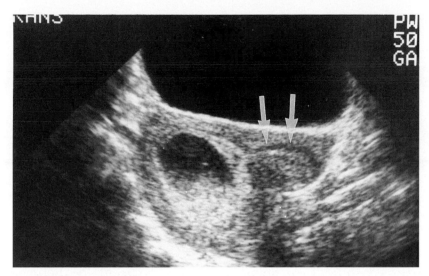

Figure 7–4. Bicornuate uterus, transverse image. Early gestational sac on right, endometrial stripe on left (*arrows*).

On ultrasound, only a cystic midline mass is seen separate from bladder and rectum. In adults, hematometras may occur from cervical carcinoma or other obstructing masses.

Tumors of the Uterus

LEIOMYOMAS

Fibroids are leiomyomas, a common benign tumor of the uterus. Estimates are that they occur in one-third of women over age 30. They are more common in blacks and dark-skinned people. They consist of smooth muscle and fibrous tissue. If there is more fibrous tissue, then the fibroid may be very echogenic, whereas, if there is more smooth muscle, then the fibroid may be relatively echolucent. Usually leiomyomas absorb sound and have poor through transmission.

Leiomyomas may undergo secondary degeneration and ultimate calcification. This will change the sonographic appearance and may lead to a calcified sonographic mass. If necrosis occurs, there may be cystic type lucencies in the center of the mass. Most women who have one leiomyoma will have others.

It is not always possible to identify leiomyomas with ultrasound as the contrast between the leiomyoma and the adjacent smooth muscle of the uterus may not be sufficient to allow definition of discrete borders. There are other secondary signs of the presence of leiomyomas that can be useful if the lesion cannot be discretely identified. The uterus may be elongated or have an increase in its anteroposterior or transverse diameter. In particular, the uterine fundus may become quite bulbous and the uterine contour may become "bumpy." These signs can be suggestive of the presence of leiomyomas. The endometrial stripe may also be bowed or displaced by a leiomyoma. This displacement also indicates the presence of an adjacent tumor. Obviously, neither of these last two signs is specific for leiomyomas. We estimate that only about 60 percent of patients with leiomyomas can be identified by ultrasound. MRI is much more sensitive, if there is an absolute need to identify a leiomyoma for excision.

In the past, it has been thought that leiomyomas increase in size and undergo degeneration during pregnancy. While these tumors are estrogen sensitive, it is disputed as to whether or not they truly increase in size during pregnancy.

Leiomyomas should not be a problem during pregnancy and delivery unless they involve the lower uterine segment (Fig. 7–5). A leiomyoma near the cervical canal can obstruct delivery of the fetus.

When the uterus is retroflexed, the fundus of the uterus may appear hypoechoic and simulate a leiomyoma. The identification of leiomyomas in this area in a retro

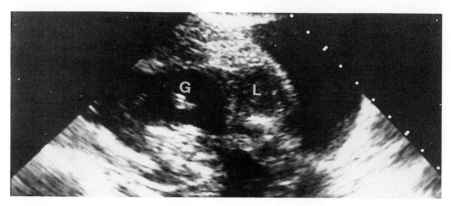

Figure 7–5. Longitudinal image. Hypoechoic leiomyoma (L) involving lower uterine segment. Early gestational sac (G).

flexed uterus is very difficult. At times, it may be useful to do endovaginal ultrasound to evaluate for leiomyomas, but fundal lesions are usually out of range of high-frequency endovaginal transducers.

There are three types of leiomyomas. The submucosal type is just under the surface of the endometrium and may actually distort the endometrial stripe. Subserosal leiomyomas are near the outside surface of the uterus. These may be pedunculated and project outside of the contour of the uterus. These can be a problem because they may simulate an adnexal mass. The most common type of leiomyoma is intramural and is within the substance of the myometrium.

After menopause, the leiomyoma should not increase in size. If a leiomyoma increases in size in an older woman, this may indicate it has transformed into a leiomyosarcoma.

LEIOMYOSARCOMAS

These are rare tumors and they are thought to be the result of sarcomatous change in a leiomyoma. They usually cause bleeding, but patients may be asymptomatic. The ultrasound appearance of a leiomyosarcoma is not significantly different from that of a leiomyoma.

ENDOMETRIAL POLYPS

These are neoplastic tissue that are a result of either hyperplastic or adenomatous change in the endometrium. They may cause uterine bleeding and sometimes will prolapse into the vagina. They most commonly occur in the perimenopausal age groups. On ultrasound these polyps cause a prominent and sometimes irregular endometrial echo complex.

ADENOMYOSIS

Adenomyosis occurs when endometrial cells penetrate into the myometrium. This tissue can bleed during menses and cause pelvic pain. Ultrasound is not sensitive for this condition but at times the diagnosis can be suggested by multiple echolucencies within the myometrium that are caused by repeated hemorrhage into the smooth muscle. Alternatively, the myometrium may be more echogenic in this region. The most common ultrasound finding is simply diffuse uterine enlargement. Focal adenomyosis may be indistinguishable from a leiomyoma. MRI is currently considered the primary means for diagnosing this condition.

ENDOMETRIAL HYPERPLASIA

Estrogen stimulation unopposed by progesterone is a common cause of uterine bleeding and leads to hyperplasia of the endometrium. This diagnosis may be suggested by ultrasound when the endometrial stripe is thicker than usual. Differential diagnosis of a broad bright endometrial stripe should include endometrial carcinoma and other entities (Table 7–1).

ENDOMETRITIS

Endometritis may be a result of a bacterial infection secondary to delivery or may

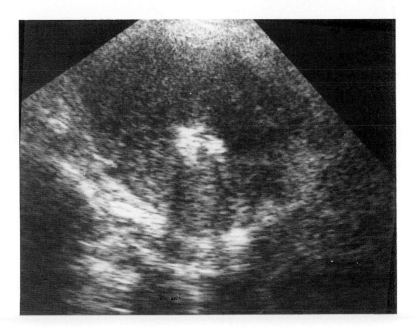

Figure 7–6. Transverse image of uterus showing thickened irregular endometrium from endometritis.

occur as an iatrogenic complication from dilatation and curettage or from a therapeutic abortion (Fig. 7–6). It can also be seen as part of pelvic inflammatory disease. On ultrasound, endometritis will produce increased echogenicity and thickening of the endometrium. A broad bright endometrial stripe will be identified (Table 7–1). Gas bubbles may sometimes be seen in the region of the endometrial canal and may cause shadowing (Table 7–4). The appearance of endometritis may not be distinguishable from endometrial hyperplasia or endometrial carcinoma or even a normal menses. Sometimes, endometritis is manifest by echolucent fluid in the endometrium (Table 7–5).

ENDOMETRIAL CARCINOMA

This neoplasm occurs in older women. They usually present with uterine bleeding. On ultrasound, there is once again a broad bright endometrial stripe secondary to the thickened endometrium indistinguishable from endometrial hyperplasia or polyps.

Intrauterine Devices (IUDs)

Ultrasound is frequently used to make certain an IUD is still in place. IUDs are very echogenic and may cause shadowing (Fig. 7–7). The shape of the IUD depends on the type. Usually the IUD is distinguishable from the normal endometrial stripe because it is much brighter than the normal stripe. Eccentric position of the IUD suggests the possibility of penetration into the myometrium. If a pregnancy is concurrent with an IUD, the IUD may be identifiable early in the pregnancy but as the pregnancy progresses, the IUD may not be found.

Table 7–4. ENDOMETRIAL SHADOWING

Gas
Intrauterine device
Calcified fibroids
Retained products of conception
Osteoid tissue

Table 7–5. ENDOMETRIAL FLUID

COMMON
Endometritis
Retained products of conception
Incomplete abortion
Pelvic inflammatory disease
Cervical obstruction

UNCOMMON
Endometrial carcinoma
Adenomyosis
After perforation
Imperforate hymen
Cervical carcinoma

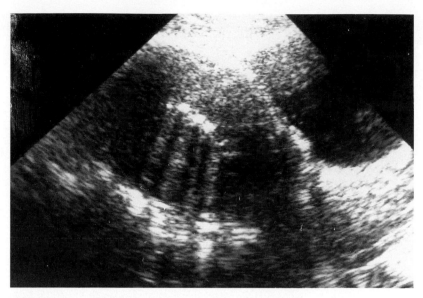

Figure 7–7. Long image of uterus shows echogenic IUD with shadowing.

Cervix

The normal cervix may be more echogenic than the remainder of the uterus due to the fact that there is more fibrous tissue in the cervix than in the uterus. Although it has been said that carcinoma of the cervix presents as a hypoechoic enlarged cervix, ultrasound is usually not utilized in the diagnosis of carcinoma of the cervix. Occasionally an enlarged cervix may be identified. Metastatic disease to pelvic lymph nodes may sometimes be seen on ultrasound.

Nabothian cysts of the cervix may sometimes be seen. They are usually several millimeters in size. Occasionally they can be up to a few centimeters in size.

Fluid in the Cul-De-Sac

Small amounts of fluid in the posterior cul-de-sac between the uterus and the rectum are a normal finding. This area, also known as the pouch of Douglas, is one of the lowest points in the body, and a few milliliters of fluid may be identifiable using sonography. The normal amounts of fluid seen in the cul-de-sac have an unknown source.

If the amount of fluid becomes more than a few milliliters, then the possibility of a pathologic etiology should be considered. Possibilities would include rupture of an ovarian cyst, pelvic inflammatory disease, generalized ascites, hemorrhage from various sources, an abscess originating from various sources, endometritis, or other forms of ovarian pathology.

Ovary

FUNCTIONAL CYSTS

Functional cysts include follicles that have not yet discharged their egg and follicular cysts that result from a failure of a follicle to develop properly and involute appropriately. After ovulation, the follicle forms a corpus luteum that secretes progesterone. If no implantation occurs, the corpus luteum involutes. If implantation does occur, the corpus luteum persists through the end of the first trimester. Corpus luteal cysts are a type of functional cyst. They may persist if involution does not occur (Fig. 7–8). Theca-lutein cysts occur when there are high levels of human chorionic gonadotropin. Classically, these are associated with gestational trophoblastic disease but also can be seen in patients who are being treated with infertility drugs. These cysts should be bilateral and can be quite large (see Fig. 8–16). They can also occur in normal pregnancies, especially twins.

Follicles can frequently be seen in ovaries, especially if transvaginal scanning is employed and if the patient is of reproduc-

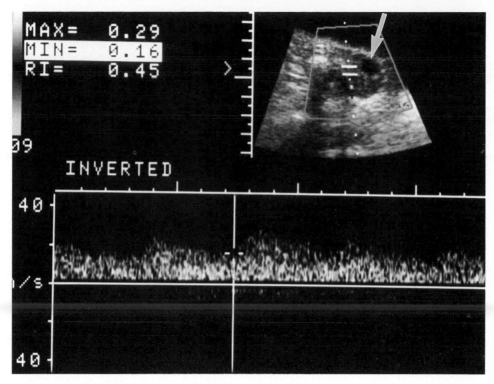

Figure 7–8. Corpus luteum cysts (*arrow*). Doppler shows high diastolic flow that is common with this type of cyst.

tive age. Follicles normally range from a few millimeters up to 2.5 cm. Follicular cysts cannot be diagnosed until they reach 2.5 cm in size since normal follicles may be up to 2.5 cm. Follicular cysts can progress to even larger sizes and can measure up to 20 cm in diameter.

All of these cysts can have internal septations. Hemorrhage can occur in all these cysts, but is most common in the corpus luteal cyst. If hemorrhage occurs, there will be many internal echoes.

These cysts will usually regress over a period of several months and one logical diagnostic step is to simply follow these patients with periodic ultrasound exams.

Polycystic ovary syndrome (PCOS) or Stein-Leventhal syndrome classically presents with symptoms of amenorrhea, hirsutism, obesity, and infertility, but the majority of patients are not "classic." Multiple follicles develop early but do not reach maturation. Many of these patients have ovaries that are enlarged, but at least one-third will have normal-sized ovaries. Attempts have been made to count the number of follicles

using endovaginal ultrasound. However, there is overlap between control subjects and those with PCOS. The diagnosis of PCOS cannot be made reliably with ultrasound, but if there are large ovaries with greater than 15 follicles, then the diagnosis can be suggested.

Follicular cysts and theca-lutein cysts may secrete estrogens while the corpus lutein cyst may secrete progesterone. The differential diagnosis of cystic or complex adnexal masses is given in Table 7–6.

PAROVARIAN CYSTS

These cysts arise from wolffian duct remnants and are found in the adnexa within the broad ligament. They may have an appearance identical to that of any other ovarian cyst and confusion may arise as to which structure is truly the ovary. The lesion should be suspected to be parovarian in origin when a second structure is identified in the adnexa, which resembles an ovary. These cysts are not cyclical and will not regress over several menstrual cycles.

Table 7–6. CYSTIC OR COMPLEX OVARY OR ADNEXAL MASS

COMMON
Follicle
Follicular cysts
Cystadenoma
Cystadenocarcinoma
Corpus luteum cyst of pregnancy/PID
Ectopic pregnancy
Pelvic lymphadenopathy

UNCOMMON
Theca-lutein cysts
Mucocele of appendix
Ovarian torsion
Fallopian tube carcinoma
Duplication cysts of bowel
Cystic mesothelioma
Ovarian varicocele
Polycystic ovaries
Pelvic varices
Arteriovenous malformation of uterus and pelvis
Peritoneal inclusion cyst
Ovarian vein thrombophlebitis
Angiomyoma of cervix
Brenner tumor of ovary
Hemorrhagic cysts
Endometrioma
Leukemic infiltration
Hydrosalpinx
Teratoma
Degenerated leiomyoma
Anterior meningocele
Pelvic kidney

ENDOMETRIOMAS

Endometriomas may take on a cystic appearance in the adnexa. Sonography is not sensitive for these lesions. However, a complex cystic to cystic mass in the adnexa may be an endometrioma (Fig. 7–9). MRI would be the test of choice for endometrioma at this time. These lesions can be a few millimeters in size to multiple centimeters. Since endometriosis commonly involves the ovary, these may simulate an ovarian cyst.

POSTMENOPAUSAL CYSTS

In older women, the development of an ovarian cyst is cause for concern since these are not physiologic. These have been called "serous inclusion cysts." If these are simple cysts and less than 5 cm in diameter, they can safely be followed by serial ultrasound exams.

TORSION OF THE OVARY

Torsion occurs when the ovary twists on its pedicle and the blood supply to the ovary is compromised. The ovary becomes edematous and congested. This condition is more common in children and adolescent females. It also occurs in conjunction with ovarian cysts or masses. The cyst or mass causes the ovary to be very lopsided with weight unevenly distributed. This predisposes the ovary to rotate. These patients present with pelvic pain. The classic finding is an enlarged ovary with multiple cysts around the periphery. These cysts are felt to be follicles that have accumulated extra fluid secondary to the edema of the ovary. In our experience, this has not been a common finding, and usually torsion simply results in enlargement of the ovary (Fig. 7–10). On ultrasound, enlargement may be either solid, complex cystic, or almost completely cystic. Color Doppler ultrasound has been used to diagnose ovarian torsion. Supposedly, flow around the periphery with lack of central flow into the ovary indicates torsion. The appearance is similar to that seen in torsion of the testicles. However, we have had several cases with central flow seen on Doppler in women whose ovaries were torsed at surgery. This may be because flow may persist with partial or intermittent torsion. Caution is advised.

OVARIAN NEOPLASMS

Ovarian neoplasms are divided into epithelial, stromal, germ cell, and metastatic tumors. Tabulations of the types of ovarian pathology would indicate that significant numbers of these tumors are bilateral. However, in our experience, bilateral tumors are much less common on ultrasound than at surgery or pathology. These tumors often present as ovarian enlargement. However, there can be many other causes of ovarian enlargement (Table 7–7).

Epithelial Tumors

Serous cystadenoma and cystadenocarcinomas are the most common types of epithelial tumors and the most common ovarian tumors in general (Fig. 7–11). These tumors may grow to be quite large and commonly measure 15 to 20 cm. Benign serous cystadenomas cannot be differentiated

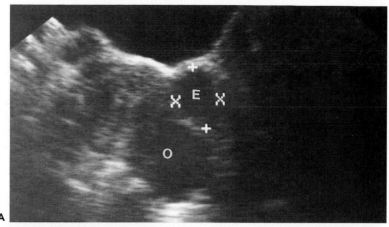

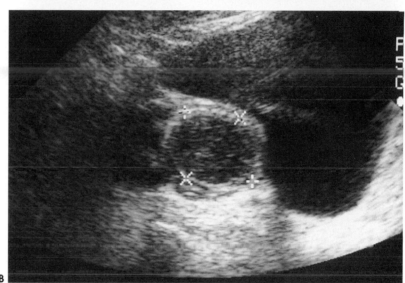

Figure 7–9. *A*, Transverse image. Ovary (O) and endometrioma (E). *B*, Different patient, long image. Endometrioma impinges on bladder.

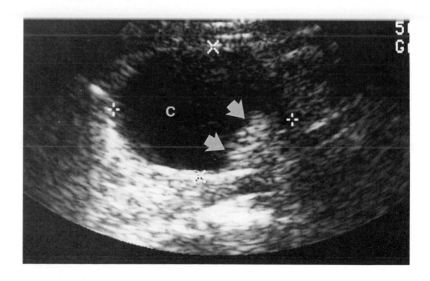

Figure 7–10. Torsion of the ovary. A large cyst is present measuring about 8 cm in diameter. The echogenic focus is a dermoid (*arrows*).

Table 7–7. ENLARGED OVARY

COMMON
Normal
Ectopic pregnancy
Follicular cysts
PID
Corpus luteum cyst of pregnancy
Carcinoma
Follicle

UNCOMMON
Polycystic ovaries
Metastases to ovary
Teratoma
Theca-lutein cysts
Ovarian torsion
Brenner tumor of ovary
Fibroma/thecoma of ovary
Dysgerminoma
Torsion of ovary
Fibrosarcoma
Leukemic infiltration
Pelvic kidney simulating ovary
Adnexal abscess adjacent to ovary
Endometrioma simulating ovary
McCune-Albright syndrome

from malignant serous cyst adenocarcinomas by ultrasound, but the larger the size the greater the likelihood the tumor is malignant.

These tumors frequently appear as multilocular cysts. They may contain solid tissue, commonly referred to as a papillary projection. There may be echogenic debris within the locules of the cyst. When these tumors are malignant, they tend to spread along peritoneal surfaces. Ascites frequently develop, and ascites in conjunction with a complex or cystic ovarian mass is an indicator of either a serous or mucinous malignancy that has spread into the peritoneum. These tumors also can metastasize to lymph nodes. Blood-borne metastases are seen only late in the development of cystadenomas or cystadenocarcinomas.

Mucinous Tumors

Mucinous cystadenomas, and cystadenocarcinomas are the second most common type of ovarian neoplasm and are indistinguishable from the serous type. Approximately 90 percent of these tumors are benign. These tumors also can be huge. There are reports of these tumors weighing several hundred pounds. On ultrasound, these tumors have a slight tendency to have more solid nodules and thicker septa than the serous form, but they cannot be definitively distinguished. These tumors also may cause ascites when they spread to peritoneal or serosal surfaces.

Endometrioid

Endometrioid carcinomas are almost always malignant. Their name comes from the fact that histologically they resemble endometrial carcinoma and are actually indistinguishable from this tumor. Originally it

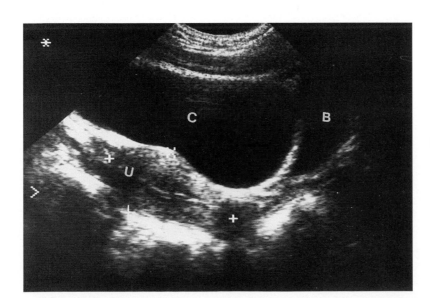

Figure 7–11. Longitudinal image. Large serous cystadenoma (C). B = Bladder, C = uterus.

was thought that endometrioid carcinomas could be metastases from endometrial carcinoma, but it is now thought that they arise separately within the substance of the ovary. Their ultrasound appearance ranges from complex cystic to solid. This is a relatively uncommon tumor.

Clear Cell Carcinomas

Clear cell carcinomas originate from the müllerian duct. They are only a small percentage of all ovarian neoplasms. Their ultrasound appearance is similar to that of the other tumors and ranges from complex cystic to solid.

Brenner Tumor

Brenner tumor is a benign type tumor and is quite uncommon. These tumors usually have multiple components and are usually solid masses. Most are benign.

Germ Cell Tumors

Germ cell tumors are divided into teratomas, dysgerminomas, and yolk sac tumors. The teratomas occur in the middle years. They are also known as dermoids or dermoid cysts because of the predominance of epidermoid-type tissue (Figs. 7–10 and 7–12). Strictly speaking, they have all the embryologic layers. They range from cystic to solid. Diagnosis can be suggested when

very echogenic components are seen in an ovary. Shadowing may be present. The echogenic components may be secondary to fat, teeth, or osseous tissue. These are generally removed surgically because they have a lifetime risk of conversion to malignancy of about 20 percent.

Struma ovarii is a type of teratoma in which thyroid tissue is present. This is quite rare. It may occur in prepubertal to teenage girls.

Dysgerminomas are undifferentiated malignant germ cell tumors. They resemble seminomas histologically. They occur more often in young females between 15 and 30 years of age. These are usually solid and echogenic by ultrasound. They are very radiosensitive and have a good survival rate.

Yolk sac tumors have a poor prognosis. They occur in girls below the age of 20. They are indistinguishable from other solid ovarian neoplasms.

Stromal Tumors

Stromal tumors consist of the granulosa cell tumor; Sertoli-Leydig cell tumor, also known as androblastoma; and thecomas and fibromas. Granulosa cell tumors occur in postmenopausal women, while Sertoli-Leydig cell tumors occur in women under age 30. These masses are usually solid.

Thecomas and fibromas sometimes have a distinctive ultrasound appearance in that they are solid and absorb sound. They tend

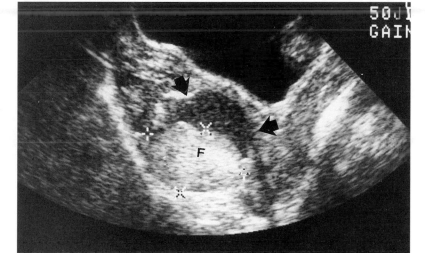

Figure 7–12. Longitudinal image. One enlarged ovary (*arrows*) with echogenic mass representing fat (F).

to be hypoechoic, with attenuation of the sound beam posteriorly.

Metastatic Tumors

Metastatic tumors usually come from the other ovary, breast, or gastrointestinal tract. Krukenberg tumors come from mucin-secreting tumors of the gastrointestinal tract. Endometrial carcinoma may metastasize to the ovary. Metastatic tumors will usually cause bilateral ovarian masses and will usually be solid on ultrasound.

DOPPLER OF ADNEXAL MASSES

Several investigators have evaluated the use of Doppler for determining whether an ovarian mass is malignant or benign. Malignant masses tend to have poorly formed capillary beds with large amounts of arteriovenous shunting and, therefore, have low diastolic resistance. Benign masses tend to have capillary beds and higher diastolic resistance. The pulsatility index and the resistive index have been used to distinguish between these two groups of tumors; however, there is some overlap. At the current time it would seem that these indices can be used as another factor in helping to distinguish whether a tumor is malignant or benign, but that they are not sufficient to make an absolute distinction.

The indexes are obtained by identifying several of the feeding vessels to the ovary and obtaining Doppler wave forms for them. A pulsatility index greater than 1.3 suggests benignity. A pulsatility index less than 1.1 is worrisome. A resistive index of less than .4 is worrisome for malignancy in reproductive-age women, and .4 to .6 is indeterminate. An index of less than .6 in postmenopausal women is worrisome. A mass with high resistance suggests a benign lesion. A low-resistance adnexal mass may result from malignancy, ectopic pregnancy, corpus luteal cysts, or inflammatory masses. Corpus luteal cysts may retain their phasicity with the cardiac cycle whereas malignant masses become less phasic.

Pelvic Inflammatory Disease

Pelvic inflammatory disease (PID) is frequently the result of a sexually transmitted disease, often gonorrhea or chlamydia. IUDs may predispose to PID with actinomycoses and other unusual organisms. Appendicitis, diverticular disease, or Crohn's disease may lead to PID with a nonsexual etiology.

Pelvic ultrasound may not reveal any abnormalities. Sometimes an abnormal quantity of debris-containing fluid may be seen in the cul-de-sac. If endometritis is present as part of the PID, then a broad bright endometrial stripe may be seen as discussed in the section on the uterus. With severe tubo-ovarian abscesses, one may see a hydrosalpinx that is manifested by a complex cystic adnexal structure often shaped like a dumbbell. These may be huge, and one should not expect to see a thin, cylindrically shaped fallopian tube. Abscess collections may develop in the adnexa around the ovary and these will be complex cystic with debris. We often use ultrasound to determine if a patient will be admitted for intravenous antibiotics since patients with discrete adnexal abscesses often require inpatient therapy.

Suggested Readings

Carter J, Saltzman A, Hartenbach E, et al. Flow characteristics in benign and malignant gynecologic tumors using transvaginal color flow Doppler. Obstet Gynecol 83:125–130, 1994.

Fleischer AC. New applications of pelvic sonography. Urol Radiol 13:9–15, 1991.

Fleischer AC, Romero R, Manning FA, et al. The Principles and Practice of Ultrasonography in Obstetrics and Gynecology, 4th ed. Norwalk, CT, Appleton & Lange, 1992.

Laing FC. Ultrasound of gynecologic pathologies. Curr Opin Radiol 4:78–84, 1992.

Rumack CM, Wilson SR, Charboneau, JW. Diagnostic Ultrasound. St. Louis, Mosby–Year Book, 1991.

Siegel MJ. Pediatric gynecologic sonography. Radiology 179:593–600, 1991.

CHAPTER 8

Obstetrical Ultrasound

Review of Embryology

In a normal pregnancy, the egg is fertilized near the distal end of the fallopian tube and the new zygote starts dividing. At approximately three days postfertilization, there is a colony of 16 cells known as a morula. At approximately four days, the zygote reaches the endometrial cavity and separates into the trophoblast portion (which becomes the chorionic membrane and the fetal part of the placenta) and an inner cell mass or embryoblast (which leads to the formation of the embryo, amnion, cord, and secondary yolk sac) (Fig. 8–1). At this point, the embryo is known as a late blastocyst. At about six days postfertilization (three weeks' menstrual age), attachment to the endometrium and implantation occur. At this time the trophoblast differentiates into an inner cell mass and an outer syncytiotrophoblast (Fig. 8–2). The syncytiotrophoblast will penetrate the endometrial epithelium.

At the time of implantation, a fluid-filled space appears between the inner cell mass and the syncytiotrophoblast. This space will become the amniotic cavity. Cells from the cytotrophoblast form an exocelomic membrane surrounding an exocelomic cavity. This becomes the primary or primitive yolk sac. By day ten, implantation is complete and the endometrium completely covers the sac. At about 14 days (Fig. 8–3) the chorion forms a chorionic sac, which surrounds the embryo, and the amniotic sac and the yolk sac form. The primitive yolk sac divides into two portions—the secondary yolk sac and the remnant of the primitive yolk sac. The secondary yolk sac is what is normally seen on ultrasound. This lies between the amnion and chorion.

Table 8–1 lists the maximum age in weeks by which certain structures should always be identifiable. If these structures are not identified by these ages, then the pregnancy is presumed to be either abnormal or ectopic (Fig. 8–4). This assumes that good-quality scans are obtained with modern high-resolution scanners. In addition, a normal intrauterine gestational sac should be identifiable when the serum human chorionic gonadotropin (hCG) reaches 1,800 International Units (Second International Standard) using the transabdominal technique or greater than 1,000 IU Units using the endovaginal technique. International Reference Prep measurement of the hCG is approximately twice that of the Second International Standard (100 mIU/ml [2nd IS] = 200 mIU/ml [IRP]).

The yolk sac seen on ultrasound is the secondary yolk sac. As indicated in Table 8–1, it should be seen by five weeks endovaginally or six-and-a-half weeks transabdominally. In the third and fourth weeks of postmenstrual life, the yolk sac has a nutrition function. It is involved in hematopoiesis during the fifth to eighth weeks. The dorsal portion of the yolk sac ultimately contributes to a portion of the primitive gut. The primordial germ cells start in the yolk sac and migrate to the sex glands so the yolk sac also has a role in reproduction.

Visible indications of problems with the yolk sac can include a solid appearance, which is an indicator of an abnormal fetus, and abnormal diameter. A yolk sac that is less than 2 mm or greater than 5.6 mm in diameter before 8 to 12 weeks indicates a bad outcome. Nonvisualization of a yolk sac also is a bad prognostic sign.

Fetal heart activity should be visible by six weeks endovaginally and seven weeks transabdominally. Before six weeks, even if an embryo is well seen, cardiac activity may

157

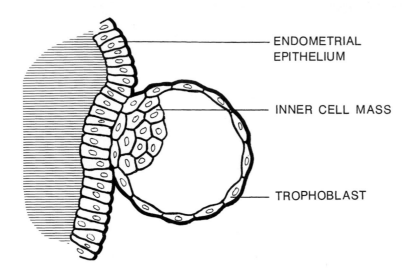

Figure 8–1. Diagram of a human embryo four days postfertilization. The inner cell mass has formed and from it will form the embryo, amnion, umbilical cord, and secondary yolk sac. (Adapted from Moore KL. The Developing Human, 5th ed. Philadelphia, WB Saunders, 1993, with permission.)

ENDOMETRIAL EPITHELIUM

INNER CELL MASS

TROPHOBLAST

not be visible because the heart may not have started beating. The heart usually starts beating between five and six weeks' menstrual age. Sometimes heart activity will be seen between three and four weeks. Nyberg, Lange, and Filly have established several sonographic criteria for determining if a gestational sac is abnormal:

Major criteria:

Greater than 25 mm average sac diameter with no embryo (Fig. 8–4)
Greater than 20 mm with no yolk sac
Distorted gestational sac shape

Minor criteria:

A thin, less than 2-mm decidual reaction
Weak decidual amplitude
Irregular contour of decidua
Absent double decidual sac sign
Low position of sac

These criteria apply to transabdominal scanning. These authors require three minor or one major criterion to indicate fetal demise. If endovaginal scanning is used, then the criteria are a sac with greater than 16 mm mean diameter and no embryo, or a mean sac diameter of 8 mm without a yolk sac.

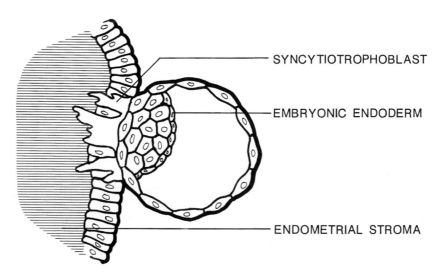

SYNCYTIOTROPHOBLAST

EMBRYONIC ENDODERM

ENDOMETRIAL STROMA

Figure 8–2. Diagram of a human egg six days postfertilization. Syncytiotrophoblast penetrates the endometrial epithelium and implantation occurs. (Adapted from Moore KL. The Developing Human, 5th ed. Philadelphia, WB Saunders, 1993, with permission.)

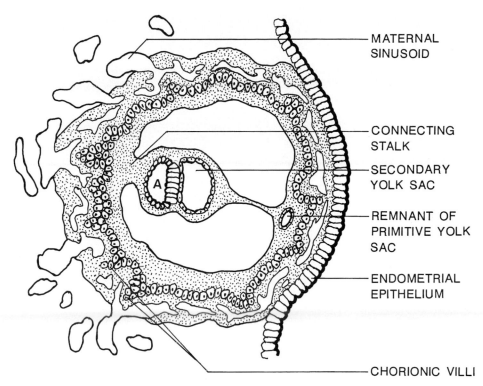

MATERNAL SINUSOID

CONNECTING STALK

SECONDARY YOLK SAC

REMNANT OF PRIMITIVE YOLK SAC

ENDOMETRIAL EPITHELIUM

CHORIONIC VILLI

Figure 8–3. Diagram of a human egg 14 days postfertilization. The secondary yolk sac has formed. This structure plus the amniotic cavity (A) form a ''double bubble'' with an embryonic disc between them. This double bubble may sometimes be seen on ultrasound. (Adapted from Moore KL. The Developing Human, 5th ed. Philadelphia, WB Saunders, 1993, with permission.)

Of all embryos that are identified as being alive at five weeks' gestation, 24 percent will die. Of all twins seen in the first trimester, 20 to 30 percent will be singleton at delivery.

AMNION AND CHORION

The amnion closely surrounds the embryo and covers the umbilical cord at the entrance of the cord into the placenta. The chorion attaches to the edge of the placenta (Fig. 8–5). A subchorionic hematoma is blood in the endometrial cavity separating decidua vera from decidua capsularis. This is an unfavorable sign that often indicates impending abortion (Fig. 8–6). Chorioamnionic fluid is fluid between the chorion and amnion and is normal until these two membranes fuse at 14 to 16 weeks. The double decidual sac sign used to help differentiate intrauterine from extrauterine gestations probably consists of decidua vera (outer ring) and chorionic villi extending around the embryo. Normally, small amounts of blood may accumulate at the

Table 8–1. MAXIMUM AGE AT WHICH STRUCTURES SHOULD BE SEEN ON ULTRASOUND: FIRST TRIMESTER

	ENDOVAGINAL AGE (wk)	TRANSABDOMINAL AGE (wk)
Gestational sac	4.5 (or when β-hCG = 1,000 IU/L)	5.0 (or when β-hCG = 1,800 IU/L)
Yolk sac	5.7 (MSD = 8 mm)	7.3 (MSD = 20 mm)
Embryo	6.7 (MSD = 16 mm)	8.0 (MSD = 25 mm)
Heart activity	CRL = 5 mm (6.2 wks)	CRL = 9.5 mm (7.0 wks)

MSD = mean sac diameter, CRL = crown-rump length.

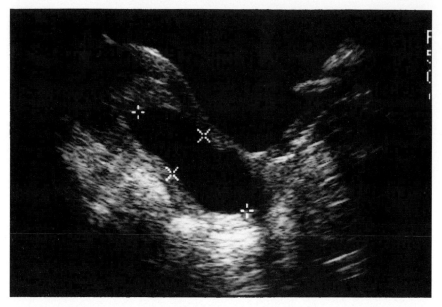

Figure 8–4. Sagittal image of the uterus with an abnormal gestational sac. Average sac diameter is 3.7 cm with no embryo and no yolk sac. The shape is also distorted (not round or elliptical). Several minor criteria for nonviability also are present: a thin decidual reaction, weak decidual amplitude, absent double sac sign, and low position of the sac.

site of implantation. This is different from a subchorionic hemorrhage and is referred to as implantational bleeding (Fig. 8–7).

First Trimester

DATING OF THE FETUS

Between five and eight and one-half weeks the fetus can be dated using a mean sac diameter. To determine this diameter, the inner-to-inner borders of the sac are measured in all three dimensions and these are averaged. Between approximately five and 12 weeks, the crown-rump length of a fetus is measured. Extremities and yolk sac should not be included in this measurement. Crown-rump length is the most accurate method of dating the embryo. Examination of crown-rump length tables

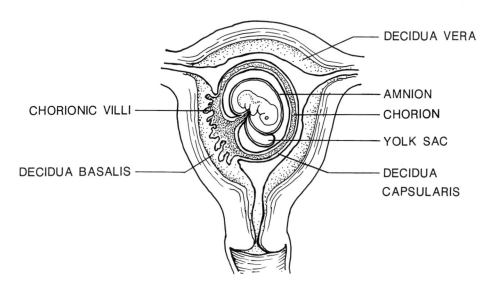

Figure 8–5. Embryo at about six weeks.

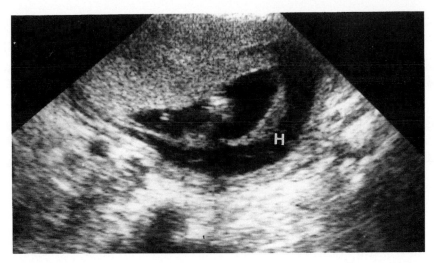

Figure 8–6. Extrachorionic (or subchorionic as it is commonly called) hematoma (H) located between the decidua vera and the decidua capsularis.

shows that a 20 or 30 percent error in measurement of the crown-rump length corresponds to only a four-day error in gestational age estimation. The embryo is growing so rapidly that even moderate errors in measurement of the crown-rump length lead to only small errors in estimates of gestational age.

After approximately 12 weeks, the biparietal diameter (BPD) is used for dating. The BPD is determined by measuring from the outer surface of the skull in the near field to the inner surface of the skull in the far field at the level of the thalamus. It is important to have a symmetric image of

the head. The head circumference can also be measured to compensate for unusual shapes of the skull. The circumference is measured along the outer margin of the calvarium. Starting at about 13 weeks, the femur can be measured. Only the longest length of the femur is used and only the diaphysis. Femoral head and distal epiphysis are not included (i.e., the ossified portion of the femur should be included in the measurement). Measurements of abdominal circumference can start at approximately 15 weeks. A transaxial view through the liver is obtained at the level of the intrahepatic portion of the umbilical vein and, ideally,

Figure 8–7. Implantation bleed. Note a small amount of hypoechoic blood collecting near the implantation site. The blood is hypoechoic. B = blood.

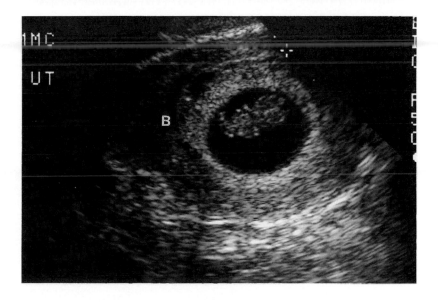

includes the stomach. The abdominal circumference is measured around the outside of the abdomen.

The most accurate dating of the fetus occurs when BPD, head circumference, femur length, and abdominal circumference are all combined in one multiple regression equation to give an estimate of gestational age.

ECTOPIC PREGNANCY

Ectopic pregnancy occurs when the fertilized egg or zygote cannot pass down the fallopian tube into the uterus. The risk factors include a previous ectopic pregnancy, pelvic inflammatory disease (PID) or a history of PID, or a history of prior tubal surgery. Increased maternal age and parity also increase risk. Also, women with a history of infertility problems are at risk for an ectopic pregnancy. A tubal problem leading to complete or partial tubal obstruction is the most likely cause of most ectopic pregnancies.

On ultrasound, if an intrauterine pregnancy can be identified, then an ectopic pregnancy is effectively ruled out. An intrauterine pregnancy certainly is present if an embryo is visible or if a gestational sac plus a yolk sac are visible. The presence of an intrauterine yolk sac indicates that division of the zygote is occurring at an intrauterine location. If no embryo or yolk sac is seen, but a gestational sac is seen, it is important to attempt to determine if there is a double decidual sac present. A double decidual sac, as illustrated in Figure 8–8, suggests an intrauterine pregnancy. A well-formed double decidual sac can be identified clearly in only about one-third of pregnancies between three-and-a-half to seven weeks of menstrual age.

An intrauterine gestational sac can be simulated by a pseudo-gestational sac. A pseudo-gestational sac is the result of fluid or secretions in the endometrial cavity forming a structure that looks like a sac. However, such fluid or secretions are the result of hormonal stimulation of the uterus caused by a pregnancy outside of the uterus. The double decidual sac sign can be very difficult to interpret. We do not rely on it as our sole means of determining intra- versus extrauterine location. Therefore, in our opinion, if no embryo or yolk sac is present in the sac, then an ectopic pregnancy has not been ruled out.

Distinguishing a double decidual sac from a pseudosac of ectopic pregnancy can be aided by color flow Doppler. Peritrophoblastic flow will be present if a true sac is present, but there will be no increase in flow around the sac if it is a pseudosac.

A live embryo in the adnexa (occurring in less than one-third of ectopic pregnancies) also indicates a definitive diagnosis of ectopic pregnancy (Fig. 8–9). An ultrasound examination is indeterminate if no intrauterine gestational sac is seen and no live embryo is seen in the adnexa. Echogenic fluid in the cul-de-sac and/or a mass in the adnexa suggest a diagnosis of ectopic

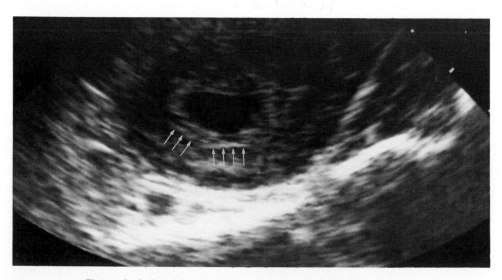

Figure 8–8. Double decidual sac. Arrows point to outer sac.

pregnancy but are not as definitive as a live embryo in the adnexa. If color Doppler shows an area of high vascularity in the adnexa, one should direct attention to that area because the high flow may indicate an ectopic gestation.

When ultrasound shows no gestational sac in the uterus and no gestational sac or embryo in the adnexa but the serum hCG is above the threshold levels (1,800 IU transabdominally, 1,000 IU endovaginally), then the possibilities are ectopic pregnancy or abortion. If quantitative hCG is not available but a pregnancy test is positive, then an intrauterine pregnancy that is too early to identify with ultrasound is a possibility.

As indicated above, we always do an endovaginal ultrasound if we do not see an intrauterine gestation transabdominally. We also do not rely on endovaginal ultrasound without transabdominal ultrasound since an ectopic may be sitting high in the pelvis out of range of the endovaginal transducer.

Although an intrauterine gestation effectively excludes an ectopic pregnancy, in reality, there is always the possibility of a coexistent intrauterine pregnancy and an ectopic pregnancy. In the past, the incidence of this was thought to be about 1:40,000. A recent study indicates an incidence of two cases in 13,554 deliveries in Boston, or an incidence of 1:6,778 pregnancies. However,

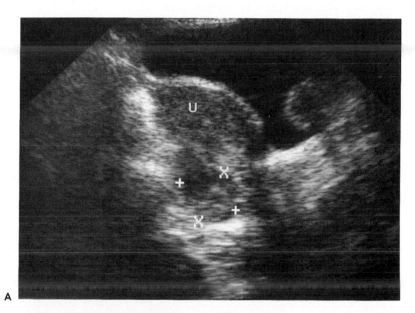

Figure 8–9. *A*, Longitudinal image of the gestational sac in the cul-de-sac (outlined by cursors). U = uterus. *B*, Magnified view shows fetal pole. Fetal heart motion (FHM) was visible.

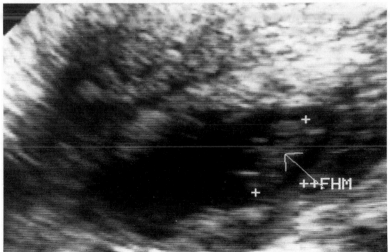

using a binomial distribution, two standard deviations around this estimation of incidence puts the true incidence somewhere between one in infinity and 1 in 2,805. Therefore, we still do not have a good estimate of this phenomenon. For all practical purposes, if the quantitative hCG level is known and it is above 1,800 IU and no intrauterine true gestational sac is identified, then a presumptive diagnosis of ectopic pregnancy can be made.

There are two less common types of ectopic pregnancies that can cause serious bleeding. One type is the interstitial or cornual ectopic pregnancy, which ruptures in the interstitial (or cornual) portion of the fallopian tube—the portion of the tube that traverses the uterus. On ultrasound, this type of ectopic pregnancy should be suspected when the gestational sac is located eccentrically away from the endometrial cavity. The second type is the cervical ectopic pregnancy in which the gestational sac is located low in the uterus in the region of the cervix. These two types of ectopic pregnancies may, at first glance, appear to be normal intrauterine pregnancies. Their location, however, puts the mother at risk. The interstitial pregnancy may rupture and cause massive bleeding. A cervical ectopic pregnancy may also lead to massive bleeding.

Second and Third Trimesters

DATING

Dating of the fetus in the second and third trimesters is best performed as described in the previous section. The dating becomes more precise as more parameters are used. The best methodology is to use BPD, head circumference, abdominal circumference, and femur length combined. Using all of these parameters, the margin of error between 15 and 19 weeks is ± 1.5 weeks. Between 20 and 29 weeks, the margin of error is approximately two weeks, and between 30 and 39 weeks, the margin of error will approach three weeks. The most accurate dating is done using the crown-rump length between six and ten weeks. The error at this time is between three and five days.

PLACENTA AND CORD

Placenta forms from the outer cell layer or trophoblast of the developing embryo. Syncytiotrophoblast invades the endometrium, and this is the site of attachment of the zygote. Placenta can sometimes be seen by eight weeks and can always be identified by twelve weeks. The umbilical cord is made up of two umbilical arteries that carry blood from the fetus to the placenta, and a single umbilical vein that carries blood from the placenta to the fetus. One percent of pregnancies will have only a single umbilical artery. Of this group, about 10 to 20 percent will have additional significant anomalies. Therefore, one should always examine the cord to see if there are three vessels. If only two vessels are seen, one must then look for other anomalies. There is a higher incidence of a single umbilical artery in diabetic mothers. Also, the normal umbilical cord should be coiled. Noncoiling of the umbilical cord greatly increases the risk of a fetal anomaly or fetal death. Color Doppler should be used to examine the cord to make certain that there is coiling (Fig. 8–10). Rarely there may be three vessels in the cord throughout most of its length but only two vessels near the placental end. This is a normal variant caused by fusion of the two umbilical arteries near the placenta.

Grading the Placenta

In the past, attempts were made to grade the placenta. All placentas have calcifications in them and the calcifications become very prominent as term approaches. Grade 0 is a homogeneous placenta. Grade 1 has small intraplacental calcifications. Grade 2 has calcifications along the base or plate of the placenta. Grade 3 has obvious septations through the placenta and is separated into cotyledons with numerous calcifications and obvious lakes throughout, which appear as hypoechoic areas (Fig. 8–11).

At one time it was hoped placental grading could be used to predict lung maturity in the infant. However, this was not found to be a reliable indicator and, therefore, placental grading is less emphasized now. Currently, if we see a Grade III placenta before 35 weeks, we suggest that the fetus may be under stress and that the placenta has "ma-

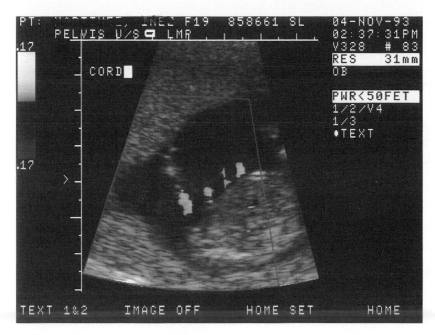

Figure 8–10. Coiled umbilical cord (normal). Noncoiling cord should raise concern for fetal anomalies. See color plate 6.

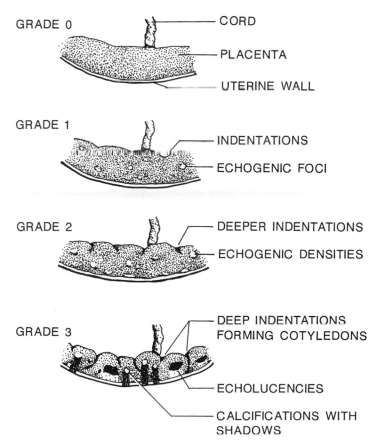

Figure 8–11. Placental grades.

tured" early, but we then try to confirm this with other indicators of fetal stress, such as the amniotic fluid index (Fig. 8–12). Oligohydramnios helps confirm that growth retardation is present.

Placentas may be described as large or small based on their thickness. A large placenta is thicker than 7 cm and a small one is thinner than 1 cm. These numbers may vary slightly between authors. Thick placentas result from hydrops either of the nonimmune or the immune type, diabetes mellitus, maternal or fetal anemia, and triploidy and other chromosomal abnormalities. A complete differential diagnosis is listed in Table 8–2. Thin placentas come about from maternal hypertension or vascular disease, toxemia of pregnancy, diabetes mellitus, cardiovascular or renal disease in the mother, congenital anomalies, and other diseases listed in Table 8–3.

Succenturiate Lobe

A succenturiate lobe of the placenta is simply an accessory lobe of placenta wherein a small portion of placenta is separated from the main part of the placenta. This accessory lobe has vessels that go through membranes to connect to the main body of the placenta. Occasionally, a rupture of these vessels may occur during delivery with ultimate fetal exsanguination. More commonly, the succenturiate lobe is retained after delivery, leading to hemorrhage and infection in the mother.

Table 8–2. THICK PLACENTA

Hydrops
Diabetes mellitus
Anemia, maternal or fetal
Rh disease
Infection
Triploidy
Chromosomal abbnormalities
Maternal heart failure
Placental hemorrhage
Neoplasms of placenta
Mole
Beckwith-Wiedemann syndrome
Sacrococcygeal teratoma

Placental Lesions

Focal placental lesions usually are seen as areas of decreased echogenicity. A complete differential diagnosis is listed in Table 8–4. These are usually referred to as "venous lakes" and simply consist of blood-filled spaces. Subchorionic fibrin deposition is thought to be a result of thrombosis of blood in the subchorionic space leading to hypoechoic areas. Perivillous fibrin deposition occurs in the intervillous space and is hypoechoic within the placenta. It involves stasis as a result of fetal bleeding into the intervillous space and is of no or minimal significance. These hypoechoic lesions are always a concern because they could be the result of placental infarct; however, infarcts are difficult to see on ultrasound. In general, infarcts have an appearance similar to the surrounding placenta. They may occasionally appear sonolucent. Placental infarcts are common and are usually of no significance unless they are large.

Placenta Percreta

Placenta percreta, increta, and accreta all refer to a placenta that grows into the myometrium with no decidua between the chorionic villi and the myometrium. Placenta

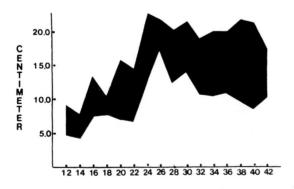

Figure 8–12. Amniotic fluid index. The largest vertical pocket of amniotic fluid in each uterine quadrant is measured and then added together. (From Phelan JP, Ahn MO, Smith CV, et al. J Reprod Med 32:601–604, 1987, with permission.)

Table 8–3. THIN PLACENTA

Maternal hypertension
Toxemia
Diabetes mellitus
Maternal cardiovascular disease
Maternal renal disease
Congenital fetal anomalies
IUGR
Infection

Table 8–4. PLACENTAL LUCENCIES

Normal subplacental complex
Intervillous thrombosis
Septal cysts
Massive subchorial thrombus
Hydatidiform change
Chorioangioma
Teratoma
Metastases
Avillous spaces
Maternal lakes
Subchorial lakes
Subchorionic fibrin deposition
Bleeding after chorionic villous sampling
Infarct
Mature placenta
Hematoma
Placenta circumvallate
Subchorionic thrombosis

accreta is an adherent placenta. Extension through the myometrium is placenta increta. Penetration all the way through the uterus to the serosa is termed percreta. On ultrasound, the hypoechoic areas that usually lie beneath the placenta, consisting of the venous lakes, will not be seen. This entity is frequently associated with placenta previa.

Placenta Previa

Placenta previa refers to a placenta covering the internal cervical os totally or partially (Fig. 8–13). In all obstetric ultrasound examinations it is important to determine the location of the placenta and to make certain that it is not covering the os. An overdistended bladder may push the placenta into a position so that it appears that it is covering the os and simulates placenta previa. Any time placenta previa is suspected, a repeat examination should be performed with the bladder empty or nearly empty. Uterine contractions may also simulate placenta previa. If a contraction is suspected, the patient should be re-examined after 20 to 30 minutes when the uterus has had time to relax. Many first- and second-trimester placenta previas or partial placenta previas will resolve before term. This "placental migration" is probably secondary to trophotropism in which the developing trophoblastic villi preferentially grow toward portions of the uterus with a better blood supply (i.e., body and fundus). When this happens, the cord origin remains fixed

and the cord may develop a marginal or velamentous insertion.

Abruptio Placenta

Abruptio placenta is a cause of vaginal bleeding associated with smoking, cocaine, and hypertension. The placenta detaches from the uterus and premature labor often follows. Various types of abruptio may occur. Marginal hematomas usually cause only mild bleeding and are associated with smoking. Retroplacental hematomas are associated with maternal hypertension. On ultrasound, the hematoma may be seen but it may also be isoechoic with adjacent placenta. The main use of ultrasound in these patients is to exclude placenta previa. A negative ultrasound does not rule out abruptio placenta, however, as the hematoma may look identical to normal placenta or it may have drained away from the placenta.

Placental Diseases

Placental tumors are usually hemangiomas (also called chorioangiomas) and, on ultrasound, they appear as a complex mass within the placenta. They have minimal significance (Fig. 8–14) unless they are large. Large tumors can result in a shunt and lead to polyhydramnios, preterm labor, and growth retardation. Table 8–5 lists the causes of placental masses.

The other placental disease of significance is gestational trophoblastic disease or hydatidiform mole. A complete mole is derived from the father and is 46XX. This occurs when an empty ovum is fertilized by a single sperm. The paternal chromosomes become duplicated to form the 46XX. Occasionally, an empty ovum will be fertilized by two haploid sperms and then 46XY occurs. The pathology includes edema and enlargement of the chorionic villi. The trophoblast that lines the chorionic villi proliferates. No fetal tissue is present.

The ultrasound appearance of trophoblastic disease may not have the classic cluster-of-grapes appearance in the first trimester (Fig. 8–15) but may simply look like an incomplete or missed abortion or an intrauterine mass. Doppler shows high flow with low resistance. Normal pregnancies have much lower flow. Late in the first tri-

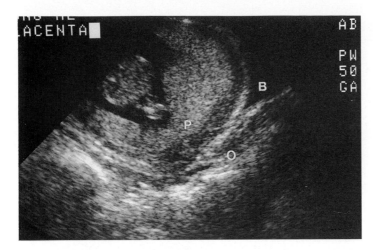

Figure 8–13. Longitudinal image. Placenta (P) completely covers os (O). B = bladder.

Table 8–5. PLACENTAL MASSES

Chorioangiomas
Teratomas
Maternal metastases
Fetal metastases
Fetal triploidy
Hematoma

mester or early in the second trimester, the classic appearance of hydropic villi with its cluster-of-grapes appearance should occur. Molar pregnancy is associated with high hCG levels, which may result in theca-lutein cysts. About one-third of patients with molar pregnancies will ultimately have

theca-lutein cysts because the ovaries are overstimulated by the high levels of hCG. The cysts are multiple, bilateral, and measure 1 to 3 cm in diameter. Theca-lutein cysts may be associated with normal pregnancies or with twins (Fig. 8–16). These cysts should disappear over several months after treatment of the molar pregnancy. About 80 percent of moles are cured by evacuation. About 15 percent ultimately lead to invasive mole in which the myometrium is penetrated by tumor, causing a risk of hemorrhage from pelvic vessels. On ultrasound, this extension of tumor may occasionally cause disorganized cystic areas in the myometrium or parametria. Five per-

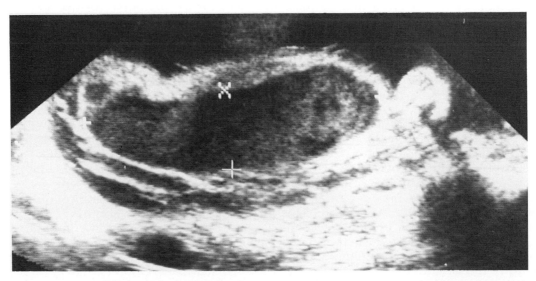

Figure 8–14. Chorioangioma measuring about 8 cm in diameter. The remainder of the placenta is not visible on this image.

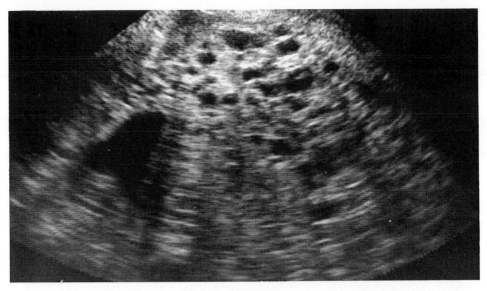

Figure 8-15. Molar pregnancy. Cluster-of-grapes appearance.

cent may develop into choriocarcinoma. These tumors may metastasize widely but patients will still have a good prognosis, probably because the tumor is recognized as "foreign" by the body's immune system.

A mole and fetus can coexist when a twin pregnancy has one normal fetus and one molar gestation. These come from two separate eggs.

Incomplete or partial mole occurs when an ovum is fertilized by two sperm, resulting in triploidy (Fig. 8-17). Pathologically,

the chorionic villi are edematous, but there is no trophoblastic proliferation. The ultrasound appearance is different from a mole. In partial mole, a dysmorphic fetus with multiple anomalies may be seen as well as a formed placenta.

Incompetent Cervix

This entity causes fetal loss in the second trimester due to painless cervical dilation.

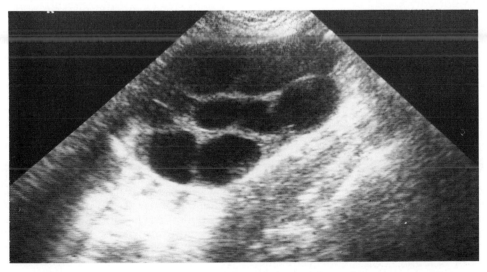

Figure 8-16. Theca-lutein cysts.

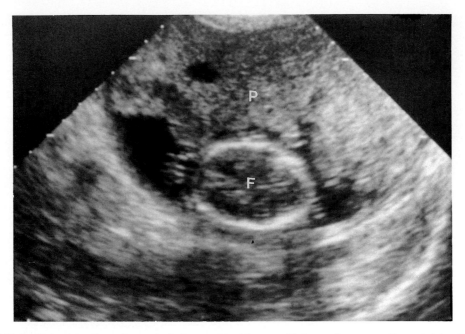

Figure 8–17. Partial mole. The placenta is formed but has multiple cystic areas. There is identifiable fetal tissue. P = placenta, F = fetal cranium. (Courtesy of E. Stamm, MD, University of Colorado, Denver, CO.)

The etiology may be prior cervical injury from dilatation and curettage, conization, or abortion. Exposure to diethylstilbestrol increases the risk of cervical incompetence. At ultrasound, this should be suspected when a dilated endocervical canal is seen. However, a full bladder can create pressure and cause the canal to appear closed, so scanning with an empty bladder (which may make visualization difficult) or with an endovaginal transducer is now advocated. The normal cervix should be at least 3 cm in length until 32 weeks' gestation. The cervix becomes shorter after this time. Cervical width should be less than 2 cm and the cervical canal should be no more than 8 mm wide. Membranes or fetal parts bulging into the canal are a bad sign. The endovaginal transducer should be gently inserted only a few centimeters.

A relatively new technique for evaluating the cervix is translabial ultrasound. The patient is placed in the lithotomy position with an empty bladder. Lubricating jelly (not irritating ultrasound gel) is placed on the labia and covered with a sheet of plastic food wrap. More gel is placed on the wrap and scanning is then performed with a 3.5-MHz sector scanner. Using this technique, the cervix should be at least 2.8 cm in length.

Evaluation for Fetal Anomalies

One should use the first-trimester ultrasound examination to document an intrauterine location for the pregnancy, assess the fetal number, determine that the fetus is living, and estimate the gestational age. Also, the adnexa should be evaluated. During the second and third trimesters, one should document the fetal lie and position of the placenta, estimate fetal weight and amniotic fluid volume, and look for fetal malformations. The fetal head and spine, chest, including heart, abdomen, and pelvis, and limbs should be examined. The cord insertion and anterior abdominal wall should also be evaluated.

BRAIN AND SPINE

At least three axial images of the fetal head at three different levels are obtained. Transthalamic, transventricular, and transcerebellar levels should all be evaluated. By the beginning of the second trimester, the lateral ventricles filled with echogenic choroid are visible. Only the frontal horns are free of choroid. Transverse measurements of the atria of the lateral ventricles are used to diagnose hydrocephalus. A normal measurement is between 6 and 10 mm throughout the second and third trimesters. In addition, the choroid plexus should almost completely fill the atrium of the lateral ventricle. Failure to do so indicates ventriculomegaly. One other helpful sign is the "dangling" choroid plexus. If the ventricle is enlarged, the choroid may be seen dangling in a pool of cerebrospinal fluid (CSF) (Fig. 8–18). A differential diagnosis of apparent hydrocephalus is given in Table 8–6.

Previously, a lateral ventricle–to–hemisphere ratio was calculated as an indicator of hydrocephalus. This method required identification and measurement of the medial and lateral wall of the lateral ventricle. It is now thought that the lateral wall of the ventricle cannot be reliably identified and that the structure actually measured was a blood vessel.

The cavum septum pellucidum is a normal CSF-containing space between the lateral ventricles that does not communicate with them. This structure develops simultaneously with other midline structures and, if it can be identified, complete agenesis of the corpus callosum is excluded as a possible diagnosis.

Hydrocephalus

Hydrocephalus is divided into communicating and noncommunicating types.

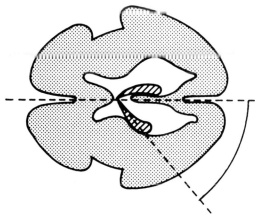

Figure 8–18. Schematic drawing of dilated ventricles shows dangling choroid plexus and increased choroid plexus angle. (From Cardoza JD, Filly RA, Podrasky AE. The dangling choroid plexus: a sonographic observation of value in excluding ventriculomegaly. AJR *151*:767–770, 1988, with permission.)

Table 8–6. HYDROCEPHALUS

Pseudohydrocephalus
Communicating
Aqueductal stenosis
Dandy-Walker syndrome
Arnold-Chiari II syndrome (associated with spina
 bifida)
Choroid plexus papilloma
Hydranencephaly
Lobar holoprosencephaly
Triploidy

Communicating hydrocephalus means that the obstruction is outside of the ventricular system, usually either in the subarachnoid space or at the level of the superior sagittal sinus and the pacchionian granulations. This condition is rare in utero. Because it leads to a failure to resorb CSF, communicating hydrocephalus should lead to enlargement of the subarachnoid spaces, but this is difficult to appreciate by fetal ultrasound. In addition, all ventricles may be enlarged, including the fourth.

Noncommunicating hydrocephalus means that there is an obstruction somewhere within the ventricular system. This is more common than communicating hydrocephalus. This condition can be at the level of the foramina of Magendie or Luschka and can lead to obstruction of the fourth ventricle. The resultant dilatation of the entire ventricular system leads to enlargement of the third ventricle and the lateral ventricles. One of the most common causes of in utero hydrocephalus is aqueductal stenosis. This can be the result of an infection, a hemorrhage, or a mass, or it may be congenital. In this condition, ultrasound shows dilatation of the lateral and third ventricles. If an obstruction occurs at the level of the foramen of Monroe, it will result in unilateral lateral ventricular enlargement.

In diagnosing hydrocephalus, one should take care to distinguish between pseudohydrocephalus and true hydrocephalus. Pseudohydrocephalus appears as a sonolucent fetal cortex and can be misinterpreted as hydrocephalus (Fig. 8–19). It is caused by inadequate gain settings with a resultant lucent appearance to the portion of brain furthest from the transducer. Acoustic noise in the near field can sometimes obscure hydrocephalus in the near ventricle and lead to a diagnosis of unilateral hydrocephalus.

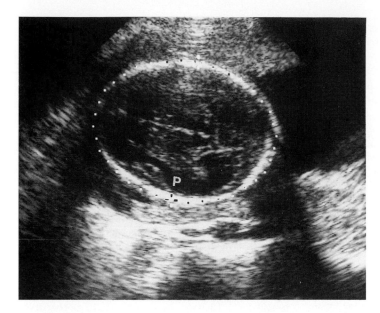

Figure 8–19. Pseudohydroce-phalus. P = sonolucent area.

Holoprosencephaly

Holoprosencephaly is relatively common. It is divided into the alobar, semilobar, and lobar types (Fig. 8–20). The alobar type has a single midline ventricle, fused thalami, and no midline structures or falx (Fig. 8–21). The semilobar type has incomplete fusion of the ventricles and may have rudimentary occipital horns. It also should have no midline structures but may have a partial falx posteriorly. The lobar type has not been diagnosed in utero and resembles very much the normal state. Holoprosencephaly has associated facial anomalies, including cyclopia, hypotelorism with a midline proboscis, cebocephaly (hypotelorism with a single nostril), median facial clefts, or bilateral facial clefts. The face must be examined carefully. Holoprosencephaly may be distinguished from hydrocephalus by the fact that in holoprosencephaly the thalami are fused, whereas in hydrocephalus the thalami are splayed.

Dandy-Walker Syndrome

Dandy-Walker syndrome is an abnormality in embryogenesis and is probably not due to obstruction of the foramina of Luschka or Magendie. It often may be detected before 20 weeks. There is complete or partial absence of the cerebellar vermis with formation of a cystic fourth ventricle (Fig. 8–22). This cyst may be quite large in the posterior fossa and it may lead to enlargement of the entire posterior fossa and

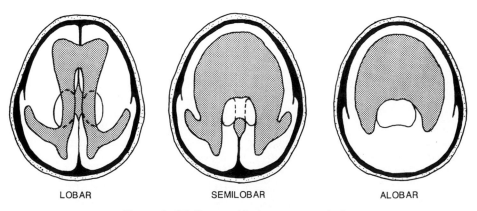

LOBAR SEMILOBAR ALOBAR

Figure 8–20. Types of holoprosencephaly.

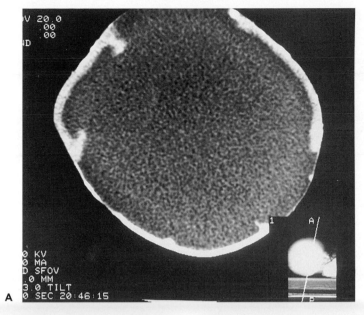

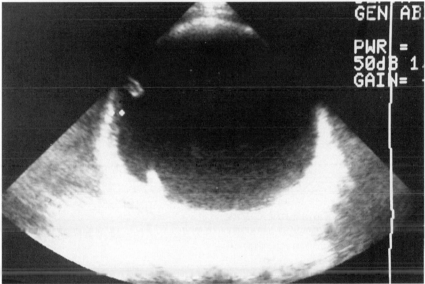

Figure 8–21. Alobar holoprosencephaly, CT (*A*) and in utero ultrasound (*B*). This case was verified at autopsy. The differential diagnosis for this condition includes hydranencephaly and severe hydrocephalus.

obstruct the third and lateral ventricles. There is a Dandy-Walker variant consisting of a smaller cyst, more cerebellar vermis and no obstructive hydrocephalus. The cerebellar hemispheres are splayed in all patients with the Dandy-Walker syndrome. In the full-blown Dandy-Walker syndrome, about two-thirds develop hydrocephalus. Agenesis of the corpus callosum also may be associated. The differential diagnosis includes a posterior fossa arachnoid cyst or a large cisterna magna. The differential diagnosis for cystic cranial masses is listed in Table 8–7.

Hydranencephaly

Hydranencephaly is the absence of cerebral hemispheres while the calvarium and meninges remain intact. This condition is thought to be secondary to severe bilateral infarctions. There may occasionally be

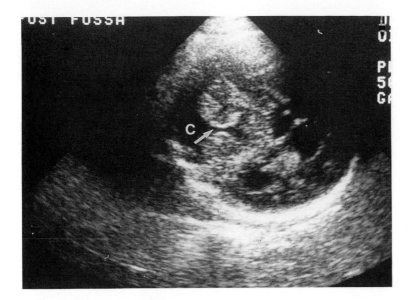

Figure 8–22. Dandy-Walker syndrome. Posterior fossa cyst (C) and communication (*arrow*) with the IVth ventricle. (Courtesy of E. Stamm, MD, University of Colorado, Denver, CO.)

small remnants of brain remaining. A falx is usually present but may be incomplete or difficult to see. These fetuses frequently have macrocephaly, and polyhydramnios is usually present. Hydranencephaly must be distinguished from severe holoprosencephaly and severe hydrocephalus. With severe hydrocephalus, a mantle of cerebral cortex will usually be seen compressed against the calvarium by the enlarged hemispheres.

Porencephaly

Porencephaly is a CSF-containing cavity within the substance of the brain, usually secondary to infarction. A common definition requires that the cavity communicate with the ventricles or subarachnoid spaces. If there is no communication, then necrotic

Table 8–7. CYSTIC MASS WITHIN CRANIUM

Dandy-Walker cyst
Porencephaly
Schizencephaly
Arachnoid cyst
Cystic tumor
Hydranencephaly
Holoprosencephaly
Choroid plexus cyst
Vein of Galen aneurysm
After in utero hemorrhage
Large cisterna magna
Colpocephaly Subdural hygroma

areas are called cystic leukomalacia. Schizencephaly is sometimes used synonymously for porencephaly, although we make a distinction. Schizencephaly is a developmental anomaly caused by failure of migration of the embryologic cerebral cortex. This causes a cleft in the brain. On magnetic resonance imaging, it is possible to see that the cleft is lined by gray matter. This gray matter is not visible on ultrasound.

Arachnoid cysts may cause hydrocephalus. They may be difficult to differentiate from a porencephalic cyst or schizencephaly.

Vein of Galen Aneurysms

Vein of Galen aneurysms are actually arteriovenous malformations that occur at the level of the quadrigeminal plate cistern. On fetal ultrasound, this causes a cystic-appearing mass (Fig. 8–23). There may be hydrocephalus due to obstruction. The arteriovenous shunt may lead to cardiomegaly and hydrops. This condition has a bad prognosis. The diagnosis can be confirmed by using Doppler to detect the high-flow state of the arteriovenous malformation.

Choroid Plexus Cysts

Choroid plexus cysts are extremely common in the second trimester, but almost always disappear by the third trimester. These cysts are usually small, less than 1 cm

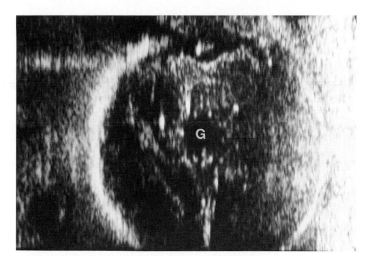

Figure 8–23. Vein of Galen aneurysm (G). Doppler ultrasound showed high flow through this lesion.

in diameter. They may be bilateral and are usually in the atria of the lateral ventricles (Fig. 8–24). Although they are of no significance, there is a possible association of these cysts with trisomy 18. However, because these cysts are so common, one should not suggest the diagnosis of trisomy 18 if other anomalies are not present.

Microcephaly

Microcephaly refers to a calvarium that is at least two standard deviations smaller than expected. It is necessary to have accurate dating to detect this anomaly. The head will be smaller than the fetal age as indicated by the abdomen or the femur. To make this diagnosis, it is best to refer to charts of head size. Common etiologies include holoprosencephaly, drug exposure, chromosomal abnormalities, radiation exposure, hypoxia, in utero infection, and encephalocele. Serial examinations should show poor growth of the cranium. There may also be associated hydrocephalus.

Agenesis of the corpus callosum may be partial or complete. If it is partial, it is usually the posterior portion that is not present. The corpus callosum forms at about 20 weeks' gestational age. An absent cavum septum pellucidum suggests the possibility of agenesis of the corpus callosum, but this structure can be difficult to see in some normal fetuses. The lateral ventricles become separated and the third ventricle moves superiorly to lie in between the two lateral ventricles. This diagnosis is difficult to make before the third trimester. Colpoce-

phaly, or dilatation of the atria of the lateral ventricles, may also be present. The differential diagnosis of a midline third ventricular cyst with agenesis of the corpus callosum should include a large cavum septum pellucidum.

Neural Tube Defects

Anencephaly, encephaloceles, and spina bifida are all considered to be types of neu-

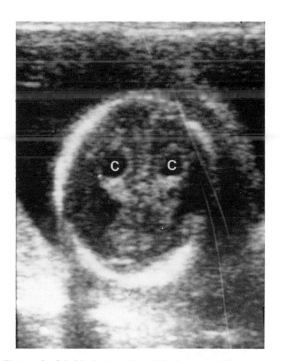

Figure 8–24. Bilateral choroid plexus cysts. C = cysts.

ral tube defects. Anencephaly has no cortex or cranium. On ultrasound, no brain is seen above the orbits (Fig. 8–25A,B). The cranial vault is also absent. This disorder may be diagnosed as early as 8 weeks. Because the sonographer cannot measure a BPD at the level of the thalami, many times he or she will attempt to make a measurement below this level erroneously. Polyhydramnios is usually associated with this disorder. The prognosis is dismal.

The second type of neural tube defect is cephalocele (Fig. 8–25C) (encephalocele). This is an imperfection in the cranium with herniation of brain and/or meninges into the sac-like defect. Meningoceles, which are herniations of meninges without brain substance, occur in 10 percent of these, while encephaloceles, which include both brain and meninges, occur in about 90 percent. Meningoceles appear cystic on ultrasound and encephaloceles have a more solid appearance. There may be associated hydrocephalus. About 10 percent of cephaloceles

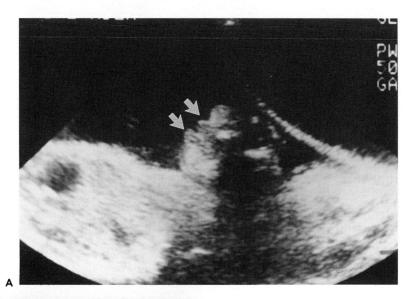

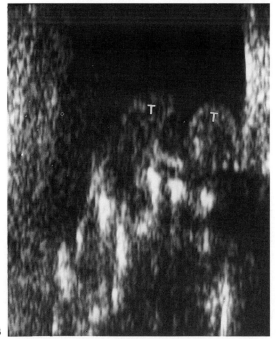

Figure 8–25. *A*, Anencephaly. Soft tissue (*arrows*) protrudes above the skull base. No cranial vault is present. *B*, Anencephaly showing the soft tissue (T) that may be mistaken for hemispheres. *Illustration continued on opposite page*

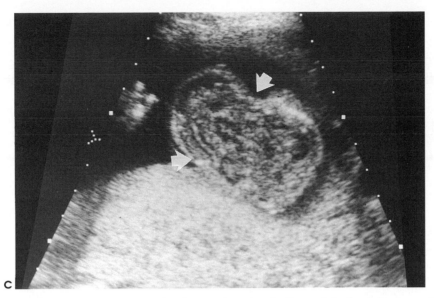

C

Figure 8–25. *Continued.* C, Encephalocele. *Arrows* demarcate the point where brain protrudes from skull. (Courtesy of Joelle Biernacki, MD, Carbondale, IL.)

are associated with spina bifida. Polyhydramnios also may be present. A differential for pericranial masses is listed in Table 8–8.

The Meckel-Gruber syndrome includes an occipital encephalocele and cystic kidneys plus polydactyly. Oligohydramnios is present in this syndrome because of the kidney disease, and it may be difficult to see the encephalocele. When cephalocele is suspected, one should try to identify the bony defect. If no bony defect is visible, then the possibility of a pericranial mass, such as a cystic hygroma or a teratoma, must be considered. Encephaloceles may also be simulated by the cranial defect that occurs with limb–body wall complex or amniotic band syndrome.

Spina bifida is the third type of neural tube defect. Most patients with spina bifida have an Arnold-Chiari type II syndrome with malformation of the posterior fossa, associated hydrocephalus, and a spina bi-

fida defect in the spine. Thirty to 40 percent of fetuses with hydrocephalus have spina bifida as a cause. Eighty percent of those with Arnold-Chiari II malformation ultimately will have hydrocephalus. It is estimated that about 80 percent of patients with spina bifida can be detected by ultrasound, although this number varies significantly because some examiners claim sensitivities above 90 percent and other examiners have reported sensitivities as low as 30 to 40 percent.

The spine has three ossification centers, a centrum and two posterior elements. Ossification occurs from cranial to caudad and begins at about eight weeks. It is finished by about twenty weeks. The spine can usually be adequately evaluated at about eighteen weeks. Before that time, failure of ossification of some of the posterior elements may make it difficult to be certain that a defect is not present. Transverse images are key. The spine must be examined carefully (transversely from cranium to sacrum) to make certain that the posterior ossification centers angle to the midline at the expected location of the spinous process (Fig. 8–26). In spina bifida they will either be parallel or splayed, with the angulation of the posterior ossification centers being away from midline (Fig. 8–27). This is the reason to obtain both axial and sagittal images during a routine examination.

Table 8–8. PERICRANIAL MASS

Encephalocele
Normal fetal hair
Hemangioma
Cystic hygroma
Scalp edema
Cephalohematoma
Subcutaneous hematoma

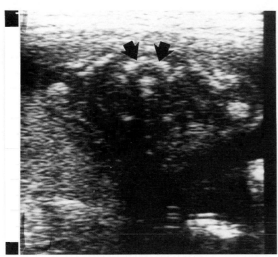

Figure 8–26. Transverse image of fetal spine. Posterior elements (*arrows*) angle toward the midline in this normal fetus.

A pseudodysraphic defect can be produced on ultrasound if the transducer is not truly perpendicular to the spine but instead is scanning obliquely in the transverse plane. We usually obtain a sagittal scan first so that we can see what the curvature of the spine is like. This helps us to keep the transducer perpendicular to the spine when we obtain our transverse images. One should look for a soft tissue mass or sac as well as splaying of the posterior elements.

Examining the cranium also requires care. As mentioned before, there may be hydrocephalus. The lemon sign consists of concavity of the frontoparietal region of the fetal head. This may be a result of low intraspinal pressure. This sign has nearly 100 percent sensitivity for spina bifida before 24 weeks. The lemon sign gradually disappears in the third trimester (Fig. 8–28*A*). About one percent of normal fetuses also may have this sign. The condition known as cloverleaf skull also can simulate a lemon sign.

Another sign of spina bifida is known as the banana sign (Fig. 8–28*B*). This refers to the shape of the cerebellar hemispheres in the small posterior fossa. The cerebellar hemispheres become banana shaped. Probably more easily recognized than the banana sign is the fact that the cisterna magna becomes obliterated. The cisterna magna should be seen in nearly 100 percent of fetuses in the second and third trimesters. Therefore, examination of the posterior fossa should be a routine part of the obstetric exam.

Other indicators of spina bifida include a head that measures small before 24 weeks of gestation. A fetus with clubfoot also suggests spina bifida. Failure to move the lower extremities also should bring this disorder to mind. However, many fetuses with spina bifida will be able to move the lower extremities.

Scoliosis of the spine will be mentioned here even though it is not strictly a neural tube defect. Scoliosis may be caused by hemivertebrae or the more serious VACTERL association (vertebral, anal, cardiac, tracheal, esophageal, renal, and limb

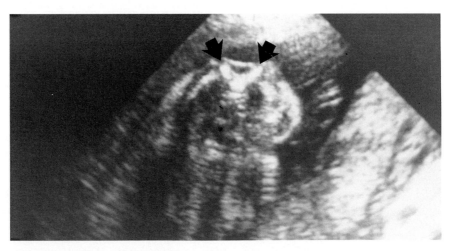

Figure 8–27. Transverse image of fetal spine. Posterior elements (*arrows*) angle laterally in this fetus with spina bifida.

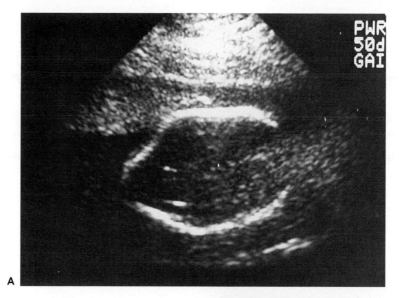

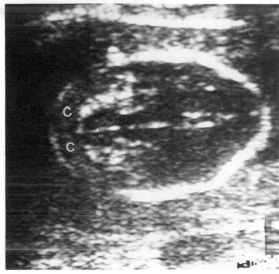

Figure 8–28. *A*, Note that the fetal cranium is concave in the frontoparietal region. This is the lemon sign. *B*, Note the banana-shaped cerebellar hemispheres (C) in the small posterior fossa and that the cisterna magna is obliterated. This is the banana sign.

anomalies). Limb–body wall complex has scoliosis as an important part of the syndrome. Neurofibromatosis and arthrogryposis are also associated with scoliosis. Scoliosis is best appreciated by coronal and sagittal imaging of the spine.

FACE AND NECK

By the end of the first trimester, fetal facial features can be identified as well as the orbits and mandible. Examination for facial clefts can be performed in the coronal plane.

Examination of the neck is important to make certain that cystic hygromas are not present (Fig. 8–29). Neck masses such as fetal goiters or teratomas may lead to polyhydramnios due to interference with fetal swallowing. Cystic hygromas are commonly seen with both Turner's syndrome and Trisomy 21 (Down's syndrome). Other causes of neck masses are given in Table 8–9.

FETAL THORAX

The fetal lungs demonstrate intermediate echogenicity similar to that of fetal liver. Lungs, heart, and thorax all grow at a similar rate; the ratio of these structures remains constant during the second and third trimesters. Abnormalities in the fetal thorax

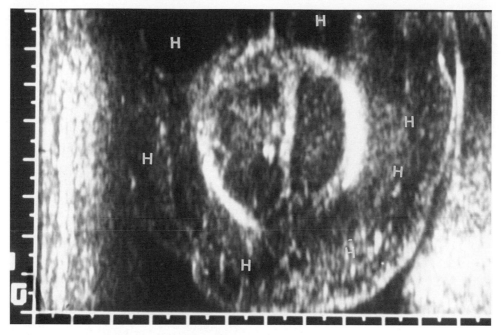

Figure 8–29. Huge cystic hygroma (H) surrounds the cranium. It extended completely around the neck. Note the low-level echoes throughout the hygroma.

are usually seen as a small thorax, a chest mass, or displacement of the heart. One should obtain a four-chamber view of the heart. This is a transverse section and the majority of the heart should lie in the anterior left quadrant. If the heart is shifted, one must search for a pleural fluid collection, thoracic mass, or hypodevelopment of one lung. Pulmonary hypoplasia may be secondary to either a space-occupying thoracic lesion or severe renal disease with associated oliguria. The oliguria leads to oli-

gohydramnios and there is a physical compression that prevents one or both lungs from developing. If pulmonary hypoplasia is suspected, then one should measure the thoracic circumference and compare it to standards from tables. The measurement is made at the level of a four-chamber view of the heart and excludes muscle and soft tissues. Causes of fetal lung masses are given in Table 8–10.

THORACIC MASSES

One thoracic mass that may cause pulmonary hypoplasia is sequestration. A sequestration is a portion of lung that develops without communication to the bronchial tree. It is fed by an artery from the aorta and usually drains into a pulmonary vein. Extralobar sequestration has its own pleural covering whereas an intralobar sequestration is contained within the visceral pleura of the normal lung. The intralobar type is more common. Both types of sequestration occur most often in lower lobes. Intralobar sequestrations occur with equal frequency on both sides, whereas extralobar sequestrations usually occur on the left. On ultrasound, there is an echogenic mass in the caudal portion of the thorax or the upper

Table 8–9. NECK MASSES

COMMON
Cystic hygroma
Nonimmune hydrops

UNCOMMON
Cervical meningocele
Cephalocele
Neck tumors
Klippel-Trenaunay-Weber syndrome
Subcutaneous edema
Goiter
Brachial cleft cysts
Hemangioma
Teratomas
Neuroblastoma of neck
Hemangioendothelioma
Twin sac of blighted ovum
Nuchal bleb

Table 8–10. LUNG MASS

Cystic adenomatoid malformation
Duplication cyst
Diaphragmatic hernia
Bronchogenic cysts
Pulmonary sequestration
Bronchopulmonary foregut malformation
Bronchial atresia
Teratomas
Enteric cysts
Rhabdomyoma
Neuroblastoma
Pleural fluid

portion of the abdomen. Color flow Doppler can sometimes be used to demonstrate the anomalous arterial supply from the aorta.

Diaphragmatic hernias are another cause of an intrathoracic mass leading to pulmonary hypoplasia (Fig. 8–30). Bochdalek hernias are usually posterior on the left with herniation of the stomach and other abdominal organs through an opening in the posterior portion of the diaphragm adjacent to the spine. Morgagni hernias are usually anterior on the right and have liver herniated into the chest.

Bronchogenic cysts occur from abnormal development of the bronchi. This cyst usually forms within the mediastinum near the carina. These cysts are lined by respiratory epithelium and may be filled with mucus. Usually a bronchogenic cyst does not com-

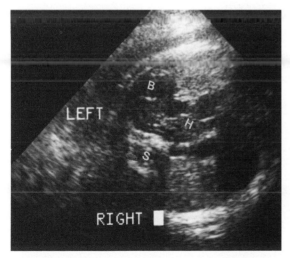

Figure 8–30. Diaphragmatic hernia on the left. Transverse image of the fetus through the chest. Loops of bowel (B) are present in the chest adjacent to the heart (H). S = spine.

municate with the trachea or bronchi. On ultrasound, this is usually a typical cystic-appearing lesion near the mediastinum.

Pleural effusion may occur from either immune or nonimmune hydrops and lead to resultant compression of a lung. Congestive heart failure, Turner's syndrome and Down's syndrome are also associated with fetal pleural fluid collections.

Cystic adenomatoid malformations are hamartomas. Type I contains large cysts. Type II has numerous smaller cysts. Type III is a large solid mass. The type III cystic adenomatoid malformations have the worst prognosis.

Fetal Heart

The fetal heart is examined for structural defects, arrhythmias, and tumors during a level I obstetric ultrasound examination. A more thorough targeted fetal heart evaluation can be performed, usually with the assistance of a pediatric cardiologist. These examinations require the use of M-mode and Doppler techniques and will not be discussed here.

Risk factors for congenital heart defects include a family history of congenital heart disease; maternal diabetes; exposure to teratogens such as alcohol, narcotics, and lithium; and possibly conception while taking birth control pills. Twenty-five percent of fetuses that are observed to have fetal hydrops will have either a structural heart defect or an arrhythmia. Of patients who are identified as having congenital heart disease, 50 percent also will have defects in another organ system.

EXAMINING THE FETAL HEART

A screening ultrasound of the fetal heart should include a four-chamber view. This is obtained by scanning transversely across the lower fetal chest. It is important to be familiar with the normal appearance of this view (Fig. 8–31). Various other views are recommended by other authors. Originally it was felt that a four-chamber view of the heart resulted in the detection of about 96 percent of cardiac defects. The current and probably more realistic estimate is that about 60 percent of cardiac defects may be picked up utilizing this view alone.

After the four-chamber view has been ob-

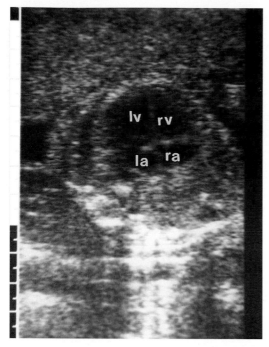

Figure 8–31. Four-chamber view of the fetal heart. Normally, the tricuspid valve sits more toward the apex than the mitral valve. la = left atrium, lv = left ventricle, ra = right atrium, rv = right ventricle.

tained, and if the transducer is angled slightly cephalad, a five-chamber view is possible. The fifth chamber is the aorta in the center of the fetal heart. By rotating the transducer to scan a plane from the infant's right shoulder through the infant's left hip parasagittally, it is possible to obtain a view of the ascending aorta. It should appear to be continuous with the left ventricle. Rotating the transducer further, into a nearly sagittal plane, one may view the pulmonary artery in continuity with the right ventricular outflow tract. These last two views will make it possible to determine if transposition of the great vessels is present.

Pitfalls in performing the fetal heart examination include the fact that the membranous ventricular septum is very thin and may simulate a ventricular septal defect (VSD). Echoes in the left ventricle may be mistaken for intraventricular masses. These probably come from papillary muscle (Fig. 8–32). Finally, a hypoechoic myocardium may simulate a pericardial effusion. Because the intraventricular and intra-atrial septa are very thin, atrial septal defects (ASDs) and VSDs are difficult to diagnose and small defects may be missed. Aortic stenosis and pulmonic stenosis are also difficult to diagnose. Total anomalous pulmonary venous return is easily missed and coarctations also are very difficult to detect.

To diagnose an ASD, it is necessary to see a discontinuity in the atrial septum. This requires a four-chamber view. The sinus venosus–type ASD is very high in the septum, near where the superior vena cava comes into the right atrium. The ostium secundum ASD is the most common type of defect and is in the midportion of the septum. The ostium primum ASD is located in

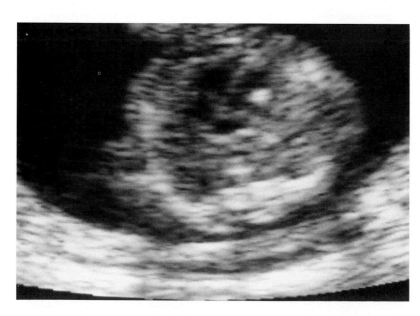

Figure 8–32. Four-chamber view of fetal heart shows aparent mass (arrow). This echogenic focus is a papillary muscle.

the low portion of the interatrial septum and frequently involves an abnormality of the mitral valve.

Most VSDs occur in the high portion of the interventricular septum or the membranous septum. Since this area is very thin, one must take care in making this diagnosis. VSDs in the muscular portion of the septum are easier to appreciate.

Cushion defects, or atrial-ventricular septal defects, involve a large, frequently prominent defect in the atrial and ventricular septa and a single atrial-ventricular valve with five leaflets.

Ebstein's anomaly is atrialization of the right ventricle. The right ventricle will be small in comparison to the right atrium.

Hypoplastic left heart syndrome depends on the demonstration of a small left ventricular cavity.

Tetralogy of Fallot has an overriding aorta with a VSD. The right ventricle may be hypertrophied, with stenosis of the right ventricular outflow tract. Usually, the right ventricular hypertrophy does not occur in utero but the large overriding aorta should be appreciated.

A truncus arteriosus should have a single large vessel that is overriding the ventricular septum with a VSD.

In transposition of the great vessels, the pulmonary artery and aorta do not spiral as they normally do. They are very straight and parallel to each other.

It also is important to make certain that the inferior vena cava and superior vena cava are entering the right atrium appropriately, and that situs is correct, with the liver on the right side and the spleen on the left side.

Arrhythmias can be diagnosed on ultrasound. A tachyarrhythmia is a heart rate greater than 180 and a bradyarrhythmia is a heart rate less than 100 beats/min. Bradycardia may be produced in the fetus transiently by pressure from the transducer, so only sustained bradycardia should be considered significant. Other arrhythmias are best evaluated with M-mode echocardiography in the presence of a pediatric cardiologist. In one study, all embryos between 5 and 8 weeks with heart rates less than 85 beats/min miscarried.

Tumors of the fetal heart (Table 8–11) include rhabdomyomas and teratomas. Rhabdomyomas are associated with tuberous

Table 8–11. HEART TUMORS

Rhabdomyoma
Teratoma
Fibroma
Myxoma
Hemangioma
Mesothelioma
Thickening of chordae tendineae
Aneurysm of foramen ovale

sclerosis and may be multiple (Fig. 8–33). Rhabdomyomas are usually in the region of the interventricular septum. Teratomas are the second most common cardiac tumor seen. They are intrapericardial in location. Fibromas are usually located in the distal interventricular septum. Endocardial fibroelastosis may be inherited or related to viral infection. This type of cardiomyopathy includes an enlarged heart and poor contractility (Fig. 8–34).

GASTROINTESTINAL TRACT, ABDOMEN, ABDOMINAL WALL

Abnormalities of the Gastrointestinal Tract and Abdomen

It is important to become familiar with normal fetal cross-sectional anatomy in order to be able to recognize abnormalities. Esophageal atresia may be seen in utero sonographically as polyhydramnios and nonvisualization of the stomach. However, these two findings are not sensitive indicators for esophageal atresia since the most common type of atresia has a fistula between the lower esophageal segment and the trachea that allows some fluid to reach the stomach. Fluid may also be secreted into the stomach. Therefore, fluid in the stomach does not exclude esophageal atresia. Nonvisualization of the stomach in conjunction with polyhydramnios can have other causes, such as central nervous system disorders that inhibit swallowing. Because esophageal atresia is associated with the VACTERL syndrome, a search for other anomalies should be done when it is suspected or found. An echogenic mass in the stomach may be from swallowed cells, swallowed blood (look for abruptio placenta), or swallowed meconium in stressed fetuses.

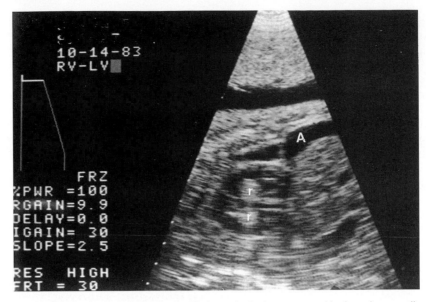

Figure 8–33. Coronal view of the fetal heart with two rhabdomyomas (r). A = descending aorta. (Courtesy of E. Stamm, MD University of Colorado, Denver, CO. Previously published in Rumack CM, Wilson SR, Charboneau JW. Diagnostic Ultrasound, vol. 2. St Louis, Mosby-Year Book, 1991, Figure 39–34.)

Duodenal atresia usually presents as a double bubble, that is, two cystic structures in the upper fetal abdomen (Fig. 8–35). A double bubble is seen in nearly 100 percent of cases with duodenal atresia. One-third of these are associated with trisomy 21. A double bubble may also be associated with a duodenal web or diaphragm, a blind pouch due to complete atresia, or an annular pancreas. Ladd's bands, which cause obstruc-

tion, may be another cause. A volvulus or duplication of bowel also may give two bubbles. Differential diagnosis for a double bubble also includes choledochal cysts, hepatic cysts, and renal cysts (Table 8–12).

Small bowel may be identified after 16 weeks and may be echogenic. Peristalsis should be visible in the third trimester. The bowel becomes sonolucent in the late second trimester. Small bowel should be less

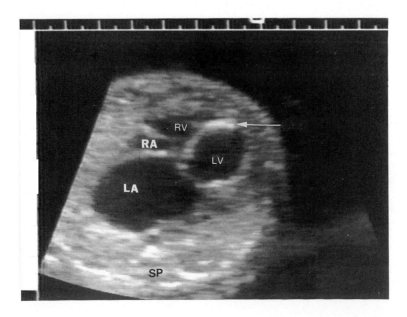

Figure 8–34. Endocardial fibroelastosis. Transverse image shows dilatation of left-sided chambers. *Arrow* points to an area of echogenic endocardium that is typical of this disease. RV = right ventricle, RA = right atrium, LV = left ventricle, LA = left atrium, SP = spine. (Courtesy of E. Stamm, M.D., University of Colorado, Denver, CO.)

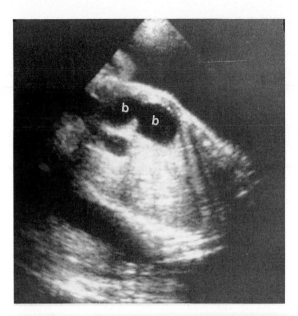

Figure 8–35. Sagittal image of a fetal head (to the right). Double-bubble sign is visible (b). Bubble on the left of the image is fluid-filled duodenum. Bubble on the right is stomach. This fetus had duodenal atresia.

than 7 mm in diameter and no continuous segment greater than 15 mm in length should be seen.

Normal colon may be up to 20 mm in diameter near term. Meconium within the bowel is a complex of sloughed cells, lanugo hairs, mucoproteins, and vernix caseosa. It is difficult to distinguish dilated small bowel from dilated large bowel. In general, large bowel is slightly greater in diameter and is located along the periphery of the abdominal cavity whereas small bowel is centrally located. One of the typical features of a bowel obstruction or bowel atresia is polyhydramnios probably because the fetus cannot continually swallow amniotic fluid if the bowel is not patent. Poly-

Table 8–12. DOUBLE BUBBLE

Duodenal atresia
Choledochal cyst
Normal stomach with prominent incisura
Congenital duplication of stomach
Duodenal web
Ladd's bands
Volvulus of bowel
Duplication of bowel
Hepatic cysts
Renal cysts

hydramnios worsens the more proximal the small bowel obstruction. Obstruction of the colon will not give polyhydramnios.

Small bowel atresias are thought to be vascular in etiology. There may be numerous dilated small bowel segments plus polyhydramnios. Ultrasound sensitivity for small bowel atresias is low. Dilated loops of bowel have a differential diagnosis of atresia, meconium ileus, volvulus, or obstructing mass.

Meconium ileus is an early clinical manifestation of cystic fibrosis. On ultrasound, dilated small bowel loops are seen and the meconium is quite echogenic. It should be emphasized that echogenic meconium is not specific for meconium ileus and can frequently be seen in normal fetuses. Polyhydramnios should be visible also.

Meconium peritonitis is the result of in utero bowel perforation, usually small bowel. This condition may be associated with numerous bowel disorders including volvulus, atresia, or meconium ileus. Meconium peritonitis is frequently thought to result from a vascular etiology. Bowel contents are spilled into the peritoneal cavity with resultant peritoneal calcification, the most common finding. This calcification is usually linear and there is associated ascites. Calcification in the scrotum indicates a peritoneal distribution. Abdominal calcifications in a fetus have a differential diagnosis of meconium peritonitis, infection, neoplasm such as in a teratoma, or anal atresia, in which case the calcifications are intraluminal in the bowel.

Other abdominal abnormalities are ovarian cysts, quite common in utero. These cysts may be the result of the enlargement of normal follicles due to stimulation by maternal hormones. Hydrometrocolpos may lead to a cystic mass in the pelvis and/or abdomen of the fetus. Hydronephrosis can lead to dilated renal pelves and ureters. Mesenteric cysts, duplication cysts, and choledochal cysts all can cause cystic lesions in the fetal abdomen (Table 8–13).

The fetal liver may appear enlarged on ultrasound. The most common cause is hydrops of either the immune or nonimmune type. However, the list of possible causes is long (Table 8–14). In utero infection is also a common cause of an enlarged liver. Likewise, splenomegaly is most often a result of either hydrops or infection.

Table 8–13. ABDOMINAL CYSTS

COMMON
Normal fetal bowel
Bowel obstruction

UNCOMMON
Duplication cysts
Intestinal atresia
Hydronephrosis
Ovarian cysts
Mesenteric cysts
Hirschsprung's disease
Omental cysts
Pancreatic cysts
Polycystic kidney disease (adult type)
Chronic chloride diarrhea
Meconium peritonitis
Urachal cysts
Volvulus of bowel
Midgut volvulus
Prenatal appendiceal abscess
Sacrococcygeal teratoma
Umbilical vein varices
Mesenteric cysts

Examining the Abdominal Wall

One must always carefully examine the anterior abdominal wall of the fetus at the cord insertion when performing ultrasound of a fetus, especially after the 12th week.

Table 8–14. HEPATOMEGALY

COMMON
Hepatitis
Cytomegalovirus infection
Rubella
Congenital hemolytic anemias, such as
  spherocytosis
Isoimmunization
Congestive heart disease

UNCOMMON
Toxoplasmosis
Syphilis
Varicella
Coxsackie virus infection
Mesenchymal hamartoma
Hemangioma
Metastatic neuroblastoma
Hepatoblastoma
Hemangiopericytoma
Galactosemia
Tyrosinemia
Alpha-1-antitrypsin deficiency
Disorders of the urea cycle
Methylmalonic acidemia
Infantile sialidosis
Beckwith-Wiedemann syndrome
Zellweger syndrome
Adult polycystic disease of liver and kidneys
Solitary cysts

Because the gut is rotating outside the abdominal cavity between 6 and 12 weeks, an anterior abdominal wall defect is of doubtful significance when detected at that time. After 12 weeks, an anterior abdominal wall defect must raise the question of an anomaly. One must note the location as to midline or off midline, whether or not any organs have protruded through the defect, and whether or not there are any other anomalies. Umbilical hernias are quite common and should not be mistaken for omphaloceles. An umbilical hernia is covered by skin and subcutaneous fat. The three most common defects and their features are listed in Table 8–15. A complete list of wall masses is given in Table 8–16.

Omphalocele is a midline protrusion through the anterior abdominal wall at the cord insertion. It should be covered by peritoneum and amnion (Fig. 8–36). Rarely, these membranes rupture in utero so that bowel will be floating free in amniotic fluid. Alpha-fetoprotein in the amniotic fluid will be low. If liver herniates through the defect, a reliable diagnosis of omphalocele is possible because liver herniation should not occur with gastroschisis (see below). One-third of fetuses with omphaloceles have polyhydramnios. The prognosis of omphalocele depends on the severity of any associated defects. The prognosis for omphalocele is not as good as the prognosis for gastroschisis.

Gastroschisis is a defect in the anterior abdominal wall that is off midline, usually on the right (Fig. 8–37). The bowel may protrude through the defect and may be quite dilated but it should not be covered by a membrane. Organs other than bowel should not protrude through the defect, generally. The defect is usually small. The bowel wall may be thickened due to its exposure to amniotic fluid. Gastroschisis has a good prognosis and is usually repaired surgically shortly after birth.

Limb–body-wall complex is a less common anomaly. It is sometimes called the body-stalk anomaly. This syndrome is thought to be related to the amniotic band syndrome, but there may also be a separate vascular etiology. Limb–body-wall complex often has severe scoliosis as one of its hallmarks and a body-wall defect that may contain eviscerated organs, including the liver. The body-wall defect may involve

Table 8–15. FEATURES OF GASTROSCHISIS, OMPHALOCELE, AND LIMB–BODY-WALL COMPLEX (LBWC)

	GASTROSCHISIS	OMPHALOCELE	LBWC
Location	Right paraumbilical	Midline	Lateral
Umbilical cord site	Normal	Apex of defect	Involved in defect
Membrane	No	Yes	Involved in defect
Liver involvement	Rare to never	Common	Common
Ascites	No	Common	Common
Bowel thickening	Common at term	Rarely (ruptured)	No
Bowel atresia	Common (15%)	Rare	Yes
Ischemia	Common (15%)	Rare	Rare
Cardiac anomalies	Rare (ASD, PDA)	Common (complex)	Common (complex)
Cranial anomalies	Rare	Occasionally	Common (encephalocele)
Limb anomalies	Rare	Occasionally	Common
Scoliosis	No	No	Common (77%)
Chromosomal abnormalities	No	Common (15%)	No

ASD = atrial septal defect; PDA= patent ductus arteriosus.
Adapted from Callen PW. Ultrasonography in Obstetrics and Gynecology, ed 2. Philadelphia, WB Saunders, 1988, with permission.

portions of the abdomen and thorax. It is frequently a large defect and is more often on the left side. There may be cranial defects and facial clefts. This complex is always fatal.

The amniotic band syndrome will be considered here because of its similarity to limb–body-wall complex. Amniotic band syndrome occurs due to fibrous strands that cause amputation of various fetal parts. It is thought to result from rupture of the amnion with protrusion of the fetal parts and entanglement of fetal parts in the chorion. Entrapment of fetal parts may lead to amputations or cleft-type defects.

Another anomaly that has a body-wall defect is bladder exstrophy. This defect occurs below the cord insertion. The bladder protrudes through the lower abdominal wall. Cloacal exstrophy has a similar appearance.

The pentalogy of Cantrell is the association of omphalocele involving the upper abdomen, an anterior diaphragmatic hernia, ectopia cordis, a defect of the lower sternum, and a deficiency of the diaphragmatic pericardium. In addition, there are usually associated intracardiac anomalies.

Beckwith-Wiedemann syndrome includes omphalocele plus macroglossia and visceromegaly.

FETAL KIDNEYS AND BLADDER

The kidneys of most fetuses can be identified sonographically by 20 weeks. They appear as ellipsoid, predominantly hypoechoic structures sitting in a paraspinous location bilaterally. Fifty percent of kidneys can be identified by 15 weeks and 90 percent at 20 weeks. The fetal bladder can be seen as early as 10 weeks and routinely by 16 weeks. The bladder is a midline cystic structure sitting in the anterior pelvis. The bladder should fill and empty approximately every 30 to 45 minutes. Ureters are not normally seen on ultrasound. The amount of amniotic fluid around the fetus is a reflection of renal function. Decreased renal function relates to decreased amniotic fluid volume. Before 16 weeks' gestational age, the kidneys are not needed to produce amniotic fluid. After 16 weeks, the kidneys

Table 8–16. ANTERIOR ABDOMINAL WALL DEFECTS OR MASSES

Omphalocele
Gastroschisis
Pentalogy of Cantrell
Beckwith-Wiedemann syndrome
Body-stalk anomaly
Bladder exstrophy
Cloacal exstrophy
Normal rotation of gut from 8 to 12 weeks
Patent urachus
Ectopia cordis
Vesicoallantoic cyst

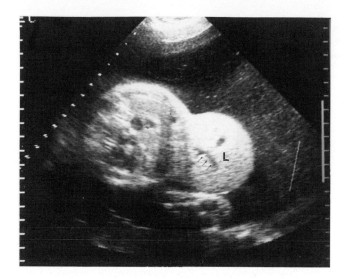

Figure 8–36. Transverse image of a fetus with a large omphalocele. The liver (L) has herniated through the defect. The lucent line is a portal vessel (arrows).

rapidly take over and account for the production of most of the amniotic fluid.

Renal Agenesis

Renal agenesis is the failure of both kidneys to develop. The result is severe oligohydramnios and no identifiable bladder. Potter's syndrome refers to bilateral renal agenesis, pulmonary hypoplasia, atypical facies with low-set ears, and skeletal abnormalities, including limb deformities, abnormal hands and feet, clubfeet, and hip dislocations. These abnormalities probably result from the severe oligohydramnios. Renal agenesis is a fatal condition.

The failure of one kidney to develop is referred to as unilateral renal agenesis or renal aplasia. If there is one normally functioning kidney, then the bladder should

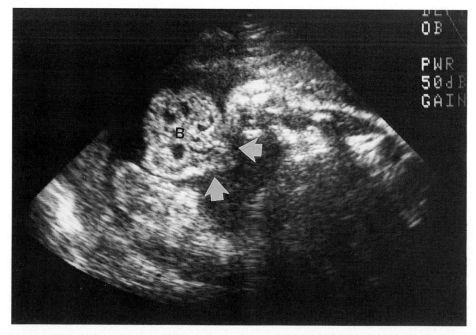

Figure 8–37. Anterior abdominal wall defect (arrows) with bowel loops (B) floating in fluid. The remainder of the fetal anatomy is not clearly depicted on this image. This is gastroschisis.

Table 8–17. HYDRONEPHROSIS

COMMON
Normal
Uteropelvic junction obstruction
Uterovesical junction obstruction
Overdistended fetal bladder
Posterior urethral valves
Vesicoureteral reflux

UNCOMMON
Primary megaureter
Prune-belly syndrome

demonstrate normal filling and emptying. It may be very difficult to determine whether or not a single kidney or both kidneys have not developed because the adrenal glands may assume a reniform shape.

If a bladder is not seen during a 60- to 90-minute examination, then a furosemide challenge test can be performed. Forty to 60 mg of furosemide is given intravenously to the mother in an attempt to induce fetal diuresis. Fluid in the bladder after administration of this drug indicates that at least one kidney is functioning. Failure to see the bladder, however, is not a reliable indicator of bilateral renal agenesis and for this reason this test has fallen from favor. Severe intrauterine growth retardation may also lead to a failure to diurese.

Dilated Collecting System

If the fetal renal pelvis is less than 5 mm in diameter, then hydronephrosis is not an appropriate diagnosis and the outcome can be expected to be good. If the renal pelvis measures between 5 and 10 mm, then hydronephrosis is a possibility and serial examinations should be performed to make sure that the condition does not worsen. A differential in this situation is given in Table 8–17. Even if the kidneys appear normal after birth, the infant who had a dilated renal pelvis in utero may have a higher risk of reflux in infancy. A voiding cystogram should be performed shortly after birth to look for reflux. However, it should not be performed on day one because the infant may be dehydrated and this may lead to a false-negative examination. If the renal pelvis measures over 10 mm, then a diagnosis of hydronephrosis is appropriate. A second method of diagnosing hydronephrosis is to determine the renal pelvis–to–renal cortex circumference ratio. It should be less than .5.

Ureteropelvic junction (UPJ) obstruction is the most common cause of neonatal hydronephrosis. This condition is usually unilateral and, when bilateral, it is asymmetric (Fig. 8–38). Unilateral UPJ obstruction may

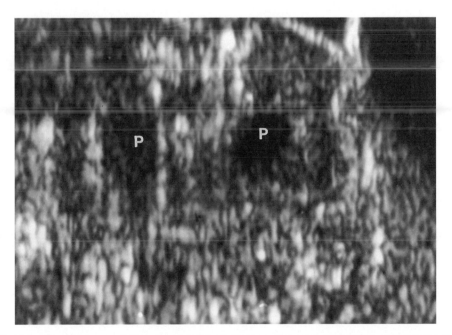

Figure 8–38. Magnified transverse image of fetal abdomen showing dilatation of both renal pelves (P).

occur with a contralateral renal agenesis or with a contralateral multicystic dysplastic kidney. UPJ obstruction may lead to a perinephric urinoma or ascites if the collecting system decompresses by rupturing.

Ureterovesical junction (UVJ) obstruction will lead to megaureter and hydronephrosis. UVJ obstruction is indistinguishable from reflux as a cause of megaureter and hydronephrosis. The megaureter usually creates a tortuous cystic-type cylinder and goes from the bladder to the kidney in an irregular course. If the structure comes in contact with the fetal spine and extends to the base of the bladder from the kidney, then that is good evidence that it is a ureter and not bowel.

Hydronephrosis may result from bladder outlet obstruction. The most common etiology is posterior urethral valves (PUV) (Fig. 8–39). PUVs are found almost exclusively in male fetuses. Urethral strictures or agenesis of the urethra may have a similar effect. A megacystic microcolon intestinal hypoperistalsis syndrome may lead to a dilated urinary tract. This usually affects females and causes abdominal distension. However, the bladder is not obstructed in this entity. Ultrasound of PUVs shows a dilated urinary bladder that fills most of the lower abdomen. The proximal urethra may be dilated and this may sometimes be seen on ultrasound as a funnel at the base of the bladder. Thickening of the wall of the bladder may sometimes be visible. PUVs may lead to megaureters and bilateral hydronephrosis. In the megacystic microcolon intestinal hypoperistalsis syndrome, the amniotic fluid volume will be normal or increased. This may allow a distinction between the other causes of urethral-level obstruction.

Prune-belly syndrome is probably related to obstruction at the level of the urethra. According to this theory, the urethral obstruction leads to a massive bladder. The bladder causes pressure on the abdominal wall musculature and resultant atrophy and/or failure of development. The testes cannot descend because of the large bladder. Prune-belly syndrome can sometimes be seen on fetal ultrasound if the bladder has decompressed and pressure can be applied to the fetal abdomen. The fetal abdomen will form a wave and will be very nonrigid.

Bladder or cloacal exstrophy can be diagnosed when the bladder is not in the usual location in the pelvis but either a solid or a cystic mass can be seen projecting from the anterior portion of the pelvis along the anterior abdominal wall. Amniotic fluid volume should be normal with bladder exstrophy. Exstrophy can be confused with an omphalocele or gastroschisis.

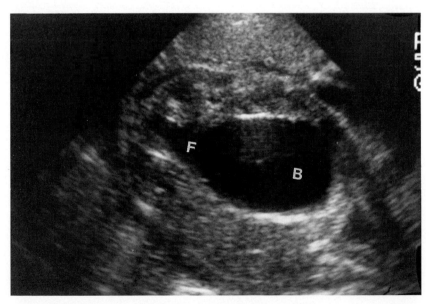

Figure 8–39. Sagittal image of fetal bladder. The outlet is funnel-shaped because of posterior urethral valves. F = funnel-shaped outlet, B = bladder.

Cystic Disease of the Kidneys

The Potter classification is used as a way to organize discussions of cystic disease of the kidney, although it is not etiologically logical. The four types of cystic disease are:

Type I—infantile polycystic kidney disease (IPKD)

Type II—multicystic dysplastic kidney disease (MDKD)

Type III—adult polycystic kidney disease (APKD)

Type IV—cystic renal dysplasia from obstruction

Potter Type I is the autosomal recessive infantile polycystic kidney disease. This disease has 1- to 2-mm cysts in place of the collecting tubules. These cysts are usually not visible on ultrasound. Instead, the kidneys are enlarged and echogenic (Fig. 8–40). Associated with this process are bile duct proliferation and fibrosis. This disease is subdivided into four types:

1. Perinatal presenting at birth—bilaterally enlarged echogenic kidneys with death within hours.
2. Neonatal—less severe renal disease but death occurs within one year.
3. Infantile form.
4. Juvenile form—both the latter present later but have more hepatic fibrosis and bile duct proliferation with longer survival.

This disease can be diagnosed as early as 20 weeks. Oligohydramnios should be present.

Potter Type II (multicystic dysplastic kidneys) is usually unilateral but can be bilateral or even segmental (Fig. 8–41). The ureteral bud fails to develop, which results in atresia of the upper ureter. The kidney becomes dysplastic and creates a mass with multiple cysts, sometimes said to resemble a cluster of grapes. The kidney is quite irregular. This condition is compatible with life as long as the other kidney functions normally. Current treatment is observation since the kidney will ultimately become atrophic and probably does not need to be removed in most cases. The other kidney may be abnormal in some respect in 40 percent of patients with multicystic dysplastic kidneys.

Adult polycystic kidney disease or autosomal dominant polycystic kidney disease is Potter Type III. This condition has occasionally been diagnosed prenatally. Multiple cysts are seen and the amniotic fluid is usually normal. The cysts may become more apparent as the gestation progresses.

Cystic renal dysplasia is Potter Type IV. Cystic renal dysplasia is thought to be sec-

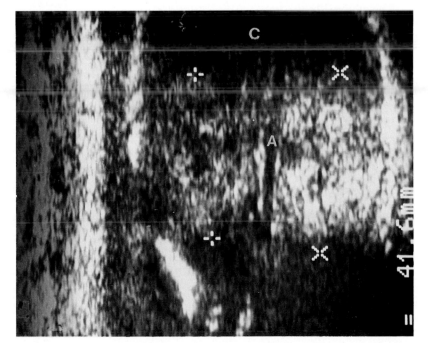

Figure 8–40. Coronal image of a fetus. The kidneys are marked by measuring calipers. The kidneys appear as large echogenic masses because of infantile polycystic kidney disease. A = aorta, C = chest.

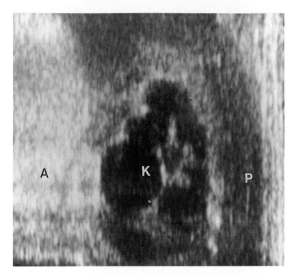

Figure 8–41. Sagittal image of a fetal abdomen. Multiple cysts are present due to multicystic dysplastic kidney (K). A = anterior, P = posterior.

ondary to urinary tract obstruction with formation of multiple cortical cysts. Potter Type IV occurs later in the development of the kidneys than the Potter Type II (multicystic dysplastic kidney). The ultrasound appearance of Potter Type IV kidneys ranges from increased echogenicity to normal echogenicity. The remainder of the urinary system should be dilated for this diagnosis to be made.

Renal cysts may be seen in several syndromes, including Jeune's, Zellweger's (see below), and the Meckel-Gruber syndrome.

Meckel-Gruber is autosomal recessive, has bilaterally enlarged kidneys with small cysts, and oligohydramnios. Most Meckel-Gruber patients have an associated encephalocele (Fig. 8–42).

Tumors

Renal tumors are only rarely identified prenatally. The most common type are mesoblastic nephromas, which are actually hamartomas. They appear as large, solid masses. These tumors are usually associated with polyhydramnios. Adrenal neuroblastomas produce a mass superior to the kidney. This mass may be hyperechoic to complex cystic, and it may be difficult to tell this mass from an adrenal hemorrhage.

SEXING

The sex of a fetus can usually be determined between 20 and 24 weeks by looking at the genitalia and determining whether labia are present or whether a penis and scrotum are present. This distinction may sometimes be difficult because the labia may appear enlarged. This is thought to be secondary to maternal hormones. We usually do not make an attempt to determine the sex unless there is a medical reason to do so.

FETAL MUSCULOSKELETAL SYSTEM

Starting at approximately 13 to 14 weeks, the fetal femur should be measured rou-

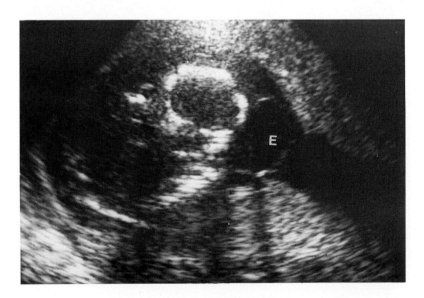

Figure 8–42. An encephalocele (E) projects posterior to the cranium in this fetus with Meckel-Gruber syndrome.

tinely and used as an aid in estimating gestational age. The femur is measured only along its ossified portion. Care should be taken to make the longest measurement and avoid foreshortening the femur; however, the nonossified cartilage at the proximal and distal end of the femur should not be included in the measurement. If the gestational age can be accurately estimated from head and abdomen measurements or from a date of last menses, then the femur should be within two standard deviations of the other measurements for a normally developing fetus. Another way to say this is that the femur measurement should be within 5 mm of the lower limit of normal for the gestational age. After 17 weeks this means the femur should be within two to three weeks of the other dating measurements. If the femur is shorter than expected, then all of the long bones should be measured and their lengths compared to normal values.

Rhizomelic shortening means that the femur and humerus are short but the tibia and ulna are normal in length. Mesomelic shortening means that the femur and humerus are normal in length but the ulna and tibia are short. Micromelic shortening means that all four measurements are short. A classification system was developed by Spirt and colleagues (Fig. 8–43). A few words about the more common syndromes that affect bone development follow.

Jeune's syndrome, or asphyxiating thoracic dystrophy, has mild micromelic shortening and a hypoplastic chest. The majority of these fetuses die of respiratory failure.

Ellis-Van Creveld syndrome, or chondroectodermal dysplasia, is a mild micromelic form of dwarfism. These fetuses have a long thorax and about 50 percent have congenital heart disease, especially atrial septal defects. About one-third die of associated cardiac problems.

Osteogenesis imperfecta (OI) Type I may not be easily diagnosed in utero. These patients have blue sclera, bone fragility, and deafness. OI Type II is lethal. The long bones show evidence of fractures with angulations and local areas of thickening secondary to callous formation. OI Type III is also difficult to diagnose in utero. OI Type IV is mild. There may be slight femoral bowing.

Hypophosphatasia is an autosomal recessive condition with demineralization of bones and low tissue alkaline phosphatase activity. This is a fatal disease. It may be recognized by marked demineralization of the calvarium. The falx may appear abnormally echogenic.

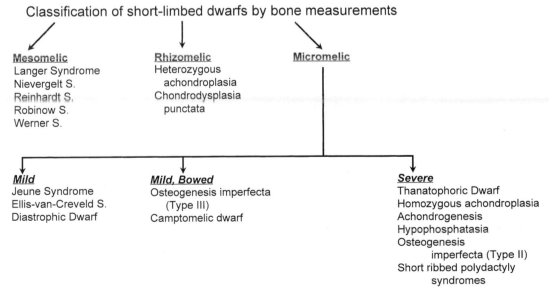

Figure 8–43. Algorithm for classification of short-limbed dwarfism on the basis of long bone measurements. S = syndrome. (From Spirt BA, Oliphant M, Gottlieb RH, Gordon LP. Prenatal sonographic elevation of short-limbed dwarfism: an algorithmic approach. Radiographics 10:217–236, 1990, with permission.)

Homozygous achondroplasia is similar to thanatophoric dwarfism. A cloverleaf skull is present. This condition is lethal (Fig. 8–44). In contrast, heterozygous achondroplasia has a good prognosis. Femur lengths become abnormal starting at about 20 weeks. The diagnosis can only be excluded after a normal femur measurement at or beyond 27 weeks.

Syndromes and Chromosomal Defects

The following section briefly reviews several other of the more common syndromes or chromosomal defects that have not been previously discussed.

Trisomy 21 (Down's Syndrome). Features are nuchal thickening, cystic hygromas, duodenal atresia, and short femurs. Ultrasound diagnosis in utero is difficult. Measurement of the thickness of the nuchal soft tissue between 14 and 20 weeks can be helpful. A measurement greater than 5 mm will be found in about 20 percent of fetuses with Down's syndrome.

This measurement is made using a transaxial image that angles through the posterior fossa and includes the cavum septi pellucidi anteriorly, and cerebellar hemispheres posteriorly. Measurements are made from outer occipital skull to outer skin. While measurements greater than 5 mm are abnormal, a significant number of normals will have a nuchal thickness greater than 5 mm. Measurements greater than 10 mm are strongly suggestive of trisomy 21.

Turner's Syndrome. Features are cystic hygromas, nonimmune hydrops, cardiovascular malformations, and genitourinary abnormalities.

Holt-Oram Syndrome. Features are cardiac abnormalities and radial abnormalities of upper extremities.

VACTERL Association. Features are vertebral anomalies, anorectal atresia, cardiac defects, tracheoesophageal fistula, renal anomalies, and limb anomalies.

Fetal Growth and Well-Being

There is no universal definition of the conditions referred to as intrauterine growth retardation (IUGR) or small for gestational age. Both of these are usually defined as a fetal body weight below the 10th percentile for the gestational age. Some define it as a fetal body weight below the 5th percentile. Likewise, there is no universal definition of macrosomia and large for gestational age (LGA). Usually macrosomia is defined as a body weight above 4 kg. LGA is defined as a body weight above the 90th percentile. It becomes very obvious that all of these definitions depend on an accurate way of assessing gestational age. With in vitro fertilization, artificial insemination, or

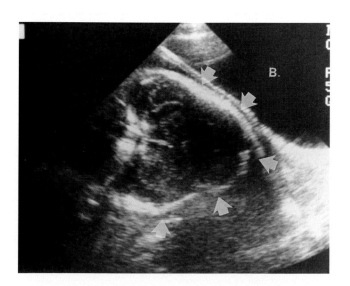

Figure 8–44. Coronal image of cloverleaf skull in homozygous achondroplasia. Margins of the skull are marked by *arrows.* B = maternal bladder. (Courtesy of E. Stamm, MD, University of Colorado, Denver, CO.)

ovulation induction, very accurate estimates of gestational age can be derived. If an ultrasound from which measurements of a crown-rump length were made early in the pregnancy is available, then gestational age can be estimated to within four or five days with a high degree of accuracy. However, if it is necessary to rely on the date of the last menstrual period or even on the measurement of a biparietal diameter, then the estimated gestational age will be much less accurate and it becomes much more difficult to determine if the weight is appropriate for the gestational age.

The presence of oligohydramnios in combination with a low fetal weight for gestational age is a good indicator of growth retardation. There are other causes for oligohydramnios, however (Table 8–18). Amniotic fluid volume can be estimated either subjectively or by using a four-quadrant quantitative technique. This technique consists of measuring the vertical depth of amniotic fluid without fetal parts and adding the four measurements together. The measurement is then compared to a graph of a normal range (see Fig. 8–12). It can be difficult to differentiate between intrauterine growth retardation with oligohydramnios and a renal problem causing oligohydramnios. The oligohydramnios is thought to result from shunting of fetal blood away from fetal kidneys and a resultant decrease in fetal urine production in IUGR (Fig. 8–45).

Amniotic fluid volume is determined also by measuring the largest pocket. If the largest pocket is smaller than 1 cm, then oligohydramnios is definitely present. If the largest pocket is less than 2 cm in depth, then oligohydramnios is probably present; conversely, if the largest pocket is greater than 7 cm, then polyhydramnios is probably present. It should be emphasized that a normal amount of amniotic fluid does not adequately exclude IUGR. IUGR is usually divided into symmetric and asymmetric varieties. The symmetric variety has small cranial measurements and a small abdominal circumference. These tend to be seen earlier, sometimes by the mid-second trimester, and are often associated with significant fetal anomalies. Asymmetric growth retardation refers to the situation in which the head measures appropriately for the gestational age but the abdomen is smaller than expected. The femur will also usually measure appropriately. This is thought to be a protective response in which the fetus shunts nutrition to the brain. The etiology probably involves the use of glycogen stores in the liver and a resultant decrease in size of the liver and decrease in size of the abdomen. Asymmetric IUGR occurs later in pregnancy, usually in the third trimester.

There is another way to assess fetal well-being and this is called an ultrasound-based fetal biophysical profile. This consists of five variables, including fetal breathing movements, fetal movements, fetal tone, fetal reactive heart rate, and qualitative amniotic fluid volume. Points are awarded for each of these during an observation period of approximately 30 minutes. The ultrasound fetal biophysical profile is not usually done routinely and is reserved for high-risk fetuses in referral centers.

DOPPLER STUDIES

Although Doppler may be an aid to evaluating fetal well-being, it is not a sensitive method as only about one half to two thirds of growth-retarded fetuses will have abnormal Doppler studies. Fetuses with other problems and/or anomalies may also have abnormal values. A ratio of peak systolic flow velocity to end-diastolic flow velocity varies with the gestational age (Fig. 8–46) when measured at the placental end of the cord in the umbilical artery. An elevated value implies increasing resistance to flow. Absent end-diastolic flow or flow reversal is a bad sign. An abnormal value may reflect IUGR, sometimes as much as four

Table 8–18. OLIGOHYDRAMNIOS

COMMON
Bilateral renal agenesis
Polycystic kidney disease (infantile or adult)
Renal obstruction
Bladder obstruction
Premature rupture of membranes
Intrauterine growth retardation

UNCOMMON
Multicystic dysplastic kidney (bilateral)
Prune-belly syndrome
Caudal regression syndrome
Absence of urethra
Triploidy
Sirenomelia
Triploid fetus

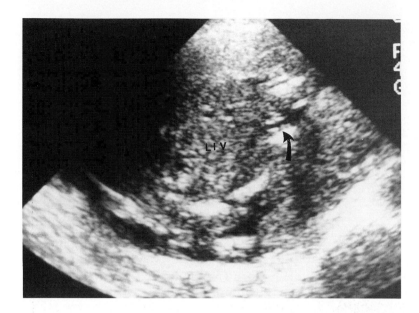

Figure 8–45. Transverse fetal abdomen. LIV = fetal liver, *curved arrow* = cord insertion. Severe oligohydramnios makes visualization of the fetal anatomy difficult. This fetus has severe IUGR.

weeks before other signs appear. Other causes of fetal distress, such as chromosomal anomalies, may give abnormal values.

HYDROPS

Fetal hydrops means that fluid has accumulated in numerous extravascular spaces. It includes anasarca, fetal ascites, pleural effusions, pericardial effusions, subcutaneous edema, and polyhydramnios. Immune hydrops fetalis occurs when maternal immunoglobulin G antibodies attack

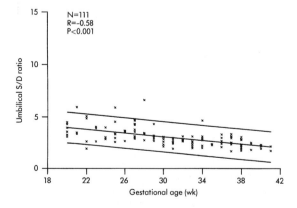

Figure 8–46. Normal systolic-diastolic (S/D) ratio in umbilical arteries. (From Cameron A, Nicholson S, Nimrod CA, et al. Duplex ultrasonography of the fetal aorta, umbilical artery, and placental arcuate artery throughout normal human pregnancy. J Can Assoc Radiol *40*: 145–149, 1989, with permission.)

fetal red cell antigens, usually the Rh antigen (Fig. 8–47). Nonimmune hydrops occurs as a result of many severe diseases and chromosomal abnormalities. Cardiac abnormalities are a common cause of nonimmune hydrops fetalis. The normal abdominal wall musculature may be hypoechoic and simulate a thin peripheral rim of ascites. Care should be used to avoid mistakenly diagnosing ascites.

Twins

In the United States, twins account for about 1.2 percent of all births but about 12 percent of neonatal deaths. Ultrasound of twins should detect the fact that more than one fetus is present, but should also determine the amnionicity and chorionicity as an indicator of the prognosis of a twin pregnancy. The ultrasonographer should be able to diagnose twins after six to seven weeks gestation.

Twins can develop from two eggs that are separately fertilized. These are fraternal twins or dizygotic twins with different genetic material. These account for 70 percent of all twin pregnancies in the United States. Monozygotic twins occur when a single egg is fertilized by a single sperm but, early in the division process, there is a separation leading to two embryos.

Dizygotic twins always have embryos that each have their own amnion immedi-

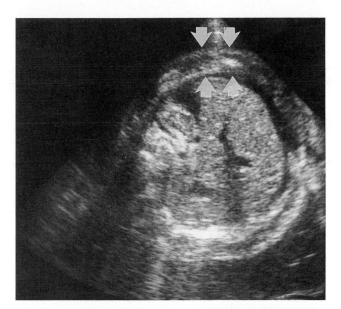

Figure 8–47. Transverse image of fetal abdomen shows ascites and body wall edema (*arrows*).

ately surrounding them and each have their own chorion (Fig. 8–48). Therefore, each embryo has its own placenta. On ultrasound, however, these placentae may fuse and appear as a single placenta. Even if the two placentae fuse, it is rare for vascular connections to occur between the placentae. Therefore, the dreaded twin-to-twin transfusion syndrome does not occur.

Monozygotic twins account for 30 percent of the twin pregnancies in the United States. If the fertilized zygote divides before four days postfertilization, then each embryo will have its own amnion and each embryo will have its own chorion just as if it had been a dizygotic pregnancy. However, just as in dizygotic twins, the placentae may fuse. If the division in the two embryos occurs between four and eight days, then each embryo will have its own amnion but a single chorion will surround both embryos. This is a monochorionic diamniotic

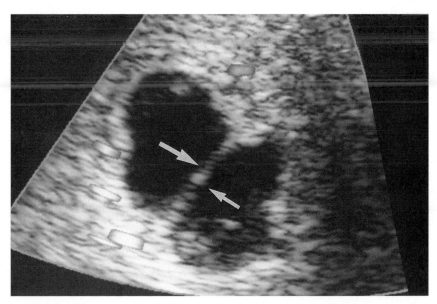

Figure 8–48. Early diamniotic, dichorionic pregnancy. The thick membrane (*arrows*) indicates that there are four layers present.

pregnancy. A single placenta will supply both embryos. Vascular connections within the placenta may lead to arteriovenous shunting and may lead to the twin-to-twin transfusion syndrome. If the separation of the monozygotic pregnancy into two embryos occurs after eight days, then there will be a single amnion surrounding both twins and a single chorion surrounding the amniotic sac. The umbilical cords and twins may become tangled and this type of pregnancy is at very high risk for complications. A monochorionic monoamniotic pregnancy accounts for only 4 percent of the total of all monozygotic pregnancies, and less than one percent of all pregnancies.

On ultrasound, the dichorionic diamniotic pregnancy early on will have two separate echogenic rings in the uterus from two gestational sacs. The monochorionic diamniotic pregnancy will have only a single echogenic ring. However, there will be two yolk sacs within the gestational sac. These two yolk sacs will be separated by an amniotic membrane (which may not be visible). A monochorionic monoamniotic pregnancy will have only a single sac with two embryos in it and no membrane. In addition to the entanglement problem mentioned above, these twins are at risk for twin-to-twin transfusion syndrome.

The separating membrane must be searched for in all twin pregnancies. If there is a separating membrane, then the ultrasonographer knows that the pregnancy is not monochorionic monoamniotic. A thick membrane implies that there are two layers of amnion and two layers of chorion and, therefore, the pregnancy is a dichorionic diamniotic. If the membrane is thin, then the implication is that there are only two layers of amnion separating the two fetuses and that it is a monochorionic diamniotic pregnancy. In the last trimester, the membranes may become thin and it may be difficult to tell if there is a thick membrane or a thin membrane.

As mentioned above, twin-to-twin transfusion syndrome occurs because of arteriovenous anastomoses in the placenta. This occurs in monochorionic pregnancies (it rarely occurs in dichorionic pregnancies). Blood is shunted from one fetus to the other fetus. The donor fetus has a closely applied amniotic membrane, oligohydramnios, and becomes "stuck." The recipient twin becomes very plethoric and hydropic. It will usually be larger than the donor twin. In the worst case, there may be reversal of blood flow from one twin to the other. The result may be an acardiac twin. This twin will have no heart, be severely deformed, and probably be missing limbs and have other severe anomalies.

One caveat: Failure to see a separating membrane does not reliably predict that there is a monoamniotic pregnancy. This is because the thin membrane of a monochorionic diamniotic pregnancy may be very difficult to detect, especially late in pregnancy. A second point is that if the twins are different genders then they are dizygotic twins and, therefore, there are two placentae present.

In the twin-to-twin transfusion syndrome, there are generally no survivors if birth occurs before 26 weeks and about a 25 percent survival if it is after 26 weeks. The mortality for the large twin in a twin-to-twin transfusion is about 88 percent and for the small twin it is about 96 percent.

To summarize, twin-to-twin transfusion should be suspected when there is a disparity in the size of the twins. While IUGR may cause such a disparity, IUGR is more commonly a problem in the third trimester. If the birth weight discrepancy between the twins is greater than 20 percent to 25 percent when calculated on the basis of sonographic parameters, then twin-to-twin transfusion syndrome should be suspected. Disparity in size of the two amniotic sacs is also an indicator of twin-to-twin transfusion. If there is hydrops in either fetus, that would be a third indicator of twin-to-twin transfusion.

AXIOMS ABOUT TWINS
(Courtesy of Jeff Seabourn, MD)

1. All dizygotic twins are dichorionic diamniotic.
2. All dichorionic gestations are also diamniotic.
3. All monochorionic twins are monozygotic.
4. Monozygotic twins can have three types of placentation
   a. Dichorionic diamniotic (18 to 36%)
   b. Monochorionic diamniotic (60 to 75%)
   c. Monochorionic monoamniotic (2 to 3%)

5. Most twins that have dichorionic diamniotic placentation are dizygotic (85 to 90%). Ten to 15 percent are monozygotic. The only way to tell zygosity of dichorionic diamniotic pregnancies is to detect different sexes or different blood groups.

6. Dichorionic diamniotic placentae may be fused or separate, but generally no vascular anastomosis exists between them.

7. Virtually all monochorionic twin gestations have placental vascular anastomoses.

8. If two placentas are seen, then the pregnancy is dichorionic diamniotic.

9. If one placenta is seen, the pregnancy may still be dichorionic diamniotic.

10. If no membrane is seen between the twins, monoamnionicity still cannot be reliably predicted.

11. If twins are facing each other, think about conjoined twins.

Alpha-Fetoprotein and Acetylcholinesterase

Alpha-fetoprotein (AFP) is a glycoprotein that can serve as a marker for neural tube defects and several other major anomalies. Low levels of AFP may be associated with increased risk for trisomy 21 and other trisomies. AFP levels are reported as multiples of the mean. The most common causes of elevated maternal serum AFP include poor dates, fetal hemorrhage, fetal demise, congenital anomalies, neural tube defects, multiple gestation, abdominal wall defects, gastrointestinal atresias, Turner's syndrome, nephrosis, abnormal chromosomes, diabetes mellitus, and maternal hepatitis. After eliminating multiple gestations and wrong dates as causes for an elevated maternal serum AFP level, about 10 percent of the remainder of patients with elevated AFP levels will have a neural tube defect. Usually amniocentesis is performed in these patients.

Acetylcholinesterase is an enzyme found in neural tissue. If amniocentesis reveals elevated AFP levels and acetylcholinesterase levels in the amniotic fluid, then there is a very high risk of a neural tube defect. If the amniotic fluid AFP level is high but the acetylcholinesterase is normal, then anomalies other than a neural tube defect should be considered.

Infertility

Ultrasound may be used either transvaginally or transabdominally to monitor the ovaries. Early in the menstrual cycle (day 5 to day 7), several follicles may usually be identified. After day 7, a dominant follicle should start to develop and may be detected. This follicle will reach a maximum diameter of 18 to 28 mm. After ovulation, the follicle will diminish in size. It may be very echogenic secondary to hemorrhage.

Ultrasound may also be used for in vitro fertilization. Initially, ultrasound is used to monitor the follicles. Ultrasound guidance is then used for oocyte retrieval.

Suggested Readings

Callen PW. Ultrasonography in Obstetrics and Gynecology. Philadelphia, WB Saunders Company, 1994.

Moore KL. The Developing Human: Clinically Oriented Embryology, ed. 4. Philadelphia, WB Saunders Company, 1988

Nyberg DA, Mahony BS, Pretorius DH. Diagnostic Ultrasound of Fetal Anomalies: Text and Atlas. Chicago, Year Book Medical Publishers, Inc., 1990.

Spirt BA, Oliphant M, Gottlieb RH, et al. Prenatal sonographic evaluation of short-limbed dwarfism: an algorithmic approach. Radiographics 10:217–236, 1990.

CHAPTER 9

Interventional and Intraoperative Ultrasound

Interventional Ultrasound

Ultrasound guidance for interventional procedures includes sonographically-guided biopsies and sonographically-guided abscess drainage. The principles for these procedures are the same; the difference is in the type of needle and/or tube that is placed into the lesion. We will also consider breast cyst aspiration, renal cyst aspiration, amniocentesis, chorionic villous sampling, and gastrostomy placement in this section.

GUIDANCE METHODS

Three basic guidance techniques can be used. One method, indirect ultrasound guidance, involves identifying the lesion being aspirated or drained, marking a spot on the skin, and inserting a needle through that spot. Needle, angle, and depth are estimated based on the ultrasound appearance, but the ultrasound transducer is not present at the time of the puncture. We frequently use this technique for thoracentesis and aspiration of ascites.

A second method is the free-hand puncture technique. The radiologist usually holds the transducer with one hand while inserting the needle with the other hand. The needle may be inserted parallel to the transducer (i.e., directly next to it). Alternatively, the needle may be inserted perpendicular to the transducer (Fig. 9–1). Visualization of the needle is somewhat easier when it is inserted perpendicular to the transducer.

A third method involves the use of a needle biopsy guide. There are dedicated transducers that have a slot for the needle in the center or in the edge. More commonly, an attachment that has a slot for the needle to slide through is placed on the transducer (Fig. 9–2). The needle slides into the ultrasound beam. Frequently, biopsy guidelines can be electronically generated on the video screen to show the approximate path of the needle. Usually, with a biopsy guide, the needle can be followed as it traverses the ultrasound image into the lesion.

NEEDLE TYPES AND VISUALIZATION

The inability to visualize the needle during ultrasound can be a significant limiting factor. If the needle cannot be seen, direct ultrasonographic guidance is not any more advantageous than indirect ultrasonographic guidance, in which the lesion is localized and angle and depth are estimated prior to puncture. Large needles are easier to see than small needles. Needles placed perpendicular to the beam are easier to see than needles placed parallel to the beam because there is more reflective surface. Needles are seen best when they are in the focal zone of the transducer. Usually the tip of the needle will return an echo and be quite bright even when the shaft of the needle is not seen. This is probably caused by the multiple surfaces of the needle tip.

Various techniques will make a needle more visible, including the use of roughened Teflon for the shaft and the placement of spiral grooves along the needle shaft, as in a Rotex needle. Other techniques to improve visualization include injecting air and

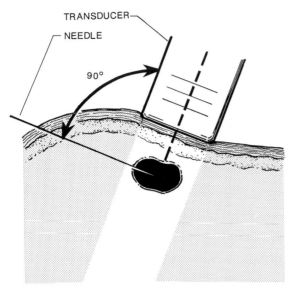

Figure 9–1. Needle is inserted perpendicular to transducer as real-time imaging is performed. Needle can be watched as it moves toward lesion.

watching for air bubbles coming out of the tip. This can actually inhibit overall visualization if the gas remains in the image and causes shadowing. The most common method of visualizing the needle tip is simply to move the needle in and out or jiggle the needle and look for the associated motion.

Needles 21- to 26-gauge in size are frequently used to aspirate for cytology or chemical fluid analysis. With larger gauge needles (14- to 19-gauge), larger pieces of

tissue can be obtained for histology. There has been a reluctance to use large-caliber needles because of a fear of increased risk of complications. However, the increase in risk is now considered minimal and is offset by the gain in information from the larger piece of tissue.

Various abscess drainage kits are available. One of the most popular is the van Sonnenberg kit. A needle is usually placed with its tip in the suspected abscess and aspiration is performed to confirm the presence of the abscess. Then, either a guide wire is inserted through the needle and a catheter placed over the guide wire, or a catheter is placed directly over the needle.

Sterile Techniques

Generally, sterile techniques should be used when using ultrasound guidance. One should place the transducer and most distal transducer cord in a sterile sheath or glove. Ultrasonic jelly is used in the glove or sheath to couple the transducer to the sheath. Sterile jelly is then used on the patient's skin as a final coupler. In the indirect ultrasonographic guidance methods and in the freehand method, where the transducer is 90° from the needle, it may not be necessary to have the transducer in a sterile sheath or glove. Sterility becomes necessary if the transducer is to be in the puncture field. In general, the transducer must be cleaned with an alcohol swab after each procedure. Most transducers cannot be ster-

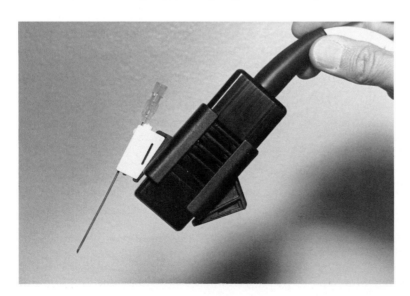

Figure 9–2. Needle guide attaches to side of transducer. Needle can be visualized as it moves through tissue, although needle is not as obvious as when it is inserted perpendicular to transducer.

ilized. In most circumstances, it is not feasible to take a transducer out of service to sterilize it.

Clotting parameters should be normal or near normal. We prefer that the prothrombin time be within 3 seconds of normal and the partial thromboplastin time be under 45 seconds. Platelets should be over 50,000. While a bleeding time may be the most accurate assessment of a patient's ability to clot, it is not feasible to do this on all patients. A bleeding time is probably not needed if the patient has no recent or remote history of bleeding problems. It is best to have an intravenous line in place. The patient may be premedicated with a mild benzodiazepine-type sedative for anxiety relief. Demerol or one of the narcotic-type drugs can be used for pain relief, depending on the situation. In children, adequate sedation is a must. Small children require general anesthesia. Intravenous pentobarbital, monitored by pulse oximeter, will work in many children and does not require an anesthesiologist.

Abscess and Fluid Aspiration

Ultrasound can be used to guide thoracentesis or fluid aspiration. A fluid collection can be identified with a patient in the upright seated position, usually a posterior intercostal approach. We usually identify the fluid collection, mark an interspace and perform the aspiration, or even return the patient to the floor for the thoracentesis. Some fluid collections will be very viscous and thick and will not be easily aspirated through a small needle. If the tap is unsuccessful, we usually recommend a switch to a larger bore 18-gauge needle and that a repeat aspiration attempt made.

Empyemas may be drained using the same technique. A large-bore 12- or 14-French pigtail catheter is usually used. If double-lumen catheters are utilized, then a pneumothorax will result unless the sump lumen is clamped.

ABDOMEN

We are frequently asked to localize ascites so that diagnostic taps can be performed. We find the largest pocket of ascites with the patient in a supine position and usually mark that spot and return the patient to the

floor. If we are performing the aspiration ourselves, we usually start with a 22-gauge needle, which can traverse bowel without serious consequences. If the fluid cannot be successfully aspirated through a 22-gauge needle, then we will attempt aspiration with a larger bore needle.

For abdominal abscess drainage, adequate access and only a single collection are needed. If multiple fluid collections are present, it is preferable that these be drained surgically.

PANCREAS AND RIGHT UPPER QUADRANT

Phlegmons are edematous inflamed soft tissue and usually do not respond to drainage. As large a catheter as possible should be used for pancreatic and right upper quadrant abscesses. After drainage, the vital signs are usually monitored closely for several hours because of the risk of septicemia. Some clinicians advocate copious irrigation of the abscess before the patient is returned to his hospital room. The catheter should be flushed twice daily. Abscesses with fistulas may require prolonged drainage before the fistula closes.

Pancreatic abscesses may be drained using techniques similar to those used in other areas of the abdomen. Biopsy of pancreatic tumors may also be performed as long as there is adequate access. For biopsies, 20- to 22-gauge needles are usually used.

Biliary drainage procedures may be guided by ultrasound. This is particularly useful when only a portion of the interhepatic biliary ductal system is dilated. The ultrasound can be used to guide the needle into the appropriate duct. Antibiotics should be administered before drainage is attempted.

Gallbladder aspiration and drainage can also be guided by ultrasound. Ultrasound can also be used to direct a gallbladder biopsy. Initially considered a high risk, gallbladder aspiration is now considered a safe procedure. Aspiration of the gallbladder has been used in an attempt to diagnose acute acalculous cholecystitis. While the specificity has been good, the sensitivity has been disappointing. Acutely inflamed gallbladders may be decompressed prior to surgical removal. Any self-retaining type of catheter, such as the McGahan catheter, may be used.

GENITOURINARY

Ultrasound can be used for cyst aspiration when a nonsimple cyst is identified in the kidney or when a patient is symptomatic from a renal cyst. Puncture is performed from either a posterior or posterior lateral position to avoid the ascending or descending colon. One should make certain that the needle enters below the costal margin. Any of the needle guidance methods discussed earlier can be used. Aspirated fluid is sent for cytology, culture and sensitivity, lactate dehydrogenase (may be a tumor marker), and protein (also a possible tumor marker) determinations. A combination of air and contrast can be instilled after aspiration of the cyst. Plain radiographs are obtained in an effort to identify mural masses.

Solid renal masses may be biopsied under ultrasound guidance. In reality, this is seldom done since the treatment of a solid renal mass is surgical removal. In some patients, surgical removal is not feasible; for example, patients with only a single kidney who have an indeterminate renal mass would be poor candidates. In the past, there was concern that seeding of the biopsy tract could occur if a renal cell carcinoma was biopsied. As there are scant reports of this phenomenon, the risk of this occurring is probably very low.

Ultrasound can be used to guide renal biopsies. For instance, patients who present with glomerulonephritis or with renal failure of unknown etiology will frequently undergo a renal biopsy. Efforts are usually made to guide the needle into a lower pole, usually of the left kidney.

Percutaneous nephrostomy for urinary diversion can be ultrasound guided. Usually, ultrasound is used in combination with fluoroscopy. The patient is placed in a prone position and the lower pole of the kidney is identified. A posterior lateral approach is used to avoid the colon. Occasionally, the bowel can be in the retroperitoneal space posterior to the kidney. One must make certain that no bowel lies between the needle insertion point and the kidney. A 22-gauge needle is usually used to puncture a lower pole collecting system.

A guide wire can then be placed through the needle, dilators are used to widen the track, and then a catheter is placed with its pigtail tip in the lower pole collecting system. Antibiotics should be administered before drainage is attempted.

GYNECOLOGY

Transvaginal ultrasound can be used for guidance of drainage of tubo-ovarian abscesses in the adnexa or in the cul-de-sac. A similar technique can be used for culdocentesis in an effort to determine if hemorrhage from an ectopic pregnancy is present. Transvaginal ultrasound can also be used for aspiration of follicles in in vitro fertilization techniques.

OBSTETRICS

Ultrasound is used to guide amniocentesis for genetic analysis of amniotic fluid. Assessment of fetal lung maturity can also be performed by analyzing the amniotic fluid for the lecithin-sphingomyelin (LS) ratio near the end of pregnancy. An LS ratio greater than 2.0 indicates mature lungs. Presence of phosphatidyglycerol is further evidence that the lungs are mature. A preliminary obstetric ultrasound should be performed and the gestation evaluated. Placenta should also be identified and the fetal lie determined. Using sterile technique, the needle is inserted alongside the transducer using the freehand or needle guide method. It is best to place the needle in the largest pocket of fluid away from the fetal head. Penetration of the placenta is acceptable but cord insertion should be avoided. A 22-gauge needle designed for amniocentesis is used. Spinal needles can also be utilized. The needle should be screwed in to avoid tenting of the membranes. The needle is placed as deeply as possible without penetrating the posterior wall. This prevents the fetus from moving and becoming punctured by the needle.

Ultrasound can also be used to guide chorionic villous sampling. This is performed between 9 and 11 weeks. Again, a preliminary obstetric ultrasound is done. Ultrasound is used to watch through the bladder while using a transcervical approach. Specialized catheters are made for this purpose. The patient is placed in the lithotomy position. The catheter is oriented with its tip in the region of the chorion frondosum of the placenta. While the sample is aspirated, the catheter is withdrawn. The procedure is contraindicated when cervical infection or cervical leiomyomata are present.

Finally, ultrasound guidance may be used for percutaneous umbilical blood sampling. This technique is used for chromosome analysis, Rh disease, in utero infection, coagulation problems, and immune disorders. The umbilical cord is punctured within a few centimeters of its placental insertion. This puncture may take place through the placenta or, if the placenta is posterior, through the amnionic sac. Usually the vein is punctured since it is larger. If the cord insertion is not accessible, then other portions of the cord can be punctured, but it is very difficult to puncture a free umbilical cord. The same technique can be used to give a fetal blood transfusion. Using this technique, a fetal blood transfusion can be given either via the cord or via the abdominal cavity of the fetus.

Intraoperative Ultrasound

CRANIAL

Ultrasound can be used in the operating room to assist with neurosurgery. Transducers between 5 and 10 MHz are usually used. A sector transducer is usually superior to a linear transducer because the opening for scanning is usually a small craniotomy. Sterile technique should be used, with the transducer gloved and sleeved. Orientation can be a problem since the ultrasonographer will not be present when the patient is being draped in the operating room. The head may be positioned in an unusual orientation so the first thing the sonographer needs to do is orient himself. The easiest way to do this is to find the two ventricles and scan transverse to them. Copious irrigation must be used during the scanning process to maintain contact with the brain. Transducer-generated, near-field artifact may interfere with scanning in the first 1 to 2 cm of the field. If a variable frequency transducer is being used, it can be worthwhile to switch back and forth between the two frequencies in an effort to eliminate this artifact. Lesions should be scanned in two planes. One use of intraoperative cranial ultrasound is to assist with the placement of ventricular shunt tubes. The shunt should not cross midline and penetrate into the opposite ventricle unless midline structures are absent. Ultrasound may also be used to assist with brain biopsy or aspiration of either solid or cystic lesions. If a brain biopsy is performed, then ultrasound can be used to monitor the biopsy location for hemorrhage for several minutes postbiopsy.

Ultrasonography of brain tumors can be useful in identifying a tumor for the neurosurgeon. Irregularly bordered tumors are usually of higher grade and are more invasive. Brain tumors are usually echogenic. In low-grade tumors the areas of increased echogenicity are viable tumor. Low-grade tumors tend to be somewhat less echogenic than high-grade tumors. Edema in the brain will also appear hyperechoic. Brain lymphoma will be echogenic and poorly marginated. One must be careful not to mistake a sulcus that is echogenic for a tumor. Tumors will usually distort the sulcus and distort surrounding structures. Solitary metastases have well-defined margins with surrounding edema.

SPINAL CORD

Ultrasound may be useful to monitor decompression of the cord. Adequate decompression has been performed when the cord no longer deviates from the normal, rounded shape and when the spinal cord and cauda equina take a normal course within the spinal canal. At times, an intraspinal mass can be identified and it is apparent when the mass has been removed.

Medullary spinal cord tumors usually cause enlargement and distortion of the cord with obliteration or effacement of central echo. They may be either isoechoic or hyperechoic. Ultrasound can be used to identify an area of tumor-related syringomyelia. Hematoma will vary in echogenicity from hypoechoic to hyperechoic depending on the age of the hematoma. The hematoma generally becomes less echogenic with time. Disk material will usually be of intermediate echogenicity and will be located adjacent to intervertebral disk. One caveat: Foam gel may interfere with scanning; therefore, if possible, all foam gel should be removed from the area that is being scanned.

Intraoperative ultrasound in the spine is also useful in the removal of bone and fragments in patients who have had fractures and the monitoring of operative reduction and stabilization during fusion or metallic rod placement procedures.

ABDOMINAL

Ultrasound can be used intraoperatively in the abdomen. It is mainly used for the liver and pancreas, although examination of the common duct can also be performed. In the liver, intraoperative ultrasound can identify lesions that are not visible or palpable on the surface of the liver so that they be resected. Intraoperative ultrasound can also be used to assist in drainage of amebic or bacterial abscesses of the liver. When performing intraoperative ultrasound in the abdomen, contact with the organ being examined is made by using copious amounts of saline. High-frequency transducers should be used, usually a 7.5- or 10-MHz. Occasionally, a 5-MHz transducer will suffice. The ultrasound transducer can be placed directly on the common duct to examine for stones. It can also be used to ex-amine intrahepatic portions of the biliary system for stones. A high-frequency transducer (10 MHz) will be necessary if the transducer is to be placed directly on the duct. Similarly, ultrasound can be used to look at and identify biliary tumors.

In the pancreas, intraoperative ultrasound is especially valuable when looking for islet cell–type tumors. These are frequently very small and may be multiple. They are usually hypoechoic. Pancreatic ultrasound, when used intraoperatively, was able to identify about 85 percent of solitary insulinomas. In the pancreas, ultrasound can also be used for small nonvisible and nonpalpable adenocarcinomas.

Suggested Readings

Fornage BD, Coan JD, David CL. Ultrasound-guided needle biopsy of the breast and other interventional procedures. Radiol Clin North Am 30:167–185, 1992.

Hall-Craggs MA. Interventional abdominal ultrasound: recent advances. Br J Hosp Med 42:176–182, 1989.

Holm HH. Interventional ultrasound. Br J Radiol 64: 379–385, 1991.

Machi J, Sigel B. Intraoperative ultrasonography. Radiol Clin North Am 30:1085–1103, 1992.

McGahan JP, Gerscovich E. Intraoperataive and interventional ultrasound. Curr Opin Radiol 2:213–222, 1990.

CHAPTER 10

Pediatric Brain, Spine, and Hip Ultrasonography

Ultrasound of the Brain

Ultrasonography of the brain is commonly performed on premature infants. If an infant weighs less than 1,500 gm or is born before 34 weeks' gestational age, there is a significant risk of an intracranial hemorrhage.

The younger the gestational age, the greater the risk of a hemorrhage. Hemorrhage and infarct also can occur in term infants, however. There is also a higher risk of hemorrhage with lower birth weights (Table 10–1).

TECHNIQUE

We use a 7.5-MHz transducer with a small foot plate. Scanning is performed through the anterior fontanelle. This fontanelle remains open until about 15 months of age. Scanning becomes difficult after about 9 to 10 months of age. Occasionally, scanning through the squamosal part of the temporal bone can be useful, especially for performing Doppler. Occasionally, the posterior fontanelle may also be used to scan the posterior fossa. As these infants are usually fragile, and frequently in an isolette, it is important to scan through the sides of the isolette so that the infant may stay warm. Warm lights may be trained on the infant. Good hand washing practices should be used. Warm sterile gel helps keep the infant clean, warm, and quiet. Transducers should be cleaned with soap and water after each examination.

Most bleeds occur within the first week of postnatal life. Therefore, screening exams should be performed between 7 and 10 days of age. Ninety-eight percent of hemorrhages will be detected. If a Grade II hemorrhage or greater is found, weekly ultrasounds are performed to observe for ventricular dilatation. If three consecutive scans show progressive ventricular dilatation, then intervention is undertaken. If the ventricles stabilize or become smaller, no intervention is done.

SCAN PLANES AND LEVELS

The infant head is scanned in the coronal and sagittal planes as a routine, with occasional scans performed in an axial plane. We obtain 12 coronal images. Six is a minimum (Fig. 10–1). The first coronal plane is anterior to the frontal horns, with each plane moving progressively posteriorly (Fig. 10–1A). Subsequent scans should be through the frontal horns just anterior to the foramen of Monroe (Fig. 10–1B), and then at the level of the foramen of Monroe (Fig. 10–1C). Additional scan planes should be through the thalami and third ventricle, through the quadrigeminal plate cistern, and then through the most posterior portion of the lateral ventricles (Fig. 10–1D). Finally, a scan can be obtained through the white matter posterior to the trigones of the lateral ventricle.

A hypoechoic cystic structure is frequently seen between the lateral ventricles superiorly. The anterior portion of this is the cavum septum pellucidum (Fig. 10–1C). The posterior portion is the cavum vergae. These structures lie in the septum pelluci-

207

Table 10–1. BIRTH WEIGHT AND HEMORRHAGE

BIRTH WEIGHT (gm)	RISK OF HEMORRHAGE (%)
500–750	63
751–1,000	57
1,001–1,500	37

dum. They are normal variants. In general, they close and become obliterated, starting posteriorly and progressing anteriorly. In most infants, the cystic structures are completely gone by six months of age. The third ventricle will frequently not be seen in normals. The quadrigeminal plate cistern is very echogenic. The cause of this increased echogenicity is not known for certain. The cerebellar vermis may be identified as an echogenic structure in the midline of the posterior fossa. The cisterna magna may be seen in the posterior fossa. Pulsations from cerebral vessels may be identified in the interhemispheric and sylvian tissues.

Sagittal images are then obtained (Fig. 10–2). The midline is imaged and each caudothalamic groove is imaged. Two additional images are taken through the body of each lateral ventricle. A minimum of five images should be obtained in the sagittal plane.

Once again, the cavum septum pellucidum and cavum vergae are identified. Corpus callosum is identified as a hypoechoic structure. The pericallosal sulcus is echogenic and contains the pericallosal arteries. The third ventricle can usually be seen on a sagittal image at the midline. Again, the quadrigeminal plate cistern is very echogenic.

The lateral ventricles are frequently asymmetric and may appear slit-like. Slit-like ventricles without any associated findings usually should not be taken as a sign of cerebral edema. Linear echoes seen in the cavum septum pellucidum are felt to represent septal veins. The cavum veli interpositi lies below and behind the cavum vergae. It is another frequently identified normal variant.

In normals, there may be a periventricular echogenic halo. This is homogeneous and not as echogenic as the choroid plexus. This is due to a technical artifact known as the anisotropic effect. One should be careful not to mistake this increased echogenicity for a cerebral hemorrhage or periventricular leukomalacia (Fig. 10–3). The latter should be considered as possible diagnoses only when the area of increased echogenicity is irregular or asymmetric in appearance.

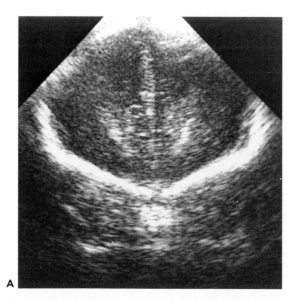

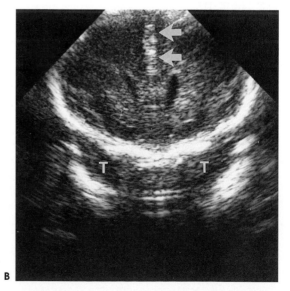

A   B

Figure 10–1 *A*, Coronal image. Frontal lobes anterior to frontal horns. *B*. Through anterior part of frontal horns. *Arrows* = interhemispheric fissure, T = temporal lobes. *Illustration continued on opposite page*

HEMORRHAGE

Intracranial Hemorrhage

Periventricular/intraventricular hemorrhage is graded based on the following classification:

Grade 1: Isolated subependymal germinal matrix hemorrhage

Grade 2: Intraventricular hemorrhage with normal-size ventricles

Grade 3: Intraventricular hemorrhage with dilated ventricles

Grade 4: Parenchymal hemorrhage

In preterm infants less than 1,550 gm birth weight, the following distribution is seen:

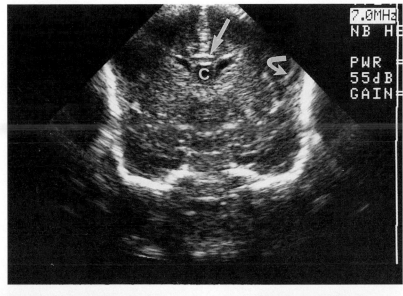

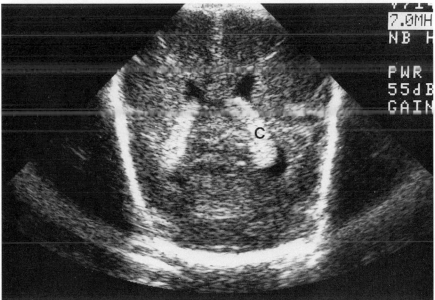

Figure 10–1 *Continued. C,* Coronal image at approximately the level of the foramen of Monroe (not seen). C = cavum septum pellucidum, *arrow* = corpus callosum, *curved arrow* = sylvian fissure. *D,* Coronal image through most posterior portion of lateral ventricles. Ventricles contain hyperechoic choroid (C).

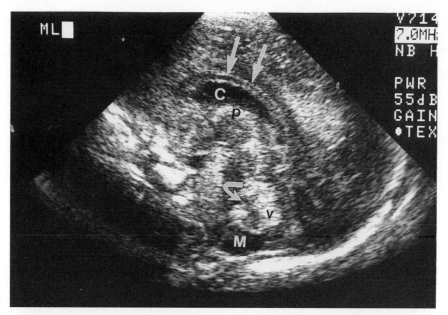

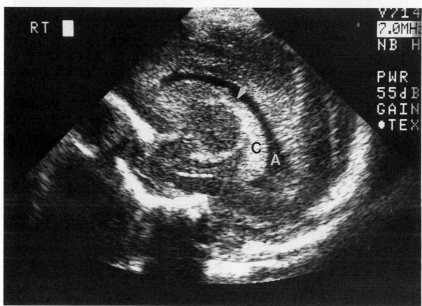

Figure 10–2. *A*, Sagittal image. Midline. C = cavum septum pellucidum and cavum vergae, *arrows* = hypoechoic corpus callosum, V = vermis, *curved arrow* = fourth ventricle, M = cisterna magna, p = choroid plexus in roof of third. *B*, Sagittal image. Slightly off midline. *Arrow* = caudothalamic groove, C = choroid, A = atrium of lateral ventricle.

Grade 1 = 40%, Grade 2 = 30%, Grade 3 = 20%, and Grade 4 = 10%.

The exact etiology of these hemorrhages is unknown. The subependymal germinal matrix is a very vascular structure. It may be that blood vessels in this area are extremely fragile in preterm infants. It is not known whether ischemic injury to capillar-ies or hypertensive rupture of capillaries leads to the hemorrhage.

Grade 1 Hemorrhage

This appears as an echogenic focus inferior and lateral to the floor of the frontal horn of the lateral ventricle. It is usually

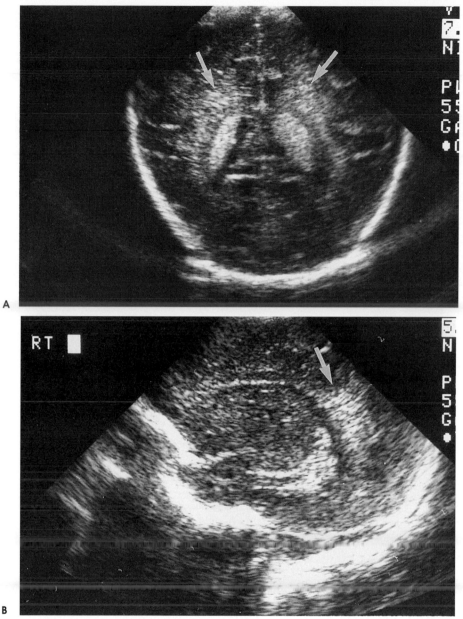

Figure 10–3. *A,* Coronal image showing anisotropic effect (*arrows*). This should not be mistaken for hemorrhage or periventricular leukomalacia. *B,* Sagittal image showing anisotropic effect (*arrow*).

near the head of the caudate nucleus and it appears as a bulge. Confusion with the normal choroid plexus can be a problem, but normally the choroid plexus tapers anteriorly and is not present anterior to the caudothalamic groove (Fig. 10–4). The differential diagnosis for these echogenic foci is given in Table 10–2. The sequela of these small hemorrhages is either a small echogenic density or a total resolution, to the point that an abnormality cannot be iden-

tified when scanned some weeks later. In a small percentage, a small subependymal cyst may form.

Grade 2 Hemorrhage

By definition, the ventricles are normal in size, and therefore it may be difficult to identify blood within the ventricles (Fig. 10–5). The differential diagnosis of intraventricular echogenic material is given in

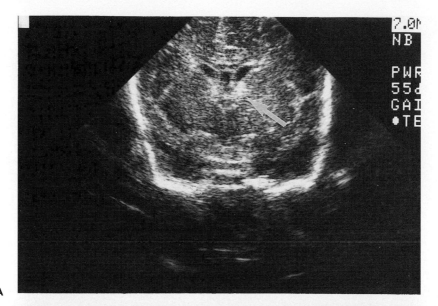

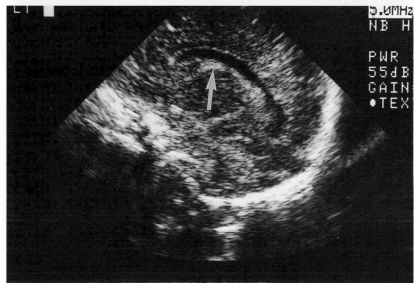

Figure 10–4. *A*, Coronal image. Asymmetric echo density near floor of left frontal horn represents Grade 1 hemorrhage (*arrow*). *B*, Sagittal image. Choroid should taper anteriorly. This focal echogenic bulge (*arrow*) anterior to the caudothalamic groove is a Grade 1 hemorrhage.

Table 10–2. ECHOGENIC AREA, REGION OF GERMINAL MATRIX

COMMON
Subependymal hemorrhage
Echogenic choroid plexus

UNCOMMON
Normal caudothalamic groove
Periventricular leukomalacia
Nonhemorrhagic infarction
Calcification
Hamartoma

Table 10–3. At times, the blood may form a complete cast of the ventricles. If these infants are followed over time, a small percentage will develop hydrocephalus. If there is intraventricular hemorrhage but no evidence of a subependymal hemorrhage, then the most likely source of blood in the ventricular system is the choroid plexus. At ultrasound it may be very difficult to recognize a choroid plexus hemorrhage because the choroid plexus is so echogenic. If the choroid plexus does not taper anteriorly,

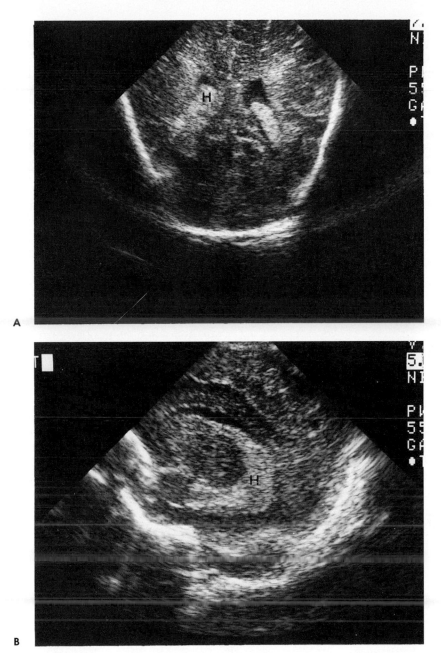

Figure 10–5. *A*, Coronal image. Hemorrhage (H) forms cast of right lateral ventricle. This is a Grade 2 bleed. *B*, Sagittal image. Hemorrhage (H) completely fills lateral ventricle.

or if there is extension of choroid plexus into the occipital horn, then the possibility of clot should be considered.

Grade 3 Hemorrhage

In this category the ventricles are dilated. This makes the recognition of intraventricular blood much easier (Fig. 10–6). The blood, once again, may form a cast of the ventricle. The blood will not necessarily be in all parts of the ventricular system, and may be confined to only one lateral ventricle. Blood/cerebrospinal fluid (CSF) levels may be seen at times. With time, the clot shrinks and resorbs. In about 50 percent of these infants the hydrocephalus will remain static or will resolve spontaneously. The other 50 percent will continue to have hy-

Table 10–3. ECHOGENIC MATERIAL WITHIN VENTRICLE OR CEREBROSPINAL FLUID

COMMON
Intraventricular hemorrhage
UNCOMMON
Meningitis
Ventriculitis
Gas

drocephalus and may require therapy. Therapy consists of either repeated lumber punctures or placement of a shunt. A pharmacologic therapy with glycerol and acetazolamide has also been attempted with some success.

Grade 4 Hemorrhage

Grade 4 hemorrhage is now referred to as "periventricular vascular infarction" by some. At ultrasound, Grade 4 hemorrhage appears as a very echogenic area near the lateral ventricle (Fig. 10–7). The differential diagnosis for echogenic parenchymal foci is given in Table 10–4. The area of hemorrhage is usually irregular and usually homogeneous. It occurs most commonly in the frontal and parietal lobes. Larger hemorrhages may result in mass effect with

shift of midline structures. At times, it can be difficult to differentiate between the hematoma in the parenchyma adjacent to a ventricle and a hematoma within the ventricle. Intraparenchymal hematomas usually have an irregular border, whereas intraventricular hemorrhage tends to have a well-defined border. Ultimately, over time, the hematoma in the parenchyma will become hypoechoic as the blood is resorbed and the clot retracts. An area of encephalomalacia will develop over several months.

Patients who are developing hydrocephalus will initially dilate only the trigonal occipital horn portions of the lateral ventricles. The frontal horns are the last portion to dilate.

Long-term Sequelae

Those with a Grade 1 hemorrhage have an incidence of major neurologic sequelae of 10% (which is the same as premature infants without hemorrhage), Grade 2 = 30%, Grade 3 = 40%, and Grade 4 = 90%.

Subarachnoid Hemorrhage

Subarachnoid hemorrhage does not usually have serious clinical sequelae. It occurs more commonly in the preterm infant than in the term infant. Ultrasound is not sensitive at detecting this abnormality. Occasion-

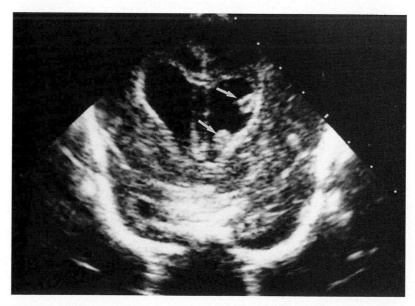

Figure 10–6. Coronal image of Grade 3 bleed. Ventricles are dilated and clots (*arrows*) can be seen within ventricles.

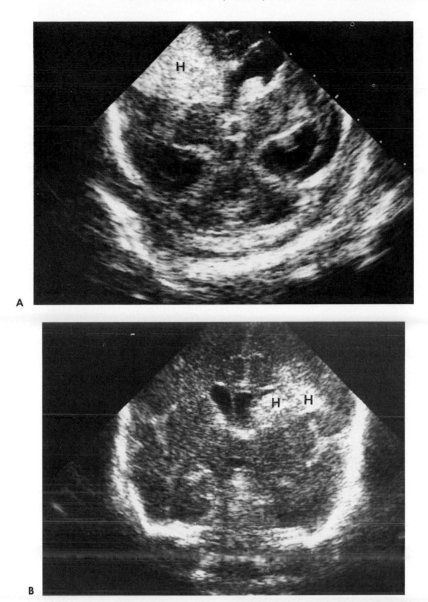

Figure 10–7. *A*, Coronal image. Large area of parenchymal hemorrhage (H) in this patient with a Grade 4 bleed. *B*, Coronal image. Different patient with Grade 4 hemorrhage (H).

ally, echogenic material may be seen in the sylvian fissures as a result of blood in this area.

Subdural Hemorrhage

This occurs in term infants more than in premature infants and is usually a result of trauma. The falx may be lacerated, resulting in a hematoma in the region of the inter-hemispheric fissure. Alternatively, laceration of bridging veins leads to hemorrhage over the hemispheres. At ultrasound these

abnormalities appear as fluid collections. Blood may be either echogenic or echo poor, depending on the age of the hematoma. Mass effect may be seen. Occasionally, subdural hematomas may be seen in the region of the tentorium and cerebellar hemispheres.

Intercerebral Hemorrhage

Intercerebral hemorrhage without hemorrhage into the region of the subependymal germinal matrix occurs occasionally in

Table 10–4. ECHOGENIC AREAS WITHIN THE BRAIN

COMMON
Hemorrhage
Normal caudothalamic groove
Brain infarct
Calcification

UNCOMMON
Tumor
Encephalitis
Edema from asphyxia
Pseudolesion
Hamartoma
Arteriovenous malformation
Air

term infants, usually as a result of trauma. Areas of abnormal hyperechoic material will be identified in the region of the hematoma.

PERIVENTRICULAR LEUKOMALACIA

Periventricular leukomalacia (PVL) is an infarction of the white matter adjacent to the frontal horns and bodies of the lateral ventricles. These lesions can be hemorrhagic. PVL occurs in preterm, low-birth-weight infants. Neonatal hypoxia or asphyxia is a predisposing event.

At ultrasound, increased echogenicity is identified in the white matter around the frontal horns and bodies of the lateral ventricles. These lesions are frequently bilat-

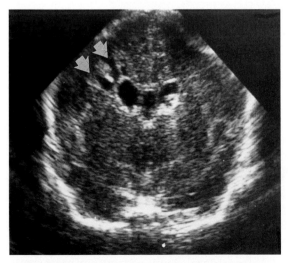

Figure 10–8. Coronal image. Cyst formation (*arrows*) as a result of periventricular leukomalacia.

eral. Cyst formation may occur as a sequela (Fig. 10–8). If the areas of increased echogenicity are small, then the chances of significant neurologic deficits are decreased. When the areas of abnormality are large and cover large amounts of white matter, then these infants frequently have significant deficits. The differential diagnosis of cystic brain lesions is given in Table 10–5.

MULTIFOCAL ISCHEMIC BRAIN INJURY

This is often called hypoxic-ischemic encephalopathy (HIE) and is a separate category of ischemia. It is felt to occur more often in term infants. HIE can affect gray matter as well as white matter. Those at risk include hypoxic infants, as well as those with congenital heart disease and those on extracorporeal membrane oxygenation. On ultrasound there are echogenic areas in both gray matter and white matter. Edema may lead to poor definition of the interfaces between gyri and sulci and there may be absent vascular pulsations. Edema may also cause compression of the ventricles. Ultimately, brain atrophy occurs with ventriculomegaly. Sometimes encephalomalacia may be seen.

CONGENITAL ABNORMALITIES

Various congenital abnormalities may be detected when neonatal head ultrasound is performed.

The vein of Galen malformation is an arteriovenous malformation. A hypoechoic mass may be identified posterior to the third ventricle. An enlarged, dilated vein can be followed into the straight sinus.

Table 10–5. CYSTIC BRAIN LESIONS

COMMON
Periventricular leukomalacia
Porencephalic cysts

UNCOMMON
Schizencephaly
Dandy-Walker cysts
Arachnoid cysts
Ventricular cysts
Arteriovenous malformations
Vein of Galen aneurysms
Alobar holoprosencephaly
Agenesis of corpus callosum with midline cyst

Color flow Doppler will allow vivid depiction of this malformation. The arteriovenous mass may lead to obstructive hydrocephalus if the aqueduct is blocked.

Tuberous sclerosis is characterized by multiple hamartomas in multiple organs. Hamartomas or tubers may be identified as echogenic foci in the walls of the lateral ventricles just beneath the ependyma. Ventricular dilatation may be seen if a tuber obstructs the foramen of Monroe. In this case the ventricular dilatation may be unilateral.

Arnold-Chiari Malformations

Arnold-Chiari type malformations are a spectrum of dystrophic disorders. Arnold-Chiari I malformation is downward displacement of the cerebellar tonsils without abnormalities of the fourth ventricle or medulla. This is frequently picked up as an incidental finding in adults and usually has no clinical significance. Chiari II malformation is the most common and is associated with spina bifida and a meningomyelocele. In this entity there will be downward herniation of the cerebellar tonsils with displacement of the pons and medulla in a caudal direction. The posterior fossa is small.

A Chiari III malformation consists of an encephalomeningocele in the highest cervical region. The medulla, fourth ventricle, and cerebellum are displaced into this sack.

Chiari IV malformation may not be a part of the same spectrum as the previously mentioned three entities. It consists of severe hypoplasia of the cerebellum, but there is no displacement of the hindbrain.

The Chiari II malformation is the most common and is frequently suspected on the basis of a meningomyelocele in the lower lumbar region. The frontal horns will be small, whereas the posterior horns of the lateral ventricles appear unusually large. The frontal horns point anteriorly and inferiorly. On the sagittal scans and coronal scans there will often be marked enlargement of the massa intermedia. The third ventricle is enlarged but may not appear enlarged, simply because so much of it is occupied by the large massa intermedia.

Dandy-Walker Malformation

The Dandy-Walker malformation has a dramatically enlarged posterior fossa with cystic dilatation of the fourth ventricle and dysgenesis or agenesis of the cerebellar vermis. A related entity, known as the Dandy-Walker variant, has only a slight enlargement of the posterior fossa and a posterior fossa cyst that connects to the fourth ventricle by a narrow tract. The Dandy-Walker variant also has dysgenesis of the cerebellar vermis. Either of these abnormalities may have hydrocephalus as a result of obstruction of the fourth ventricle. Hydrocephalus is usually not present at birth but develops in infancy. At ultrasound, one sees a posterior fossa cyst with hypoplasia of the cerebellar hemispheres and partial or complete absence of the cerebellar vermis. Differential diagnosis would include a mega cisterna magna or an arachnoid cyst in the posterior fossa.

Holoprosencephaly

The initial single ventricle of the prosencephalon does not divide into two lateral ventricles. The most severe form of this abnormality is the alobar holoprosencephaly. This has a very poor prognosis and has associated cebocephaly (hypotelorism and proboscis), cyclopia, and a midline proboscis. Trisomy 13 may be present as well. A single midline ventricle is identified. The two cerebral hemispheres and the thalami are fused and no falx is identified. In the semilobar variety, a single ventricle is present with separate occipital horns. There may be an incomplete falx and an interhemispheric fissure in the region of the occiput. There is usually absence of the corpus callosum. Mild hypotelorism and trigonencephaly may exist as well as cleft lip and palate. The lobar form of holoprosencephaly has fused frontal horns but two lateral ventricles. The frontal horns have a square shape. The bodies of the lateral ventricles lie close to one another. An interhemispheric fissure and falx are usually present posteriorly and may be present anteriorly, but are less prominent anteriorly (see Fig. 8–20).

Other Disorders

Lissencephaly has a smooth cortical surface without obvious sulci or gyri. The subarachnoid space and sylvian fissures are enlarged; the ventricular system is also enlarged.

Schizencephaly has large irregular clefts extending from the lateral ventricles to the cortical surface of the brain. These clefts are lined by gray matter. Magnetic resonance imaging (MRI) can be very helpful in making this diagnosis and in distinguishing between schizencephaly and encephalomalacia. If gray matter lines these clefts on MRI, a diagnosis of schizencephaly is made. On ultrasound, large clefts show up as fluid-filled spaces. There may be partial absence of the septum pellucidum resulting in squared frontal horns.

Agenesis of the corpus callosum has lateral ventricles that are more widely spaced than usual. The medial side of each lateral ventricle is either concave or more straight than usual. The third ventricle may be more superior than normal and extend up in between the two lateral ventricles. The frontal horns will be narrow while the posterior horns will be enlarged. This is called colpocephaly.

Hydranencephaly has long been thought to represent bilateral cerebral infarctions from bilateral occlusion of the internal carotid arteries in utero. At ultrasound the cranial vault is filled with CSF. This entity can be difficult to distinguish from severe hydrocephalus, in which the cerebral cortex is compressed against the inner table of the skull. Doppler of the carotid arteries should show absent flow. If a falx is present, it may be hydranencephaly or severe hydrocephalus, but this essentially rules out alobar holoprosencephaly as a possible diagnosis. If the falx is absent or incomplete, then it may be holoprosencephaly, but hydranencephaly can also have an incomplete falx. The thalamus should also be normal in hydranencephaly.

HYDROCEPHALUS

Hydrocephalus may be the result of obstruction to the flow of CSF at the level of the foramen of Monroe, the third ventricle, the aqueduct of Sylvius, the foramina of Magendie and Luschka in the fourth ventricle, or anywhere along the subarachnoid space where CSF must flow (Fig. 10–9) (Table 10–6). Normally, CSF will flow through the basal cisterns and up over the convexities. Hydrocephalus is usually classified as intraventricular or extraventricular. The intraventricular form has a block somewhere between the fourth ventricle and lateral ventricles; the extraventricular form has a block at the level of the convexities or at the level of the superior sagittal sinus. Hydrocephalus can sometimes result from overproduction of CSF due to a choroid plexus papilloma or from venus obstruction, either at the level of the superior vena cava or the superior sagittal sinus. Arteriovenous malformations can sometimes also cause hydrocephalus.

Ventricular size can be followed by measuring the ratio of the ventricle to the hemispheric width at the level of the caudate nucleus and at the level of the atria.

Subjectively, the frontal horns become rounded and dilated. This is the earliest sign of hydrocephalus.

In scanning hydrocephalus, a sonographer must determine which ventricle is normal and which is abnormal. If the obstruction is at the level of the foramen of Monroe, then one ventricle may be larger than the other ventricle in the frontal horn region. With aqueductal stenosis, both the third and lateral ventricles will be enlarged with a normal-sized fourth ventricle. The fourth ventricle may even be small. If the obstruction is at the level of the foramina of Luschka or Magendie, there may be dilatation of the fourth ventricle with lesser degrees of dilatation of the third and lateral ventricles. If the obstruction is over the convexities, or at the level of superior sagittal sinus, then the lateral ventricles and third ventricles will be enlarged. The fourth ventricle may or may not be enlarged. In general, the fourth ventricle may not dilate even if logically it seems as though it should.

ULTRASOUND IN INFECTIONS

In acute meningitis, there may be echogenic sulci and areas of increased parenchymal echogenicity mixed with areas of decreased parenchymal echogenicity and extra-axial fluid collections with ventriculomegaly. All of these signs appear with variable frequency and may or may not be seen. In meningitis, effusions may develop either in subdural or subarachnoid locations. Linear echogenic bands may be seen in the ventricles. These are an indication of

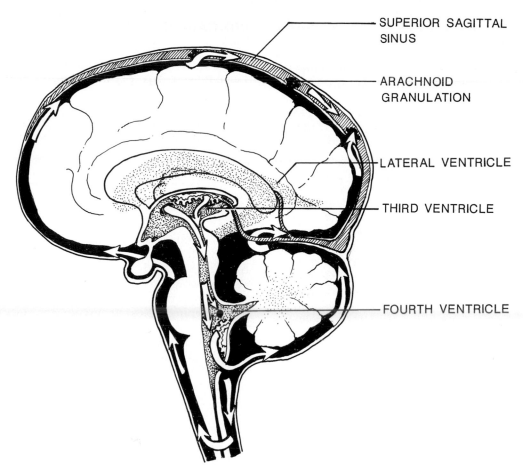

Figure 10-9. Diagram of flow of CSF. *Arrows* in third ventricle represent flow from the foramina of Monroe and from production of CSF by choroid plexus. Flow then goes down the cerebral aqueduct to the fourth ventricle.

ventriculitis. In addition, ependymal septic debris may be identified in the ventricles and the ependymal lining of the ventricles may be very echogenic. Increased echogenicity of the sulci may be seen but does not have prognostic significance and usually resolves.

Congenital infections are usually of the TORCH variety (toxoplasmosis, other [syphilis, hepatitis, Zoster], rubella, cytomegalovirus, and herpes simplex). Cytomegalovirus is the most common. There may be calcifications around the ventricle at ultrasound. These are usually punctate and diffuse. Subependymal cysts and microcephaly may occur.

In toxoplasmosis, the ultrasound findings are scattered calcifications with more in the basal ganglia. Some of these calcifications may be quite large. In this disease, calcifications in many other areas of the brain may also develop. Finally, encephalomalacia and porencephaly can sometimes be seen. Hydrocephalus may result from obstruction of the flow of CSF.

Table 10-6. DILATED VENTRICLES

COMMON
After hemorrhage
Obstructing mass
Aqueductal stenosis
Obstruction over convexities
Obstruction at level of superior sagittal sinus

UNCOMMON
Semilobar holoprosencephaly
Associated with meningomyelocele
Dandy-Walker cyst
Ventriculitis
Simulated by hydranencephaly

Herpes infections may lead to intracranial calcifications and also encephalomalacia. The herpes simplex type 2 is the most common herpesvirus to cause congenital infection. Calcifications and brain atrophy may occur.

Rubella, likewise, can lead to calcifications and subependymal cysts.

DOPPLER OF THE PEDIATRIC BRAIN

The anterior cerebral artery can be approached via the anterior fontanelle. The middle and posterior cerebral arteries are best evaluated through a transtemporal approach. Usually the resistive index is used to evaluate these vessels since this parameter is not angle dependent. The resistive index decreases progressively as gestational age increases, meaning that the vessels are flowing against less resistance. As the neonate becomes older, the velocities increase. This is true for most systolic and diastolic velocities. Infants with hydrocephalus have an elevated resistive index. This is a nonspecific finding and may be present in diseases other than hydrocephalus. Serial Doppler studies may be used in an effort to track hydrocephalus both before and after shunting.

With brain death there is reversal of diastolic flow. However, a small percentage of brain-dead infants may have normal resistive indices, so the technique appears to be specific but not 100% sensitive. Increased flow velocities have been seen with bacterial meningitis. Arteriovenous malformations also have increased flow.

Ultrasound of the Pediatric Spine

Because the posterior elements are not completely ossified at birth, ultrasound may be used to examine the spinal cord. The spinous process of the lumbar vertebral bodies begins to ossify first. After a few months of age, only transverse scanning can be accomplished in between spinous processes. If spina bifida is present, there may be an opening in the bony elements allowing scanning in older children.

INDICATIONS

The examination is usually performed to identify the level of the conus medullaris. The inferior tip of the conus normally should not be below the L2-L3 interspace. If it is lower than the L3 vertebral body, then a diagnosis of tethered cord is made. Patients with dimples, masses, sinus tracts, and patches of hair in the lumbar region are frequently screened because of the associated cord-tethering that may occur. A tethered cord is fixed so that the conus medullaris is lower in the spinal canal than usual. As the child's spine grows, traction on the conus stretches the conus and the cord, with resultant neurologic dysfunction. Also, infants with neurologic or orthopedic abnormalities such as neurogenic bladder or equinovarus are often screened. Patients with meningoceles or myelomeningoceles can be examined to look for cord position and associated tumors. Patients who have already undergone a primary operation for myelomeningocele shortly after birth, but who present later in infancy with new neurologic findings, can be re-examined to look for adherence of the cord to the myelomeningocele repair site.

Children with malformations of the anus and rectum, as well as those with caudal regression and bony abnormalities of the sacrum, may have associated cord abnormalities. These patients should also be examined by ultrasound.

TECHNIQUE

The patient is usually placed in a prone or decubitus position. It can be useful to place a pillow or a pad under the abdomen so that the infant is flexed in a kyphotic position. This will tend to open up the spinous processes and increase visualization of the cord. We use a variable-frequency transducer ranging between 5 and 7 MHz. A linear transducer is used in infants. As a child gets older, a sector transducer can be used.

NORMAL ANATOMY

As indicated previously, the cord should end at approximately the L2-L3 level. If the cord is below this, a diagnosis of tethered cord can be made. Identification of the cord level can be made by counting vertebral bodies or by identifying the iliac crest and realizing that it is usually at L4 and then counting up. Finally, if there is doubt about the level at which the cord is located, then a marker can be placed at the cord location and a plain radiograph obtained.

The cord is hypoechoic (Fig. 10–10). A central echogenic area is referred to as the central echo complex. In the past, this has been felt to be the central canal, but it probably is the result of an interface between myelinated ventral white commissure and the central end of the anterior median fissure. This interface is slightly anterior to the central canal. This central echo complex will be a linear line on sagittal images and will be a dot or a double dot on transverse images. In the cervical region the cord is round and large, compared to the thoracic region, where the cord is relatively small. In the lumbar area the cord expands again and is larger. In the region of the conus the cord may become more elliptical in shape. The nerve roots of the cauda equina are linear echogenic bands radiating from the region of the conus medullarus. The filum terminale projects from the conus down to the sacral region. The filum is usually less than 2 mm in diameter in a normal patient. The filum should be quite echogenic.

The normal cord should pulsate with cardiac activity and move with breathing and crying. Normally, the cord will be against the ventral wall of the spinal canal. A cord that is plastered against a dorsal wall of the spinal canal is suspicious for tethering or fixation to that wall.

TETHERED SPINAL CORD

A tethered spinal cord simply means that the tip of the cord, the conus medullarus, is in an abnormally low position so that the cord is stretched mechanically. This may progress as a child grows, with progressive neurologic deficits. Several different mechanisms can lead to tethering. A filum terminale that is greater than 2 mm in diameter may lead to tethering. In this case, the short, thick filum holds the cord at an abnormally low level. In addition to an abnormally thick filum, the pulsations of the conus will be decreased. The cord will often be in a dorsal location within the spinal canal. Intraspinal tumors, such as a lipoma, can lead to tethering of the cord. A lipoma will be identified as an echogenic mass. Diastematomyelia may occur. This is a bony or fibrous band that separates the lower cord into two portions. Two distinct cords can be identified at ultrasound with two central echo complexes (Fig. 10–11).

If a patient has a meningocele on physical examination, ultrasound may be performed to determine if this is a meningocele or a myelomeningocele. The latter has elements of the cord within it. Lipomas may coexist with a myelomeningocele; this then becomes a lipomyelomeningocele.

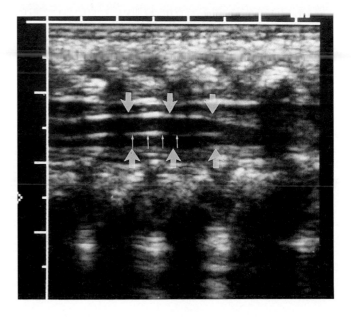

Figure 10–10. Normal cord. *Large arrows* mark boundaries of the cord. *Small arrows* point to the central echo complex.

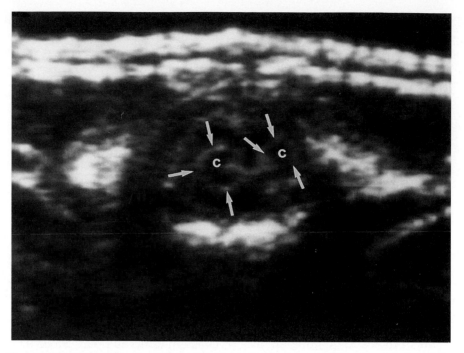

Figure 10–11. Diastematomyelia. C = each of two cords. *Arrows* mark the boundaries of the cord.

After myelomeningocele repair, if there are progressive neurologic deficits, the cord can be re-examined to look for retethering. This may be secondary to scarring at the operative site. In this case the cord will lie in a dorsal position. There will be decreased or absent pulsations in the distal cord.

Patients with myelomeningocele should also be examined for hydromyelia. This may be seen as part of the Arnold-Chiari Type II malformation. A dilated central canal would be the finding at ultrasound.

Ultrasound of the Pediatric Hip

Ultrasound of the pediatric hip is performed in those infants who are suspected of having developmental dysplasia of the hip based on a physical examination. If developmental dysplasia of the hip is treated early, then most of the sequelae can be prevented. The dynamic sonographic technique for evaluating the infant hip is based on the Barlow test, which is a test for hip dislocation. The hip is flexed with the thigh adducted. Then the femur is pushed posteriorly in an attempt to cause the femoral head to move out of the acetabulum. The

Ortolani test determines if a dislocated hip can be reduced. The dislocated hip is taken from the flexed position described in the Barlow test and abducted. A vibration or quiver may be felt by the examiner's hand when the femoral head relocates.

The hip is considered to be subluxed when the femoral head is partially in contact with the acetabulum. It is dislocated when the femoral head is positioned such that there is no coverage by the acetabulum.

Scanning is performed with either a 5- or 7.5-MHz linear transducer. Bone is echogenic. Cartilage is hypoechoic in comparison to soft tissue. The ilium, ischium, and pubis form a Y that is known as the triradiate cartilage. The labrum is made of cartilage and extends outward from the acetabulum, forming a cup. The outer portions of the labrum are formed of fibrocartilage instead of hyaline cartilage and have more echogenicity than other cartilage in the hip. The proximal ossification center of the femoral head is seen between 2 and 8 months radiographically. This is reflected in the sonographic appearance. Once this ossification center is fully developed at about 1 year of age, sonographic evaluation for developmental dysplasia of the hip is precluded.

TECHNIQUE

The examiner stands at the infant's feet. To examine the left hip, the examiner's left hand is placed on the infant's left leg while the right hand manipulates the transducer. To examine the infant's right hip, the transducer is shifted to the examiner's left hand. The infant starts in a supine position. Beginning with the lateral portion of the hip, the transducer is oriented transversely (Fig. 10–12). One scans until one has located the round femoral head of the proximal femur. The femoral head should be centered on the hypoechoic triradiate cartilage. If the hip is subluxed or dislocated, it will either be moved posteriorly in respect to the acetabulum or moved completely out of the acetabulum. The femur can then be flexed to 90° while scanning is performed. The femoral head should remain in contact with the acetabulum. The flexed hip should be moved from maximal adduction to abduction (frog-leg).

The hip is then scanned in a coronal plane (Fig. 10–13). The hip should be maintained in 90° of flexion. The femoral head should remain seated in the acetabulum. The subluxed femoral head will be slightly

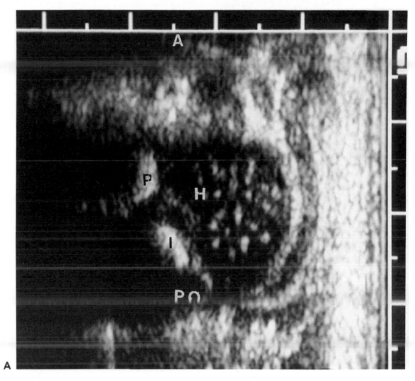

Figure 10–12. *A*, Transverse image of hip showing orientation of transducer. A = anterior, H = femoral head, I = ischium, P = pubis, PO = posterior. *B*, Schematic of infant hip. Image is oriented so that transducer is on the right.

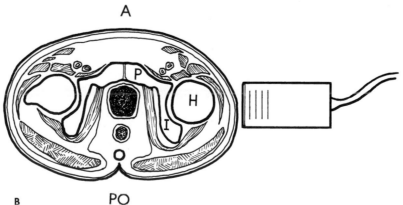

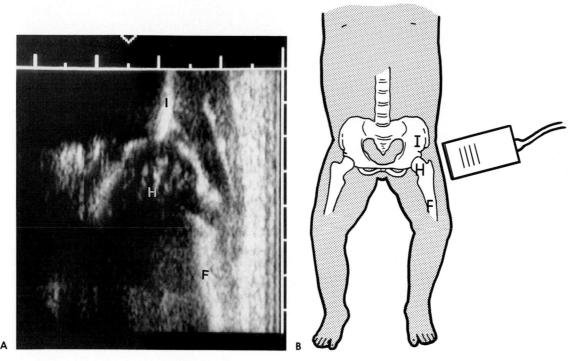

Figure 10–13. *A*, Coronal image of left hip. F = femoral shaft, H = femoral head, I = ileum. *B*, Coronal depiction of hip. Image is oriented so that transducer is on the right.

displaced laterally or posteriorly. In dislocation, the femoral head will be completely out of the acetabulum. While scanning is performed, the infant's knee is pushed posteriorly while the hip is flexed. In this coronal scanning plane, the acetabulum can be evaluated for proper shape and depth. A normal acetabulum will have a "ball-on-a-spoon" appearance.

HIP EFFUSION

Ultrasound can also be used to diagnose a hip joint effusion. This can be done after one year of age when sonography for evaluation of developmental dysplasia of the hip is no longer possible. To look for a joint effusion, the patient should be supine with the hips nonflexed. Once again, a high-frequency linear transducer is used. The hip is scanned from an anterior position, with the long axis of the transducer going along the long axis of the femoral neck. Normally, the

joint capsule will have a concave shape. The joint capsule should be between 2 and 5 mm thick. The hip capsule should be symmetric when one side is compared to the other. With an effusion, the hip capsule becomes distended and convex. The abnormal side will have a joint capsule that is more than 2 mm thicker than the normal side.

Suggested Readings

Brain
Rumack CM, Wilson SR, Charboneau JW. Diagnostic Ultrasound, Vol. 2. St. Louis, Mosby–Year Book, 1991, p. 1009.

Spine
Rumack CM, Wilson SR, Charboneau JW. Diagnostic Ultrasound, Vol. 2. St. Louis, Mosby–Year Book, 1991, p. 1045.

Hip
Rumack CM, Wilson SR, Charboneau JW. Diagnostic Ultrasound, Vol. 2. St. Louis, Mosby–Year Book, 1991, p. 1242.

CHAPTER 11

Quality Control

Quality control is the process of checking ultrasound equipment to make certain that it is functioning properly. Quality assurance includes quality control but is a more comprehensive process. Quality assurance examines image interpretation of the ultrasound reporting process and the ultimate effect on the patient.

Quality control may be divided into imaging quality control and Doppler quality control.

Imaging Quality Control

The quality control process for imaging instruments evaluates the performance of the entire system, including transducers, main console of the machine, and camera.

Quality control tests use test objects or phantoms. Many devices are available (Table 11–1). Included here are pictures of the American Institute of Ultrasound in Medicine (AIUM) "Standard Test Object" and the Nuclear Associates (NA) "Multipurpose Tissue/Cyst Phantom" (Figs. 11–1 and 11–2). In general, these devices consist of a substance that transmits sound at 1,540 m/sec to simulate human tissue. They also attenuate sound at about 0.7 dB/cm/MHz, which also simulates human tissue.

Rows of wires or rods are positioned as reflectors. Cysts are simulated by low-attenuating cylinders or spheres.

Nine quality assurance checks should be performed on real-time machines (Table 11–2).

We test each transducer every two months. Each time these tests are performed, the machine settings (time gain compensation, gain, etc.) should be the same. Results should be recorded in a log book. This log book is useful in identifying long-term changes in machine performance. It is also useful during evaluations by accrediting organizations such as the Joint Commission on Accreditation of Hospitals (JCAH).

PARAMETERS TO BE TESTED

Sensitivity

The sensitivity of a system is the maximum depth at which echoes from scatterers can be detected. It is a reflection of the performance of the entire system. Sensitivity may deteriorate slowly as a machine ages.

This test should be performed with one or two transducers. The machine is set for maximal penetration. The deepest reflector is recorded. An alternate method uses one rod in the phantom each time the machine is tested. The gain setting necessary to detect this rod is recorded.

Distance Calibration

A vertical and a horizontal arrangement of rods (groups A and B in AIUM test object) are scanned and photographed. Calipers are used to measure the distance between rods on film. The distance between the first and last rods should be 100 mm. This distance should measure 98 to 102 mm or ±2%. The individual rods should be 20 mm apart. The test should be performed for vertically and horizontally placed rods.

Caliper Calibration

The electronic calipers are used to measure the distance between rods. This measurement can be done on group A or B of the AIUM test object and should measure ±2%.

Dead Zone

The top row of rods, group D, in the AIUM test object is scanned to see which

Table 11–1. AVAILABLE TEST DEVICES FOR USE IN A DIAGNOSTIC ULTRASOUND QUALITY CONTROL PROGRAM (SUPPLIER*)

TEST OBJECTS
American Institute of Ultrasound in Medicine (AIUM) Test Object
Dynamic Doppler Flow System (NA)
Beam Shape Phantom (NA)
Sensitivity, Uniformity, and Axial Resolution Phantom (NA, RMI)
Scan Thickness Phantom (RMI)

PHANTOMS
Multi-purpose Tissue/Cyst Phantom (NA)
Tissue-Equivalent Phantom (NA)
Contrast/Detail Phantom (NA)
Prostate Phantom (NA)
Particle Image Resolution Test Object (NA)
Tissue Mimicking Phantom, five models (RMI)
Doppler Phantom/Flow Control System (RMI)

*NA = Nuclear Associates, RMI = Radiation Measurements Inc.

rods are visible. Four millimeters is the maximal dead zone. Pulse-length changes may increase the dead zone.

Axial Resolution

Rod group E of the AIUM test object is imaged. Rods that are barely distinguishable indicate axial resolution.

Lateral Resolution

Group C rods of the AIUM test object are scanned through the axial C surface and the A surface. Scanned through surface A, the rods are 150 mm deep; through surface C, they are 50 mm deep. This allows lateral resolution to be checked at different depths. It may be necessary to check focused transducers with a stand-off pad. Once again, rods that are clearly identifiable as separate indicate the lateral resolution at both depths.

Time Gain Compensation (TGC)

One should scan group A through surface D initially with TGC "off." The gain

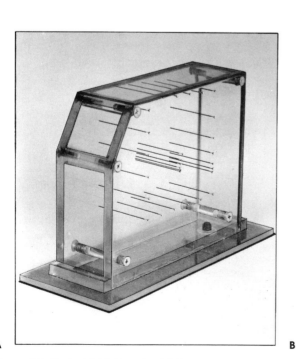

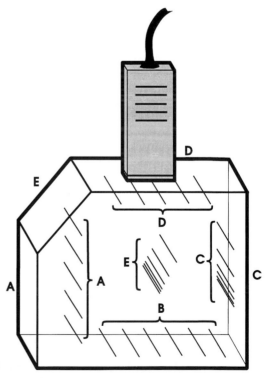

Figure 11–1. *A*, AIUM Standard 100-mm test object. *B*, Schematic has each surface and each row of pins identified by labels. (Courtesy of Nuclear Associates, Division of Victoreen, 100 Voice Road, Carle Place, NY 11514.)

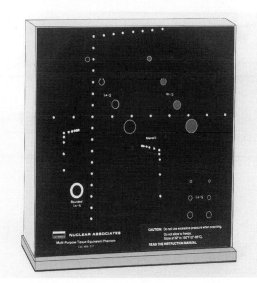

Figure 11–2. Nuclear Associates ''Multipurpose Tissue/Cyst Ultrasound Phantom''. (Courtesy of Nuclear Associates, Division of Victoreen, 100 Voice Road, Carle Place, NY 11514.)

setting to detect each rod is noted. Scanning is then done with TGC set up properly. Gain settings to just detect each rod are noted. The difference between the two gain settings indicates the amount of TGC at each depth. These settings are unique for each transducer.

Display Characteristics

This is a subjective test. A liver (or a phantom) is scanned and filmed. The film is compared to a monitor. Film processing may significantly affect the appearance of the image. A faint finding such as sludge in

Table 11–2. QUALITY ASSURANCE THAT SHOULD BE ROUTINELY PERFORMED WITH THE AIUM TEST OBJECT

1. System sensitivity
2. Distance or time calibration
3. Accuracy of distance caliper
4. Evaluation of misregistration
5. Determination of dead zone depth
6. Evaluation of axial resolution
7. Evaluation of lateral resolution
8. Determination of time gain characteristics
9. Evaluation of display system—CRT, hardcopy camera, processor
10. Visual inspection of all components

the gallbladder may also be filmed and compared to the monitor image to determine if the film is capable of printing faint, poorly seen structures.

Visual Inspection

The operator should look for problems with cord and wire integrity as well as cracks and bubbles in the transducer.

Other

Cysts (in a tissue equivalent phantom) should be imaged to make sure that they appear echo free.

FOCAL ZONE VERIFICATION

For focused transducers, the location of the focal zone can be checked by scanning vertical rods. Each rod produces a line and the length of the line reflects the width of the beam. Rods should be shortest within the manufacturer's stated focal zone.

Doppler Quality Control

Several commercially available devices are available for checking the performance of Doppler instruments. These may use a blood substitute such as dextrose patterns in liquid or polystyrene microspheres or a moving string or wire. We have seen a phantom made of tomato soup pumped through tubing by an intravenous pump. The constancy or reproducibility of Doppler measurements may be checked. Sensitivity may be evaluated by checking the maximum depth at which flow is detected and also by checking the slowest velocity that can be measured. Finally, velocity measurements by the instruments may be checked at several rates.

Suggested Readings

Bushong SC, Archer BR. Diagnostic Ultrasound: Physics, Biology, and Instrumentation. St. Louis, Mosby –Year Book, 1991.
Kremkau FW. Doppler Ultrasound: Principles and Instruments. Philadelphia, WB Saunders Company, 1990.
McDicken WN. Diagnostic Ultrasonics: Principles and Use of Instruments, ed. 3. Edinburgh, Churchill Livingstone, 1991.

CHAPTER 12

Bioeffects of Ultrasound

The American Institute of Ultrasound in Medicine (AIUM) has concluded that there is no confirmed proof of biologic effects on patients or instrument operators at typical intensities produced by present ultrasound instruments.[1] However, because effects may be discovered in the future, patient exposure should be minimized by keeping gain settings and examination time to a minimum.

Mechanism of Bioeffects

Two possible mechanisms of bioeffects in living tissue have been inferred: heating and cavitation. Heating of tissues occurs because of the absorption of energy. In general, it has been concluded that increases in body temperature of 1°C or less are not harmful.[2] However, elevation of the body temperature 2.5°C or more has been shown to cause abortions or fetal abnormalities in multiple species.[2] The amount of heating produced by any given ultrasound machine depends on beam profile characteristics, transducer size, transducer frequency, characteristics of intervening tissue, whether continuous-wave or pulsed equipment is used, and overall power output. Large transducers cause less heating than smaller ones. Focused transducers cause more heating in the area of beam focusing; higher frequency transducers also cause more heating. Bone has a higher absorption coefficient than other tissues, thereby absorbing more heat. Continuous-wave instruments cause more heating than pulsed instruments. It is unlikely that heating of more than 1°C would occur during a proper examination performed by a skilled operator, but patient exposure should be minimized during any examination.

Cavitation occurs when an acoustic wave interacts with microscopic gas bubbles. These microscopic gas bubbles must be present in the tissue before exposure to the acoustic wave. There is little known about the conditions for existence, location, and physical properties of gas microbubbles in human tissues. However, it must be assumed that such bubbles do periodically occur in humans.[3] These bubbles may resonate if exposed to sound of an appropriate frequency. If bubbles are smaller than the resonance size of the sound wave, they may grow when stimulated by the sound. When resonating in an acoustic field, these bubbles may absorb more acoustic power than would be predicted by their size. The bubbles will then oscillate, resulting in shear stresses and microstreaming. The bubbles may also expand and collapse violently, leading to shock waves. These processes are less likely to occur with short pulses than with longer pulses or continuous wave. They are also more likely to occur at high power settings. At the current time, there is little evidence to indicate that cavitation causes significant tissue damage in humans. There is evidence that cavitation can affect *Drosophila*, other insects, and plants. Once again, patient exposure should be minimized because of the possibility of effects that have yet to be identified.

Epidemiology

The National Council on Radiation Protection and Measurements has reviewed the epidemiology of ultrasound without finding significant evidence for a deleterious effect.[4] Because in utero exposure of mice to ultrasound has been shown to cause a decrease in birth weight, numerous studies have looked for such an effect in humans. In prospective and retrospective studies, investigators have found no effect on birth weight.[5] A study by Moore et al.[6] did suggest an effect of ultrasound on birth weight, but the study design made it impossible to evaluate whether or not those fetuses exposed to ultrasound were at risk for being low birth weight independent of the ultrasound exposure.

Several studies have attempted to find an association between generation of fetal structural anomalies and exposure to ultrasound. Currently there is little evidence of such an association.

Stark et al.[7] found that children exposed in utero to ultrasound were more likely to have dyslexia. The dyslexic children were also of lower birth weight. This study has not been confirmed but cannot be totally dismissed. No association between ultrasound and cancer has been found.

The AIUM has concluded that no convincing proof of a significant effect has been shown. They have also pointed out that detection of a harmful effect is dependent upon the natural occurrence of the event, the percentage increase in the incidence after exposure, and sample size. Sample sizes of hundreds of thousands may be required to detect subtle effects.

Other Indicators of Damage

In searching for bioeffects of ultrasound, other endpoints may be examined.

CHROMOSOME EFFECTS

A 1970 report by MacIntosh and Davey[8] concluded that chromosomal abnormalities in lymphocytes were caused by ultrasound. However, the authors repeated their work in 1975 and this time blinded themselves as to which slide preparations were controls and which were treated. This time they found no significant evidence of chromosome aberrations. Numerous other authors have attempted to demonstrate chromosomal effects and for the most part have been unsuccessful. The prevailing opinion is that there is little evidence to suggest any chromosomal effects.

Sister-Chromatid Exchange

A sister-chromatid exchange (SCE) occurs when portions of chromosomes in a chromosome pair are exchanged. An increase in SCEs indicates chromosome damage, but these exchanges correlate poorly or not at all with production of mutations or carcinomas. Therefore, it is uncertain that these exchanges have any significance for human subjects.

In 1979, a single paper reported a small increase in SCE.[9] Two subsequent studies have confirmed this effect; 11 have contradicted it.[10]

In 1984, the AIUM Bioeffects Committee[1] concluded that any SCE effects are small if they exist at all, that they occur only under unusual conditions, and that they have uncertain significance.

Nuclear Effects

In 1979, Liebeskind reported that tissue culture cells exposed to pulsed ultrasound showed findings suggesting the presence of single stranded or denatured DNA.[9] However, use of yeast and bacteria as study subjects has shown no evidence of increased mutations. These rapidly replicating organisms should show evidence of mutations quickly. It is doubtful that any significant effect occurs.

Conclusion

As with other diagnostic and therapeutic interventions, a favorable risk-to-benefit ratio should be present before ultrasound is used. There is little evidence to suggest a significant harmful effect, but the possibility of such effects cannot be totally dismissed.

References

1. AIUM. Bioeffects considerations for the safety of diagnostic ultrasound. J Ultrasound Med 7(suppl 9):S1–S38, 1988.
2. National Council on Radiation Protection and Measurements. NCPR Report No. 113: Exposure

Criteria for Medical Diagnostic Ultrasound: I. Criteria Based on Thermal Mechanisms. Bethesda, MD, National Council on Radiation Protection and Measurements, 1992.

3. Wells PNT. The safety of diagnostic ultrasound: Report of a British Institute Radiology Working Group, 1987. Br J Radiol 19:(suppl 20):

4. National Council on Radiation Protection and Measurements. NCPR Report No. 74: Biological Effects of Ultrasound: Mechanisms and Clinical Implications. Bethesda, MD, National Council on Radiation Protection and Measurements, 1983.

5. Scheidt PC, Stanley F, Bryla DA. One-year follow-up of infants exposed to ultrasound in utero. Am J Obstet Gynecol 131:743, 1978.

6. Moore RM, Barrick MK, Hamilton PM. Ultrasound exposure during gestation and birth weight. Presented at the 15th annual meeting of the Society for Epidemiologic Research, Cincinnati, Ohio, June 16–18, 1982.

7. Stark C, Orleans M, Haverkamp A, Murphy J. Short- and long-term risks after exposure to diagnostic ultrasound in utero. Obstet Gynecol 63: 194, 1984.

8. MacIntosh IJC, Davey DA. Chromosome aberrations induced by an ultrasonic fetal pulse detector. Br Med J 4:712–722, 1970.

9. Liebeskind D, Bases R, Mendez F, et al. Sister chromatid exchanges in human lymphocytes after exposure to diagnostic ultrasound. Science 205:1273, 1979.

10. Martin A. Can ultrasound cause genetic damage? J Clin Ultrasound 12:11–20, 1984.

Suggested Readings

AIUM. Bioeffects considerations for the safety of diagnostic ultrasound. J Ultrasound Med 7(suppl 9): s1–s38, 1988.

National Council on Radiation Protection and Measurements. NCPR Report No. 113: Exposure Criteria for Medical Diagnostic Ultrasound: I. Criteria Based on Thermal Mechanisms. Bethesda, MD, National Council on Radiation Protection and Measurements, 1992.

World Health Organization: Environmental Health Criteria 22: Ultrasound 65, 1982.

Appendix Tables

Appendix Table I. GESTATIONAL SAC MEASUREMENT

MEAN PREDICTED GESTATIONAL SAC (cm)	GESTATIONAL AGE (wk)	MEAN PREDICTED GESTATIONAL SAC (cm)	GESTATIONAL AGE (wk)
1.0	5.0	3.6	8.8
1.1	5.2	3.7	8.9
1.2	5.3	3.8	9.0
1.3	5.5	3.9	9.2
1.4	5.6	4.0	9.3
1.5	5.8	4.1	9.5
1.6	5.9	4.2	9.6
1.7	6.0	4.3	9.7
1.8	6.2	4.4	9.9
1.9	6.3	4.5	10.0
2.0	6.5	4.6	10.2
2.1	6.6	4.7	10.3
2.2	6.8	4.8	10.5
2.3	6.9	4.9	10.6
2.4	7.0	5.0	10.7
2.5	7.2	5.1	10.9
2.6	7.3	5.2	11.0
2.7	7.5	5.3	11.2
2.8	7.6	5.4	11.3
2.9	7.8	5.5	11.5
3.0	7.9	5.6	11.6
3.1	8.0	5.7	11.7
3.2	8.2	5.8	11.9
3.3	8.3	5.9	12.0
3.4	8.5	6.0	12.2
3.5	8.6		

From Hellman LM, Kobayashi M, Fillisti L, et al. Growth and development of the human fetus prior to the twentieth week of gestation. Am J Obstet Gynecol *103*:789, 1969, with permission.

Appendix Table II. RELATION BETWEEN MEAN SAC DIAMETER AND HUMAN CHORIONIC GONADOTROPIN

MEAN GESTATIONAL SAC DIAMETER (mm)	PREDICTED hCG (MIU/mL) RANGE = 95% CI
2	1,164 (629–2,188)
3	1,377 (771–2,589)
4	1,629 (863–3,036)
5	1,932 (1,026–3,636)
6	2.165 (1,226–4,256)
7	2,704 (1,465–4,990)
8	3,199 (1,749–5,852)
9	3,785 (2,085–6,870)
10	4,478 (2,483–8,075)
11	5,297 (2,952–9,508)
12	6,267 (3,502–11,218)
13	7,415 (4,145–13,266)
14	8,773 (4,894–15,726)
15	10,379 (5,766–18,682)
16	12,270 (6,776–22,235)
17	14,528 (7,964–26,501)
18	17,188 (9,343–31,621)
19	20,337 (10,951–37,761)
20	24,060 (12,820–45,130)
21	28,464 (15,020–53,970)
22	33,675 (17,560–64,570)
23	39,843 (20,573–77,164)
24	47,138 (24,067–93,325)

From Nyberg DA, Filly RA, Filho DL, et al. Abnormal pregnancy: Early diagnosis by US and serum gonadotropin levels. Radiology 158:393, 1986, with permission; hCG calibrated against the Second International Standard.

Appendix Table III. RELATION BETWEEN MEAN SAC DIAMETER AND MENSTRUAL AGE

MEAN GESTATIONAL SAC DIAMETER	PREDICTED AGE (wk) RANGE = 95% CI
2	5.0 (4.5–5.5)
3	5.1 (4.6–5.6)
4	5.2 (4.8–5.7)
5	5.4 (4.9–5.8)
6	5.5 (5.0–6.0)
7	5.6 (5.1–6.1)
8	5.7 (5.3–6.2)
9	5.9 (5.4–6.3)
10	6.0 (5.5–6.5)
11	6.1 (5.6–6.6)
12	6.2 (5.8–6.7)
13	6.4 (5.9–6.8)
14	6.5 (6.0–7.0)
15	6.6 (6.2–7.1)
16	6.7 (6.2–7.2)
17	6.9 (6.4–7.3)
18	7.0 (6.5–7.5)
19	7.1 (6.6–7.6)
20	7.3 (6.8–7.7)
21	7.4 (6.9–7.8)
22	7.5 (7.0–8.0)
23	7.6 (7.2–8.1)
24	7.8 (7.3–8.2)

From Daya S, Woods S, Ward S, et al. Early pregnancy assessment with transvaginal ultrasound scanning. Can Med Assoc J *144*:441, 1991, with permission.

Appendix Table IV. PREDICTED MENSTRUAL AGE (MA) IN WEEKS FROM CROWN-RUMP LENGTH (CRL) MEASUREMENTS (cm)*

CRL	MA	CRL	MA	CRL	MA	CRL	MA	CRL	MA	CRL	MA
0.2	5.7	2.2	8.9	4.2	11.1	6.2	12.6	8.2	14.0	10.2	16.1
0.3	5.9	2.3	9.0	4.3	11.2	6.3	12.7	8.3	14.2	10.3	16.2
0.4	6.1	2.4	9.1	4.4	11.2	6.4	12.8	8.4	14.3	10.4	16.3
0.5	6.2	2.5	9.2	4.5	11.3	6.5	12.8	8.5	14.4	10.5	16.4
0.6	6.4	2.6	9.4	4.6	11.4	6.6	12.9	8.6	14.5	10.6	16.5
0.7	6.6	2.7	9.5	4.7	11.5	6.7	13.0	8.7	14.6	10.7	16.6
0.8	6.7	2.8	9.6	4.8	11.6	6.8	13.1	8.8	14.7	10.8	16.7
0.9	6.9	2.9	9.7	4.9	11.7	6.9	13.1	8.9	14.8	10.9	16.8
1.0	7.2	3.0	9.9	5.0	11.7	7.0	13.2	9.0	14.9	11.0	16.9
1.1	7.2	3.1	10.0	5.1	11.8	7.1	13.3	9.1	15.0	11.1	17.0
1.2	7.4	3.2	10.1	5.2	11.9	7.2	13.4	9.2	15.1	11.2	17.1
1.3	7.5	3.3	10.2	5.3	12.0	7.3	13.4	9.3	15.2	11.3	17.2
1.4	7.7	3.4	10.3	5.4	12.0	7.4	13.5	9.4	15.3	11.4	17.3
1.5	7.9	3.5	10.4	5.5	12.1	7.5	13.6	9.5	15.3	11.5	17.4
1.6	8.0	3.6	10.5	5.6	12.2	7.6	13.7	9.6	15.4	11.6	17.5
1.7	8.1	3.7	10.6	5.7	12.3	7.7	13.8	9.7	15.5	11.7	17.6
1.8	8.3	3.8	10.7	5.8	12.3	7.8	13.8	9.8	15.6	11.8	17.7
1.9	8.4	3.9	10.8	5.9	12.4	7.9	13.9	9.9	15.7	11.9	17.8
2.0	8.6	4.0	10.9	6.0	12.5	8.0	14.0	10.0	15.9	12.0	17.9
2.1	8.7	4.1	11.0	6.1	12.6	8.1	14.1	10.1	16.0	12.1	18.0

*The 95% confidence interval is ±8% of the predicted age.

From Hadlock FP, Shah YP, Kanon DJ, Lindsey JV. Fetal crown-rump length: Reevaluation of relation to menstrual age (5–8 weeks) with high-resolution real-time US. Radiology *182*:501–505, 1992, with permission.

Appendix Table V. PREDICTED MENSTRUAL AGE FOR BIPARIETAL DIAMETER MEASUREMENTS (2.6–9.7 cm)

BPD (cm)	MENSTRUAL AGE (wk)	BPD (cm)	MENSTRUAL AGE (wk)
2.6	13.9	6.2	25.3
2.7	14.2	6.3	25.7
2.8	14.5	6.4	26.1
2.9	14.7	6.5	26.4
3.0	15.0	6.6	26.8
3.1	15.3	6.7	27.2
3.2	15.6	6.8	27.6
3.3	15.9	6.9	28.0
3.4	16.2	7.0	28.3
3.5	16.5	7.1	28.7
3.6	16.8	7.2	29.1
3.7	17.1	7.3	29.5
3.8	17.4	7.4	29.9
3.9	17.7	7.5	30.4
4.0	18.0	7.6	30.8
4.1	18.3	7.7	31.2
4.2	18.6	7.8	31.6
4.3	18.9	7.9	32.0
4.4	19.2	8.0	32.5
4.5	19.5	8.1	32.9
4.6	19.9	8.3	33.3
4.7	20.2	8.3	33.8
4.8	20.5	8.4	34.2
4.9	20.8	8.5	34.7
5.0	21.2	8.6	35.1
5.1	21.5	8.7	35.6
5.2	21.8	8.8	36.1
5.3	22.2	8.9	36.5
5.4	22.5	9.0	37.0
5.5	22.8	9.1	37.5
5.6	23.2	9.2	38.0
5.7	23.5	9.3	38.5
5.8	23.9	9.4	38.9
5.9	24.2	9.5	39.4
6.0	24.6	9.6	39.9
6.1	25.0	9.7	40.5

Variability Estimates (±2 SD)

12–18 wk	±1.2 wk
18–24 wk	±1.7 wk
24–30 wk	±2.2 wk
30–36 wk	±3.1 wk
36–42 wk	±3.2 wk

Data from Hadlock FP, Deter RL, Harrist RB, et al. Fetal biparietal diameter: A critical reevaluation of the relation to menstrual age by means of realtime ultrasound. J Ultrasound Med 1:97, 1982; and Hadlock FP, Deter LR, Harrist RB, Park SK: Estimating fetal age: Computer-assisted analysis of multiple fetal growth parameters. Radiology 152:497, 1984.

Appendix Table VI. PREDICTED MENSTRUAL AGE
FOR HEAD CIRCUMFERENCE
MEASUREMENTS (8.5–36.0 cm)

HEAD CIRCUMFERENCE (cm)	MENSTRUAL AGE (wk)	HEAD CIRCUMFERENCE (cm)	MENSTRUAL AGE (wk)
8.5	13.7	22.5	24.4
9.0	14.0	23.0	24.9
9.5	14.3	23.5	25.4
10.0	14.6	24.0	25.9
10.5	15.0	24.5	26.4
11.0	15.3	25.0	26.9
11.5	15.6	25.5	27.5
12.0	15.9	26.0	28.0
12.5	16.3	26.5	28.6
13.0	16.6	27.0	29.2
13.5	17.0	27.5	29.8
14.0	17.3	28.0	30.3
14.5	17.7	28.5	31.0
15.0	18.1	29.0	31.6
15.5	18.4	29.5	32.2
16.0	18.8	30.0	32.8
16.5	19.2	30.5	33.5
17.0	19.6	31.0	34.2
17.5	20.0	31.5	34.9
18.0	20.4	32.0	35.5
18.5	20.8	32.5	36.3
19.0	21.2	33.0	37.0
19.5	21.6	33.5	37.7
20.0	22.1	34.0	38.5
20.5	22.5	34.5	39.2
21.0	23.0	35.0	40.0
21.5	23.4	35.5	40.8
22.0	23.9	36.0	41.6

Variability Estimates (±2 SD)

12–18 wk	±1.3 wk
18–24 wk	±1.6 wk
24–30 wk	±2.3 wk
30–36 wk	±2.7 wk
34–42 wk	±3.4 wk

From Hadlock FP, Deter RL, Harrist RB, Park SK. Fetal head circumference: Relation to menstrual age. AJR *138*:649, 1982, with permission.

Appendix Table VII. PREDICTED MENSTRUAL AGE FOR ABDOMINAL CIRCUMFERENCE MEASUREMENTS (10–36 cm)

ABDOMINAL CIRCUMFERENCE (cm)	MENSTRUAL AGE (wk)	ABDOMINAL CIRCUMFERENCE (cm)	MENSTRUAL AGE (wk)
10.0	15.6	23.5	27.7
10.5	16.1	24.0	28.2
11.0	16.5	24.5	28.7
11.5	16.9	25.0	29.2
12.0	17.3	25.5	29.7
12.5	17.8	26.0	30.1
13.0	18.2	26.5	30.6
13.5	18.6	27.0	31.1
14.0	19.1	27.5	31.6
14.5	19.5	28.0	32.1
15.0	20.0	28.5	32.6
15.5	20.4	29.0	33.1
16.0	20.8	29.5	33.6
16.5	21.3	30.0	34.1
17.0	21.7	30.5	34.6
17.5	22.2	31.0	35.1
18.0	22.6	31.5	35.6
18.5	23.1	32.0	36.1
19.0	23.6	32.5	36.6
19.5	24.0	33.0	37.1
20.0	24.5	33.5	37.6
20.5	24.9	34.0	38.1
21.0	25.4	34.5	38.7
21.5	25.9	35.0	39.2
22.10	26.3	35.5	39.7
22.5	26.8	36.0	40.2
23.0	27.3		

Variability Estimates (±2 SD)

12–18 wk	±1.9 wk
18–24 wk	±2.0 wk
24–30 wk	±2.2 wk
30–36 wk	±3.0 wk
36–42 wk	±2.5 wk

From Hadlock FP, Deter RL, Harrist RB, Park SK. Fetal abdominal circumference as a predictor of mentrual age. AJR *139*:367, 1982, with permission.

Appendix Table VIII. PREDICTED MENSTRUAL AGE FOR FEMUR LENGTH (1.0–7.9 cm)

FEMUR LENGTH (cm)	MENSTRUAL AGE (wk)	FEMUR LENGTH (cm)	MENSTRUAL AGE (wk)
1.0	12.8	4.5	24.5
1.1	13.1	4.6	24.9
1.2	13.4	4.7	25.3
1.3	13.6	4.8	25.7
1.4	13.9	4.9	26.1
1.5	14.2	5.0	26.5
1.6	14.5	5.1	27.0
1.7	14.8	5.2	27.4
1.8	15.1	5.3	27.8
1.9	15.4	5.4	28.2
2.0	15.7	5.5	28.7
2.1	16.0	5.6	29.1
2.2	16.3	5.7	29.6
2.3	16.6	5.8	30.0
2.4	16.9	5.9	30.5
2.5	17.2	6.0	30.9
2.6	17.6	6.1	31.4
2.7	17.9	6.2	31.9
2.8	18.2	6.3	32.3
2.9	18.6	6.4	32.8
3.0	18.9	6.5	33.3
3.1	19.2	6.6	33.8
3.2	19.6	6.7	34.2
3.3	19.9	6.8	34.7
3.4	20.3	6.9	35.2
3.5	20.7	7.0	35.7
3.6	21.0	7.1	36.2
3.7	21.4	7.2	36.7
3.8	21.8	7.3	37.2
3.9	22.1	7.4	37.7
4.0	22.5	7.5	38.3
4.1	22.9	7.6	38.8
4.2	23.3	7.7	39.3
4.3	23.7	7.8	39.8
4.4	24.1	7.9	40.4

Variability Estimates (±2 SD)

12–18 wk	±1.0 wk
18–24 wk	±1.8 wk
24–30 wk	±2.0 wk
30–36 wk	±2.4 wk
36–42 wk	±3.2 wk

From Hadlock FP, Deter RL, Harrist RB, Park SK. Fetal femur length as a predictor of menstrual age: Sonographically measured. AJR *138*:875, 1982, with permission.

Appendix Table IX. LENGTH OF FETAL LONG BONES (mm)

WEEK NO.	HUMERUS PERCENTILE			ULNA PERCENTILE			RADIUS PERCENTILE			FEMUR PERCENTILE			TIBIA PERCENTILE			FIBULA PERCENTILE		
	5	50	95	5	50	95	5	50	95	5	50	95	5	50	95	5	50	95
11	—	6	—	—	5	—	—	5	—	—	6	—	—	4	—	—	2	—
12	3	9	10	—	8	—	—	7	—	—	9	—	—	7	—	—	5	—
13	5	13	20	3	11	18	—	10	—	6	12	19	4	10	17	—	8	—
14	5	16	20	4	13	17	8	13	12	5	15	19	2	13	19	6	11	10
15	11	18	26	10	16	22	12	15	19	11	19	26	5	16	27	10	14	18
16	12	21	25	8	19	24	9	18	21	13	22	24	7	19	25	6	17	22
17	19	24	29	11	21	32	11	20	29	20	25	29	15	22	29	7	19	31
18	18	27	30	13	24	30	14	22	26	19	28	31	14	24	29	10	22	28
19	22	29	36	20	26	32	20	24	29	23	31	38	19	27	35	18	24	30
20	23	32	36	21	29	32	21	27	28	22	33	39	19	29	35	18	27	30
21	28	34	40	25	31	36	25	29	32	27	36	45	24	32	39	24	29	34
22	28	36	40	24	33	37	24	31	34	29	39	44	25	34	39	21	31	37
23	32	38	45	27	35	43	26	32	39	35	41	48	30	36	43	23	33	44
24	31	41	46	29	37	41	27	34	38	34	44	49	28	39	45	26	35	41
25	35	43	51	34	39	44	31	36	40	38	46	54	31	41	50	33	37	42
26	36	45	49	34	41	44	30	37	41	39	49	53	33	43	49	32	39	43
27	42	46	51	37	43	48	33	39	45	45	51	57	39	45	51	35	41	47
28	41	48	52	37	44	48	33	40	45	45	53	57	38	47	52	36	43	47
29	44	52	56	40	46	51	36	42	47	49	56	62	40	49	57	40	45	50
30	44	52	56	38	47	54	34	43	49	49	58	62	41	51	56	38	47	52
31	47	53	59	39	49	59	34	44	53	53	60	67	46	52	58	40	48	57
32	47	55	59	40	50	58	37	45	51	53	62	67	46	54	59	40	50	56
33	50	56	62	43	52	60	41	46	51	56	64	71	49	56	62	43	51	59
34	50	57	62	44	53	59	39	47	53	57	65	70	47	57	64	46	52	56
35	52	58	65	47	54	61	38	48	57	61	67	73	48	59	69	51	54	57
36	53	60	63	47	55	61	41	48	54	61	69	74	49	60	68	51	55	56
37	57	61	64	49	56	62	45	49	53	64	71	77	52	61	71	55	56	58
38	55	61	66	48	57	63	45	49	53	62	72	79	54	62	69	54	57	59
39	56	62	69	49	57	66	46	50	54	64	74	83	58	64	69	55	58	62
40	56	63	69	50	58	65	46	50	54	66	75	81	58	65	69	54	59	62

From Jeanty P. Fetal limb biometry (Letter). Radiology *147*:602, 1983, with permission.

Appendix Table X. FETAL MEASUREMENTS BY GESTATIONAL AGE

MENSTRUAL AGE (wk)	BPD (mm)	HEAD CIRCUMFERENCE (mm)	FEMUR LENGTH (mm)	ABDOMINAL CIRCUMFERENCE (mm)
12		68	7	
13		82	11	
14	27	97	14	
15	30	111	17	93
16	33	124	21	105
17	37	138	24	117
18	40	151	27	129
19	43	164	30	141
20	46	177	33	152
21	49	189	36	164
22	53	201	38	175
23	56	213	41	186
24	58	224	44	197
25	61	235	46	208
26	64	246	49	219
27	67	256	51	229
28	69	266	54	240
29	72	275	56	250
30	75	284	58	260
31	77	293	61	270
32	79	301	63	280
33	82	308	65	290
34	84	315	67	299
35	86	322	69	309
36	88	328	71	318
37	90	333	72	327
38	91	338	74	336
39	93	342	76	345
40	95	346	77	354

Measurement	SD		5th%–95th%
BPD	3	mm	5 mm
Head circumference	10	mm	16.5 mm
Femur length	3	mm	5 mm
Abdominal circumference	12.3	mm	20.2 mm

Data from Hadlock FP, Deter RL, Harrist RB, Park SK. Fetal biparietal diameter: a critical re-evaluation of the relation to menstrual age by means of real-time ultrasound. J. Ultrasound Med 1:97–104, 1982; Hadlock FP, Deter RL, Harrist RB, Park SK. Fetal head circumference: relation to menstrual age. AJR 138:649–653, 1982; Hadlock FP, Deter RL, Harrist RB, Park SK. Fetal abdominal circumference as a predictor of menstrual age. AJR 139: 367–370, 1982; and Hadlock FP, Deter RL, Harrist RB, Park SK. Estimating fetal age: computer-assisted analysis of multiple fetal growth parameters. Radiology 12:497–501, 1984.

Appendix Table XI. FETAL THORACIC CIRCUMFERENCE MEASUREMENTS (cm)

GESTATIONAL AGE (wk)	No.	PREDICTIVE PERCENTILES								
		2.5	5	10	25	50	75	90	95	97.5
16	6	5.9	6.4	7.0	8.0	9.1	10.3	11.3	11.9	12.4
17	22	6.8	7.3	7.9	8.9	10.0	11.2	12.2	12.8	13.3
18	31	7.7	8.2	8.8	9.8	11.0	12.1	13.1	13.7	14.2
19	21	8.6	9.1	9.7	10.7	11.9	13.0	14.0	14.6	15.1
20	20	9.5	10.0	10.6	11.7	12.8	13.9	15.0	15.5	16.0
21	30	10.4	11.0	11.6	12.6	13.7	14.8	15.8	16.4	16.9
22	18	11.3	11.9	12.5	13.5	14.6	15.7	16.7	17.3	17.8
23	21	12.2	12.8	13.4	14.4	15.5	16.6	17.6	18.2	18.8
24	27	13.2	13.7	14.3	15.3	16.4	17.5	18.5	19.1	19.7
25	20	14.1	14.6	15.2	16.2	17.3	18.4	19.4	20.0	20.6
26	25	15.0	15.5	16.1	17.1	18.2	19.3	20.3	21.0	21.5
27	24	15.9	16.4	17.0	18.0	19.1	20.2	21.3	21.9	22.4
28	24	16.8	17.3	17.9	18.9	20.0	21.2	22.2	22.8	23.3
29	24	17.7	18.2	18.8	19.8	21.0	22.1	23.1	23.7	24.2
30	27	18.6	19.1	19.7	20.7	21.9	23.0	24.0	24.6	25.1
31	24	19.5	20.0	20.6	21.6	22.8	23.9	24.9	25.5	26.0
32	28	20.4	20.9	21.5	22.6	23.7	24.8	25.8	26.4	26.9
33	27	21.3	21.8	22.5	23.5	24.6	25.7	26.7	27.3	27.8
34	25	22.2	22.8	23.4	24.4	25.5	26.6	27.6	28.2	28.7
35	20	23.1	23.7	24.3	25.3	26.4	27.5	28.5	29.1	29.6
36	23	24.0	24.6	25.2	26.2	27.3	28.4	29.4	30.0	30.6
37	22	24.9	25.5	26.1	27.1	28.2	29.3	30.3	30.9	31.5
38	21	25.9	26.4	27.0	28.0	29.1	30.2	31.2	31.9	32.4
39	7	26.8	27.3	27.9	28.9	30.0	31.1	32.2	32.8	33.3
40	6	27.7	28.2	28.8	29.8	30.9	32.1	33.1	33.7	34.2

From Chitkara U, Rosenberg J, Chervenak FA, et al. Prenatal sonographic assessment of the fetal thorax: normal values. Am J Obstet Gynecol 156:1069, 1987.

Appendix Table XII. IN UTERO FETAL SONOGRAPHIC WEIGHT STANDARDS

MENSTRUAL WEEKS	ESTIMATED FETAL WEIGHT (gm) BY PERCENTILE				
	3rd	*10th*	*50th*	*90th*	*97th*
10	26	29	35	41	44
11	34	37	45	53	56
12	43	48	58	68	73
13	55	61	73	85	91
14	70	77	93	109	116
15	88	97	117	137	146
16	110	121	146	171	183
17	136	150	181	212	226
18	167	185	223	261	279
19	205	227	273	319	341
20	248	275	331	387	414
21	299	331	399	467	499
22	359	398	478	559	598
23	426	471	568	665	710
24	503	556	670	784	838
25	589	652	785	918	981
26	685	758	913	1068	1141
27	791	876	1055	1234	1319
28	908	1004	1210	1416	1513
29	1034	1145	1379	1613	1724
30	1169	1294	1559	1824	1949
31	1313	1453	1751	2049	2189
32	1465	1621	1953	2285	2441
33	1622	1794	2162	2530	2703
34	1783	1973	2377	2781	2971
35	1946	2154	2595	3036	3244
36	2110	2335	2813	3291	3516
37	2271	2513	3028	3543	3785
38	2427	2686	3236	3786	4045
39	2576	2851	3435	4019	4294
40	2714	3004	3619	4234	4524

From Hadlock FP, Harrist RB, Martinez-Poyer J. In utero analysis of fetal growth: a sonographic weight standard. Radiology *181*:129–133, 1991, with permission.

Appendix Table XIII. NOMOGRAM OF ESTIMATED FETAL WEIGHT IN TWIN GESTATIONS

GESTATIONAL AGE (wk)	ESTIMATED FETAL WEIGHT (gm) BY PERCENTILE				
	5th	*25th*	*50th*	*75th*	*95th*
16	132	141	154	189	207
17	173	194	215	239	249
18	214	248	276	289	291
19	223	253	300	333	412
20	232	259	324	378	534
21	275	355	432	482	705
22	319	452	540	586	876
23	347	497	598	684	880
24	376	543	656	783	885
25	549	677	793	916	1118
26	722	812	931	1049	1352
27	755	978	1087	1193	1563
28	789	1145	1244	1337	1774
29	900	1266	1395	1509	1883
30	1011	1387	1546	1682	1992
31	1198	1532	1693	1875	2392
32	1385	1677	1840	2068	2793
33	1491	1771	2032	2334	3000
34	1597	1866	2224	2601	3208
35	1703	2093	2427	2716	3336
26	1809	2321	2631	2832	3465
37	2239	2540	2824	3035	3679
38	2669	2760	3017	3239	3894

From Yarkoni S, Reece EA, Holford T, et al. Estimated fetal weight in the evaluation of growth in twin gestations: A prospective longitudinal study. Obstet Gynecol 69:636, 1987. Reprinted with permission from The American College of Obstetricians and Gynecologists.

Appendix Table XIV. BIRTH WEIGHT BASED ON BPD AND ABDOMINAL CIRCUMFERENCE

BPD (mm)	ABDOMINAL CIRCUMFERENCE (mm)															
	70	80	90	100	110	120	130	140	150	160	170	180	190	200	210	220
40	145	158	171	186	202	219	237	257	279	303	329	357	387	420	456	494
42		169	183	198	215	233	252	273	296	321	348	377	408	442	479	519
44		180	195	211	229	247	268	290	314	340	368	398	431	466	504	546
46			208	225	244	263	285	308	333	359	389	420	454	491	531	575
48				240	256	280	302	326	352	381	411	444	479	517	558	603
50				256	276	298	321	346	374	403	434	468	505	545	587	633
52					294	317	341	368	396	426	459	495	533	574	618	666
54						337	363	390	420	451	486	522	562	605	650	700

BPD (mm)	ABDOMINAL CIRCUMFERENCE (mm)															
	120	130	140	150	160	170	180	190	200	210	220	230	240	250	260	270	280
56	359	385	414	445	478	513	552	593	637	684	735	790	849	912	980	1200	1284
58		409	439	471	506	543	583	625	671	720	773	829	890	955	1025	1253	1340
60			466	500	536	574	615	659	707	758	812	870	933	1000	1072	1309	1398
62				530	567	607	650	696	745	797	853	913	978	1047	1121	1367	1458
64				561	600	642	686	734	784	839	897	959	1025	1096	1172	1428	1521
66					635	678	725	774	826	882	942	1006	1075	1148	1226	1491	1587
68					673	717	765	816	870	928	990	1056	1127	1202	1282	1558	1656
70					712	758	808	861	917	977	1041	1109	1181	1258	1340	1627	1727
72					754	802	853	908	966	1028	1094	1164	1238	1317	1402	1700	1802

BPD (mm)	ABDOMINAL CIRCUMFERENCE (mm)																
	190	200	210	220	230	240	250	260	270	280	290	300	310	320	330	340	350	360
74	958	1018	1081	1149	1221	1298	1379	1466	1558	1656	1759	1870	1987	2112	2244	2385	2534	2693
76	1010	1072	1138	1208	1282	1361	1444	1533	1627	1727	1833	1946	2065	2192	2327	2470	2622	2783
48	1065	1129	1197	1269	1346	1426	1512	1603	1700	1802	1910	2025	2147	2276	2413	2558	2712	2875
80	1124	1190	1260	1334	1412	1495	1583	1677	1775	1880	1990	2107	2231	2363	2502	2594	2805	2970
82	1185	1253	1325	1402	1482	1568	1658	1758	1864	1961	2074	2193	2319	2453	2594	2743	2901	3068
84	1250	1320	1395	1473	1556	1643	1736	1834	1937	2046	2161	2282	2411	2547	2690	2841	3001	3170
86	1318	1391	1467	1548	1633	1723	1818	1918	2023	2134	2252	2375	2506	2644	2789	2942	3104	3275
88	1391	1465	1544	1627	1714	1806	1903	2005	2113	2227	2346	2472	2605	2745	2892	3047	3211	3383
90	1467	1544	1624	1710	1799	1893	1993	2097	2207	2323	2445	2573	2707	2849	2999	3158	3321	3495
92	1547	1626	1709	1797	1888	1985	2087	2193	2305	2423	2547	2677	2814	2958	3109	3268	3435	3611
94	1632	1713	1798	1888	1982	2081	2185	2294	2408	2528	2654	2786	2925	3071	3224	3385	3554	3731

BPD (mm)	ABDOMINAL CIRCUMFERENCE (mm)													
	260	270	280	290	300	310	320	330	340	350	360	370	380	390
92	2193	2305	2423	2547	2677	2814	2958	3109	3268	3435	3611	3796	3990	4194
94	2294	2408	2528	2654	2786	2925	3071	3224	3385	3554	3731	3917	4112	4317
96	2399	2515	2637	2765	2900	3041	3188	3343	3505	3676	3854	4041	4238	4444
98	2508	2627	2751	2881	3018	3160	3310	3466	3630	3802	3982	4170	4367	4574
100	2623	2744	2870	3002	3141	3285	3436	3594	3760	3933	4114	4303	4501	4708

Adapted from Shepard MJ, Richards VA, Berkowitz RL. An evaluation of two equations for predicting fetal weight by ultrasound. Am J Obstet Gynecol 142:47–54, 1982, with permission.

Appendix Table XV. AMNIOTIC FLUID INDEX VALUES IN NORMAL PREGNANCY

WEEK	AMNIOTIC FLUID PERCENTILE VALUES (mm)				
	3rd	5th	50th	95th	97th
16	73	79	121	185	201
17	77	83	127	194	211
18	80	87	133	202	220
19	83	90	137	207	225
20	86	93	141	212	230
21	88	95	143	214	233
22	89	97	145	216	235
23	90	98	146	218	237
24	90	98	147	219	238
25	89	97	147	221	240
26	89	97	147	223	242
27	85	95	146	226	245
28	86	94	146	228	249
29	84	92	145	231	254
20	82	90	145	234	258
31	79	88	144	238	263
32	77	86	144	242	269
33	74	83	143	245	274
34	72	81	142	248	278
35	70	79	140	249	279
36	68	77	138	249	279
37	66	75	135	244	275
38	65	73	132	239	269
39	64	72	127	226	255
40	63	71	123	214	240
41	63	70	116	194	216
42	63	69	110	175	192

Adapted from Moore TR, Cayle JE. The amniotic fluid index in normal human pregnancy. Am J Obstet Gynecol 162:1168, 1990, with permission.

INDEX

Note: Page numbers in *italics* refer to illustrations; page numbers followed by t refer to tables.

ISBN 0-7216-6642-6